The Nature of Theoretical Thinking in Nursing

Third Edition

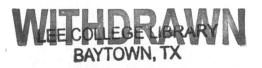

Hesook Suzie Kim, PhD, RN, has been professor at the University of Rhode Island since 1979 and Professor II at the Institute of Nursing Science, Faculty of Medicine, University of Oslo in Norway from 1992 to 2003. She is professor emerita of nursing at the University of Rhode Island, from which she retired in 2004, and has held the professorship at Buskerud University College in Norway from 2004 to 2008. Currently she is a research project director at Buskerud University College. Dr. Kim began teaching at the University of Rhode Island in 1973 and was dean of the College of Nursing there from 1983 to 1988. She holds a doctorate in sociology from Brown University, and nursing degrees (BS and MS) from Indiana University. She has published extensively in the area of nursing epistemology, theory development in nursing, the nature of nursing practice, and collaborative decision making in nursing practice as well as in various areas of clinical nursing research. She is also the coeditor with Dr. Ingrid Kollak of Berlin, Germany, of the book, *Nursing Theories: Conceptual and Philosophical Foundations*, the first edition of which was published both in English and in German in 1999 and the second edition (in English) in 2006.

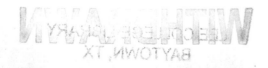

The Nature of Theoretical Thinking in Nursing

Third Edition

HESOOK SUZIE KIM, PhD, RN

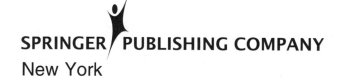

SPRINGER PUBLISHING COMPANY
New York

Springer Publishing Company, LLC
11 West 42nd Street
New York, NY 10036
www.springerpub.com

Acquisitions Editor: Allan Graubard
Senior Editor: Rose Mary Piscitelli
Cover design: Steve Pisano
Composition: International Graphic Services

ISBN: 978-0-8261-0587-5

Ebook ISBN: 978-0-8261-0588-2

10 11 12 13 / 5 4 3 2 1

Library of Congress Cataloging-in-Publication Data

Kim, Hesook Suzie.
  The nature of theoretical thinking in nursing / Hesook Suzie Kim.—3rd ed.
    p. ; cm.
  Includes bibliographical references and index.
  ISBN 978-0-8261-0587-5 (alk. paper)
  1. Nursing—Philosophy.
  I. Title. [DNLM: 1. Nursing Theory. 2. Models, Nursing. 3. Philosophy, Nursing. WY 86 K49n 2010]
  RT84.5.K545 2010
  610.73'01—dc22
                     2010012488

Printed in the United States of America by Hamilton Printing

For Hyung

Contents

Preface

It has been more than 25 years since the publication of the first edition, and nearly 10 years since the second edition of this work. During this period, nursing as a scientific discipline has achieved a great deal in terms of the development of knowledge. There especially has been a tremendous growth and enrichment in nursing's theoretical work. Several grand theories and conceptual models that were initially presented by the early 1980s have been revised, reformulated, and refined either by the original theorists or by their followers.

A great deal of nursing's theoretical work also has focused on the development of middle-level theories. In addition, there has been a significant growth in the delineation, clarification, and refinement of concepts in nursing from various perspectives. Furthermore, during the last 2 decades serious debates and discussions on the epistemological and other philosophical underpinnings of the development of knowledge in nursing began in earnest. As a discipline, nursing is evolving into a mature knowledge system that is clarifying its subject matter and the problems it faces as a science.

However, because nursing, as a knowledge system, has embraced pluralism not necessarily by design but *de facto*, it continues to struggle with what this means, especially in terms of making nursing knowledge relevant to nursing practice. My hope here, in this third edition, is to shed some light on how we are dealing with pluralism as well as addressing theoretical issues in nursing.

Although we have advanced in developing nursing concepts and theories, we are still engaged with the theoretical clarification of essential features of the phenomena of interest to nursing, with their conceptualizations, and with theorizing about them. There still are enough tensions in the field that call for an integrated approach to theoretical thinking in nursing. As has been my position from the first edition of this book, I intend to provide conceptual tools for use in delineating the world of nursing in theoretical terms.

Any serious student or scholar concerned with theoretical work in nursing would ask, at one time or another: "What is nursing concerned with in a theoretical sense?" It seems that for one to answer this question satisfactorily, it is necessary to have a systematic framework for the analysis of theoretical elements in the field of nursing.

In this book, I propose a systematic framework that can be used to examine elements in the field of nursing and to posit important concepts in a system of order and within a boundary of specific meaning. The purpose is to enhance understanding about how conceptualizations and theoretical statements are developed and refined in nursing while offering, at the same time, a typology of conceptual domains that can be used to delineate theoretical elements essential to nursing. In this third edition, I have retained the previous typology of four domains—*the domain of client, the client–nurse domain, the domain of practice, and the environment domain*—as the way to structure conceptual fields for nursing, incorporating further clarifications and current advances. I believe this typology, as a conceptual mapping device, is a useful analytic tool for delineating and theorizing about phenomena of interest to nursing, as it has done for many students and scholars in nursing since its initial publication.

I have added a new chapter on the nature of nursing epistemology, to address critical issues pertaining to pluralism in knowledge development in nursing. In the 21st century, we must work toward theoretical advances in nursing within a synthesizing framework that can consolidate and sort out the multifaceted and complex nature of knowledge required for nursing as a discipline and a practice. Taken together, the framework for nursing epistemology, as presented here, and the typology of four domains should become a map for developing and systematizing theoretical works in nursing. This is especially important in providing nursing knowledge with a critical heuristic value for nursing practice.

The book is primarily designed for graduate students in nursing who are struggling with conceptualization and the theoretical analysis of nursing phenomena. However, many colleagues have shown that it is also useful in introducing undergraduate students to nursing conceptualizations. I believe it is important to introduce senior-level nursing students to theoretical thinking in nursing, so that they are able to appreciate and recognize nursing knowledge as a systematized work for nursing practice. My goal is to show how empirical elements in the world of nursing are translated into theoretical terms and, in turn, how theoretical concepts articulate the real world of nursing.

As such, the specification of concept delineation is proposed along with the typology. The book also shows how various forms of theoretical expositions may be used in theoretical thinking in nursing.

Although I discuss and analyze many conceptual and theoretical ideas expressed by nursing theorists, namely, Rogers, Roy, Johnson, Orem, and King, I do not make systematic evaluations of the values and applicabilities of their theoretical systems. I have attempted neither to evaluate nor to criticize theories, whether in nursing or from other fields, in a systematic or comprehensive manner, as that is not my aim in this book. I have included those appropriate aspects of nursing (and other) theories mainly to illustrate, expand, and apply the ideas under discussion. Again, this book does not purport to examine the adequacies and inadequacies of theories for nursing *qua* science. On the other hand, the book does show how such theories either approximate to or differ from each other in their uses of abstraction, conceptualization, and theoretical approaches.

I focus on delineating and describing essential features of concepts in nursing that are thought to be important for development of theoretical systems. I contrast similarities and differences in conceptualization of nursing and elements in nursing to show how the same elements and phenomena are perceived differently from various perspectives, and how the same ideas encompass many different conceptual disguises. Furthermore, I have no specific "clinical" orientation, which reflects my conviction that theoretical development in nursing should follow universally applicable conceptual strategies, regardless of the specific ways nursing problems are classified. The main emphasis is on the *how to* and *what of* theoretical analysis in nursing.

In this edition, I have carried out a comprehensive literature review and have updated or supplemented my expositions with new and current material. However, I have retained many references that go back several decades, as these remain relevant, with many such references providing the critical historical background necessary to understand the issues addressed.

I have been fortunate to be associated with many colleagues and graduate students who have stimulated my thinking on this typology over the years. Many serendipitous ideas and insights were gained from working with them. Among them, I must acknowledge continued support from colleagues at the University of Rhode Island, even after my retirement from the College of Nursing, and many classes of doctoral students who were often exposed to my "underbaked" ideas. With them, I was never hesitant to grapple with even the most elementary theoretical questions.

I owe much gratitude to Professor Donna Schwartz-Barcott, who has spent endless hours debating and questioning with me many of the ideas presented in the book. Likewise, the faculty at the Institute of Nursing Science, University of Oslo, have continuously encouraged me to pursue the line of thinking that I was discussing with them. Many nursing faculty members of universities in Korea, especially Seoul National University and Yonsei University, have also given me encouragement as well as new insights for theoretical thinking. In addition, over the years, many well-established scholars who studied with me for their doctoral work at the University of Rhode Island have given me their unwavering support in this work. Their support especially has given me the courage and hope in putting myself through this revision. The Japanese translation of the second edition by Dr. Shigemi (Sato) Kamitsuru and Ms. Hiroko Harada gave me an added incentive to work on this edition.

For granting me the most scholarly and enhancing atmosphere that any scholar could want, I am most grateful to the succession of Deans at the College of Nursing, University of Rhode Island, especially during the period of the publication of the first and second editions. Dr. Barbara L. Tate was the staunchest supporter of my effort during the initial period. I believe it was this atmosphere of creative warmth, more than anything else, that enabled me to write the first two editions of this book. As with most good things in life that need special grace, my interest in theoretical thinking initially received a push from Professor Martin U. Martel of Brown University during my doctoral study in sociology there so many years ago. I thank him for showing me the way to question theoretically.

In writing this type of book, one must draw a great deal of support from one's personal resources. I have had the most wonderful support from my family and friends over the years. Most of all, my husband, Hyung, has been the true source of support for the mental energy that was so necessary and critical for the writing of the second edition and has continued to be so during my work with this revision.

My appreciation goes to Allan Graubard, Senior Acquisitions Editor at Springer Publishing, who pursued me to write this revision.

I hope this book can provide readers with insights and ideas that propel them to venture into deep theoretical thinking and work, challenging them to forge toward the systematization of nursing knowledge.

HESOOK SUZIE KIM
Haymarket, Virginia

1 Introduction

The nursing profession has gone through more than 5 decades of struggle, both internally and externally directed, to finally gain recognition and legitimacy as a profession and as a scientific discipline. The nursing profession of the 21st century is a product of various stages of development and change, paralleling changes that have come about in culture and society at large as well as in particular sectors of society, such as health care, science and technology, and other professions. It has moved into its maturity, coming out of its jubilant, energetic, but confused pubescence into a more self-examining, responsible adulthood. The political forces within the nursing profession that have influenced its development during this period were rooted in the spirit of self-determination, in the professionalization of work, and in the equal rights and feminist movements.

The profession of nursing is an organized mechanism for the nursing role encompassing its *central core, nursing practice,* which is supported by three interlocking, related components: (a) what its practice is based on, *nursing knowledge;* (b) what its background is, *nursing tradition;* and (c) how it prepares its role players, *nursing education.* This view of the nursing profession is broader in its conceptualization than the concept of the nursing discipline as an area of study in a generic sense (Donaldson & Crowley, 1978) and the concept of nursing as a role from a social perspective. Because the nursing role is a response to societal needs for a specific type of health care profession, and because the characteristics of this role do not remain static but evolve in relation to its internal development and in its interaction with external forces, this characterization is subject to evolutionary development and transformation.

The most epitomized early definition of the nursing role is one by Henderson to the effect that "the unique function of the nurse is to assist the individual, sick or well, in the performance of those activities contributing to health or its recovery (or to peaceful death) that he would perform unaided if he had the necessary strength, will or knowledge, and to do this in such a way as to help him gain independence as rapidly as possible" (1961, p. 42). With Henderson's definition as the background and in view of the then-current situation of health care and nursing, the WHO (World Health Organization) Expert Committee on Nursing Practice convened in Geneva in 1995 and proposed the following as "a functional definition of nursing":

> Nursing helps individuals, families and groups to determine and achieve their physical, mental and social potential, and to do so within the challenging context of the environment in which they live and work. The nurse requires competence to develop and perform functions that promote and maintain health as well as prevent ill-health. Nursing also includes the planning and giving of care during illness and rehabilitation, and encompasses the physical, mental and social aspects of life as they affect health, illness, disability and dying.

> Nursing promotes the active involvement of the individual and his or her family, friends, social group and community, as appropriate, in all aspects of health care, thus encouraging self-reliance and self-determination while promoting a healthy environment.

> Nursing is both an art and a science. It requires the understanding and application of specific knowledge and skills, and it draws on knowledge and techniques derived from the humanities and the physical, social, medical and biological sciences. (WHO, 1996, p. 4)

In a general perspective similar to these two definitions, the Social Policy Statement initially developed in 1980 by the American Nurses' Association, revised in 1995, and recapitulated in 2003 offers the following definition of nursing:

> Nursing, a profession based on knowledge, is the protection, promotion, and restoration of health, prevention of illness and injury, alleviation of suffering through the diagnosis and treatment of human responses. (ANA, 1995)

These definitions embrace nursing's role as helping and providing unique services to people in the context of health. Although nursing has been firmly established in our society as a role assuming responsibilities for specific aspects of health care, the profession is still in a struggle to define itself, as the images of nursing continue to represent a confusion viewed from both inside and out (Kitson, 1997). Kitson goes further, stating that nursing as a profession needs to "refocus on those essential elements, those universal principles that give nursing its structure, character, presence, and strength in a turbulent health care environment" (1997, p. 111), and suggests that nursing must reconcile its two sides—the scientific, technical base and the authentic, care base—so that it meets the social and professional expectation of viable contribution to people's health through "innovative schemes" in "empowering, enabling, educating people to take control of their lives" (1997, p. 115). Herdman (2001) insists in another way that nursing has not been effective in positioning itself in relation to "the moral, the aesthetic and the ecological" because of its alliance with professionalization, scientism, and "Western centrism." Such disagreements and controversies create a mind-set that pits science against art, cure against care, and technology against humanism, as though nursing has to embrace one of the two alternatives.

This controversy has been complicated in recent decades by: (a) the need to "cost in" nursing within the health care financing system (Lang, 1988); (b) the presence of diversity in the patterns of educational preparation of nurses (Reed, 2000); (c) different roles, positions, and responsibilities available in nursing within health care settings; and (d) different directions in which nursing knowledge has been developed without an apparent integration. While some of these forces are either external to the profession itself or policy-oriented (thus requiring political responses by the profession), the most critical and central issue the nursing profession must address internally is the issue of knowledge development in nursing.

Furthermore, various definitions of nursing were able to furnish only a weak foundation for the generation of nursing knowledge, notwithstanding their positive impact on society and the profession. As a matter of fact, such definitions were the ones exactly needed as general guides for understanding what nursing is all about as a social role in the mind of the public as well as in the mind of the profession itself. A rigorous and exact definition of nursing as a role and as a scientific discipline is necessary specifically when it is used as the conceptual basis for the development of nursing knowledge. This points to the need to continue our journey to clarify what sorts of knowledge we need to develop and how we develop that knowledge.

Many eminent voices of earlier times have provided a base from which nursing leaders and scholars of more recent decades have been able to extract the characteristics and essences of the discipline of nursing as a knowledge system. In addition, the conceptual and cognitive foundations of nursing had their origins in the writings of early scholars. Florence Nightingale (1859, 1992), with pioneering foresight, insisted on a formal training for nurses, which became an impetus for building a body of knowledge for nursing. Virginia Henderson's ideals, on the other hand, have sustained nursing's emphasis on humanizing care (Henderson, 1966). Similarly, Rozella Schlotfeldt and Rosemary Ellis were important advocates in strengthening nursing's quest for scientization: Schlotfeldt (1978, 1987) insisted early on that nursing should become an independent academic field of study, whereas Ellis (1970), who abhorred casualness in scholarly pursuits, instilled analytic seriousness into nursing studies.

The image of nursing as a science has been in the making for the past several decades, and nursing is emerging as a field rich in theoretical and empirical knowledge. However, it is continuing to struggle to define its proper subject matter and the approaches with which nursing can develop the knowledge it needs. The beginnings of nursing knowledge as a specific movement can be traced to just after World War II. The journey from the 1950s to the current decade can be divided into four phases: the first period, from the 1950s to 1960s, as the *declaration of independence phase*; the second period, from the 1970s to the early part of the 1980s, as the *formative phase*; the third period, from the middle of the 1980s to the end of the 20th century, as the *reformatory phase*; and the first decade of the current century, as the *diversifying phase*.

The first phase, the *declaration of independence phase,* which spans the 1950s and 1960s, was forged by nursing leaders to carve out the uniqueness of nursing as a role with a different focus than that of medicine. During this phase there were two threads with which nursing leaders and scholars declared the nature of nursing and nursing knowledge: (a) the focus on the relationship between nurse and patient as the pivotal and unique characteristic of nursing; and (b) the focus on the patient's problems, to which nurses must attend.

The first focus on the patient–nurse relationship was issued by writers such as Peplau (1952), Orlando (1961), Travelbee (1964), and Wiedenbach (1964), who offered various frameworks in which nurse–patient relationships can be understood, examined, and studied with the intention of producing nursing approaches that are guided by theories or frameworks of interpersonal relationships. This was an effort to emphasize nursing's unique position in patient care, that is, nurses' constant presence with patients and nursing's focus on the person rather than on his/her medical problems. These scholars therefore did not specify or address the specific nature of patients' problems that nursing needed to address.

On the other hand, the second focus, with the view that nursing should deal with patients' problems that are different from those of medicine, was addressed in a textbook by Henderson and Harmer (first published in 1955) that identified 14 areas of basic human needs as the major areas of nursing responsibilities; by Abdellah, Beland, Martin, and Matheney (1960), who proposed a typology of 21 nursing problems for patient-centered nursing as areas for nursing care; and by Levin (1966), who, in a somewhat different perspective, introduced the concept of adaptation as the basis for understanding and assessing patients' problems. These proposals were the first wave of conceptual frameworks that separated nursing's orientation from that of disease. However, these were not developed by adopting specific theoretical strategies, did not have specific theoretical contents, and were loose in their linkages to philosophical or theoretical frameworks.

Along with these two sorts of theoretical proposals during this phase, the discipline of nursing began to align itself with the mainstream scientific culture of the time by embracing scientific rationalism and positivism. The concept of nursing process, which epitomizes scientific rationalism and embraces causality, was initially proposed by Orlando (1961), was accepted and integrated into practice and education by nursing leaders, educators, and practitioners in full force, and, by the end of this period, became the major tool for carrying out nursing care. In addition, during this phase many nursing leaders and scholars proclaimed the need for nursing to become a scientific discipline (Johnson, 1959; Leininger, 1969; Moore, 1968; Schlotfeldt, 1960; Rogers, 1963, among many others). This discourse was supplemented by proposals that offered guidelines, frameworks, and processes for developing scientific theories in nursing (Dickoff & James, 1968; Dickoff, James, & Wiedenbach, 1968a, 1968b; Ellis, 1968; Johnson, 1968). Nursing knowledge, synonymously identified as nursing science, was to be developed through theories and research in the prevailing tradition of positivistic sciences. The stage was beginning to be set for the development of nursing as a scientific discipline differentiated from other fields, especially from medicine. The 1965 position statement of the American Nurses Association, which declared the proper educational preparation of nurses to be at the collegiate level, became the impetus also for forging ahead with the scientization of the discipline.

The second phase, the *formative phase,* from the 1970s to the early part of the 1980s, is the period during which fervent efforts were made to develop and systematize nursing knowledge. Three specific stages of development can be identified for this phase: (a) grand theories of nursing; (b) translation and adoption of theories from other disciplines and development of new models to address clinical nursing questions; and (c) empirical research. Several grand theories and conceptual frameworks were proposed to provide nursing perspectives in the study of nursing's clients and practice. These include Rogers's initial work (1970), which later evolved into a science of unitary humans, Roy's adaptation model (1970), Orem's self-care model (1971), King's theory of goal attainment (1971), and Neuman's systems model (1974). These models (some scholars have labeled them conceptual frameworks, others called them theoretical frameworks) aimed to provide unique perspectives from which nursing clients should be understood and studied, and to address the full range of theoretical and empirical questions regarding clients and practice.

These models were used to describe in general three points: (a) with what aspect or aspects of the human condition the discipline is concerned; (b) in what ways we can understand and/or explain the key phenomena of concern; and (c) what the members of the discipline do as the practitioners of a scientific field. Because of the pan-disciplinary focus of these frameworks, they have been labeled as "grand theories" of nursing. Following their introduction in the early 1970s, these models went through some revisions, were supplemented with additional conceptual clarifications, and in some cases were fleshed out with detailed theoretical statements (see, for example: King, 1992; Neuman, 1998; Orem, 1995; Rogers, 1990; Roy & Andrews, 1991 [latest revisions all]).

In addition to these grand theories that were introduced in the early 1970s, two other grand theories were presented initially during the later part of this (the formative) phase—Watson's theory of human care (1979, 1985a, 1988), and Parse's "human becoming" theory (1981, 1992, 1997a). Although there were efforts to apply these theoretical/conceptual frameworks in carrying out empirical research, they were more frequently used to guide the development of nursing curricula or to frame nursing process. The development of these grand theories was instrumental in putting into place a signpost for the direction to which nursing knowledge development would advance. In addition, these grand theories, having different ontological and epistemological orientations, became the initial base from which nursing knowledge began to embrace pluralism.

Parallel to the advancement of these grand theories was the development of different sorts of theoretical work and empirical research, a development influenced by the strong invocation of clinically oriented research in nursing. This was also influenced by the production of a cadre of nurse scientists with doctoral degrees in fields such as psychology, sociology, anthropology, and biology during the 1970s through the federal program aimed at increasing the number of nurse scientists.

As these nurse scientists assumed the leadership roles in education and research, especially within the growing number of master's and doctoral programs in nursing, they were engaged, not only through their own theoretical work and research but also through their students' work, in clinical nursing research seeking theoretical understanding from the nursing perspective and at the same time applying theories developed in other disciplines. Their generative, reconstructive, and revisional approaches along with the adoption of the empirical research tradition resulted in knowledge production in nursing that was quite different from the efforts based on the grand theories (see, for example, Barnard, 1973, 1983, on infant development; Benoliel, 1977, 1985, on dying; Johnson, Christman, & Stitt, 1985; Johnson & Rice, 1974; Johnson, Rice, Fuller, & Endress, 1978, on pain and pain management; McCorkle, 1974, 1976, 1981, on cancer and dying experiences; Mercer, 1974, 1981, on maternal role development; and Woods, 1980, 1885; Woods & Earp, 1978, on women's health). These advancements were results of an active pursuit of empirical nursing research. The mainstream methods of scientific research, including various quantitative research methods, such as instrument development and experimental and intervention research, were used in many research programs that were being established at many universities.

This period was followed by the third phase, the *reformatory phase*, from the middle 1980s to the close of the 20th century, which was burgeoning with knowledge development at the conceptual, empirical, and theoretical levels from multiple philosophical orientations. Although nursing knowledge development during the second phase was valuable for advancing the nursing discipline toward becoming a legitimate scientific field, by the end of this second period many nursing scholars began to question the lack of conceptual and theoretical clarity in theoretical works, the predominance of the positivistic philosophy among the scientists, and the development of nursing interventions that were not firmly grounded in theory. In response to such questioning, the work during this third period advanced with three distinct movements: (a) adoption of alternative philosophies for scientific work in nursing; (b) concept development and middle-range theory development; and (c) nursing therapeutics work.

American social sciences, during the period from the 1960s to the 1970s, had gone through tumultuous self-questioning about their epistemology and philosophy, in the wake of debates in the philosophy of science over the death of the received view (Suppe, 1977), Kuhns' work (1962, 1970) on paradigmatic sciences and scientific revolution, and debates on scientific realism versus relativism. This resulted in the emergence and establishment of various schools of thought and theoretical orientations representing phenomenology, hermeneutic philosophy, critical philosophy, and postmodernism in the social sciences during that period. As the third period of development for nursing ensued, nursing scholars on the coattails of this broadening in the social sciences also began to seek out alternative philosophies and approaches to nursing knowledge development.

The literature shows that phenomenology, not only as a philosophy but also representing specific scientific methods, was applied in studying nursing phenomena beginning in the early 1980s with the initial proposals by Oiler (1982) and Omery (1983). Nursing scholars were into transcendental, existential, and hermeneutic phenomenology, drawing especially upon developments not only in philosophy proper but also in psychology and sociology. Hermeneutic philosophy and critical theory were also debated within nursing, as in the human sciences, and nursing scholars also joined in the discourse of postmodernism in questioning the fallibility of knowledge, the role of language and power in knowledge development (especially from the feminist critique), and scientism's effects on nursing practice (Allen, 1985; Chinn, 1985; Thompson, 1985; Thompson, Allen, & Rodrigues-Fisher, 1992).

Philosophical and methodological pluralism thus became the context of and a key issue in nursing knowledge development. Many nursing scholars pointed out that nursing knowledge was developing under different philosophical orientations and paradigms (Fawcett, 1993; Newman, 1992; Parse, 1987; Stevenson & Woods, 1986; Suppe & Jacox, 1985), and the pros and cons of pluralism were debated (Gortner, 1993; Gortner & Schultz, 1988; Kim, 1993a; Norbeck, 1987). The textbooks edited by Omery, Kasper and Page (1995), and Kim and Kollak (2006) presented various philosophical orientations that could be applied in developing knowledge in nursing, showing the range of perspectives from postpositivism and pragmatism to postmodernism. The annual knowledge development symposia held at the University of Rhode Island from 1990 to 1994 and at Boston College from 1996 to 2001 (Roy & Jones, 2007; University of Rhode Island, 1996) also examined the relationships between/among philosophy, theory, methods, and practice brought on by pluralism. These symposia were the follow-up to the Nursing Science Colloquia held at Boston University from 1984 to 1987, addressing strategies for theory development in nursing. Thus, by the end of this third phase, the field of nursing knowledge was fully infused with pluralism in philosophy, paradigm, and scientific methodology, resulting in the development of theories from various perspectives and carrying out research applying diverse methodological orientations.

At the same time, from the content perspective, this period was truly reformatory, as the theoretical and research attention was shifted from the big-picture orientation (i.e., the grand schemes) to the practice orientation. Concept development work became the cornerstone for this period through the development of new concepts and by refining and revising existing concepts. This was especially spurred by the need to formulate theoretically useful concepts that could be applied to the development of middle-range theories. Furthermore, nursing diagnosis classification work, which began in the later part of the 1970s and gathered steam during the 1980s, followed by the classification work for nursing interventions and outcomes, seemed to press for the need for concept development in nursing. Concepts were developed, reexamined, and refined, applying several methods of concept analysis and development, which were proposed specifically in nursing (Rodgers & Knafl, 1993, 2000). In addition, theory development workers lost interest in developing new grand theories, and instead focused on developing middle-range theories, applying inductive, deductive, and interpretive methods. Smith and Liehr (2003) identified 22 middle-range theories published in nursing between 1988 and 1998 and 14 additional ones published from 1998 to 2001.

In conjunction with the development of middle-range theories, a heightened interest in developing nursing interventions grounded on theories through research emerged. This interest was partly a response to the political force within the health care system to "cost out" all aspects of patient care. The movement for evidence-based practice in health care that began in the 1990s also added to the urgency with which nursing felt the need to develop nursing-specific therapeutics.

By the dawning of the new century, the key players engaged in nursing knowledge development were getting into debates about globalization versus local needs, nursing as science versus nursing as art, nursing's focus on health versus illness, quality control in practice, and standardization versus creativity. On one hand, the knowledge development has continued along the same path of pluralism established during the earlier decades; on the other hand, there has been a growing angst related to the legitimacy of the current pursuits. Thus, this first decade of the 21st century is labeled as the *diversifying phase* for nursing knowledge development. Knowledge development in nursing, as reflected in professional publications during recent years, is replete with works representing biobehavioral and bio-psycho-social perspectives as well as those from the interpretive, critical, and postmodern camps. Skirmishes still break out in the nursing literature between the camp advocating for the dominant scientific culture (i.e., the so-called value-free science) and the "opposing" force mostly engaged in postmodern power critiques, each camp claiming to be the true representative of nursing. The apparent differences between these two camps regarding the approach to knowledge development as well as understanding of the nature of nursing sometimes propelled the discipline along bifurcated roads, making reconciliation and integration difficult or problematic (Holmes & Gastaldo, 2004; Pitre & Myrick, 2007). However, according to Georges, nursing is beginning to carry on an "intertextual discourse" of "epistemic diversity" by which a diversity in nursing scholarship is valued as the only way for nursing to make "a positive difference in a global community informed by multiple lived realities" (2003, p. 50).

This journey, then, has put us in the midst of continuous questioning not only in terms of what the nature of nursing knowledge is—and should entail—but also as to how that knowledge needs to be developed for practice. Although nursing practice from the 1980s onward has forged a firm alliance with the culture of scientific knowledge and technological advances that are aimed at controlling health problems, a strong sentiment has been expressed in the recent discourse in nursing to the effect that nursing needs to stand apart from that culture. Nursing practice encompasses *both* the scientific, problem-solving orientation *and* the human-practice orientation. Nurses are not only dealing with and seeking solutions for clients' health problems, but are also concerned about how to help clients in their "living" in health-related situations. This means that the essential features of nursing knowledge required for practice must embrace the science of control and therapy as well as the knowledge of understanding and care. This also means that nursing as a scientific discipline must delineate its specific nature as a "human practice" science, distinguished not only from the natural and social sciences, but also from the so-called human sciences. This points to the need to develop and clarify approaches to knowledge development that cover these complexities, the complexities in the disciplinary matrix for nursing as a human practice discipline.

One of the major confusions in the discussions regarding nursing knowledge is the ambiguity with which scholars treat the differences between knowledge possessed by individual practicing nurses and that of the discipline of nursing as a whole. Knowledge thus exists in two sectors—as *private* knowledge and *public* knowledge—in the discipline of nursing because, in practice disciplines, practitioners are not only the users of knowledge of the discipline, but also the possessors of certain sets of knowledge. Hence, there is knowledge that is held by practitioners as private knowledge, and there is knowledge that belongs, as it were, to the public domain (i.e., to the discipline). While there is an intimate connection between these two sectors of knowledge, nursing knowledge development basically is for the knowledge at the disciplinary sector (i.e., the "public" knowledge). Confusion exists because, often, nursing scholars are both practitioners and scientists, who contribute to the development of the public knowledge while at the same time generating their own private knowledge.

One can view this partitioning from Popper's epistemology of "world 2" and "world 3" (Popper, 1985). Popper proposed three "worlds" within the universe: "world 1," referring to the physical world; "world 2," referring to the world of states of consciousness that belong to specific subjective humans; and "world 3," referring to "the world of objective contents of thought" (Popper, 1985, p. 58). From this, two types of epistemology are considered: one originating from world 2 as knowledge in the subjective sense, and the other belonging to world 3 as objective knowledge consisting of theories, objective problems, and objective arguments. Scientific knowledge thus is considered to belong to world 3 and is not tied to specific, individual knowing subjects. Scientists are concerned with the growth of knowledge in world 3, but are dependent upon processes of world 2 as the basis for that growth. Drawing from these notions advanced by Popper, it is possible to partition nursing knowledge into two sectors, private and public. Private knowledge refers to the knowledge that belongs to specific individuals gained through one's consciousness and mental processing of experiences and responses; it thus belongs to Popper's world 2. Public knowledge, on the other hand, aligns well with Popper's world 3 as knowledge that exists at large. Public knowledge, although gained through the private processes of scientists, is objective and is oriented towards systematization.

Benner's work (1984, 1996b) has especially created the somewhat comforting idea that nurses can come to possess that holistic knowledge of clinical situations through experience and exposure to problem-solving situations. Each practicing nurse is a possessor and generator of knowledge, and each nurse possesses and generates a unique set of knowledge that is different from all others' private knowledge. Each nurse has a private nursing knowledge that is generative and dynamic as well as idiographic. At the same time, some parts of nurses' private knowledge have shared elements with other nurses' private knowledge and with the disciplinary knowledge at large (that is, the public nursing knowledge). Knowledge considered from this private, personal perspective points to the workings of processes individual nurses are engaged in that either expand or stagnate their private knowledge. Hence, what constitutes nurses' private knowledge and how it becomes constituted and generated are questions not of epistemology (that is, of philosophy) but of experientially based cognition, requiring answers from specific types of inquiry. Benner, Tanner, and Chesla (1992) have attempted to provide answers to such questions from the perspective of phenomenological hermeneutics, while others are considering these questions from the perspective of cognitivism or of social structuralism. On the other hand, Silva and her colleagues (Silva, Sorrell, & Sorrell, 1995) have adopted an ontological orientation in addressing such questions, focusing on knowledge of reality, meaning, and being.

Professional education, certainly, is the starting point at which each student or trainee gains access to the public knowledge of a discipline and moves to build a private knowledge that initially is more standardized than unique. Enrichment of private knowledge can be from personal experiences, from self-referential and reflexive constructing at individual levels, or may draw from the knowledge in the public "sector" that is continuously enriched through activities within nursing's scientific community. Conceptually, thus, the private knowledge that refers to knowledge held by and generated through individual nurses is different from what Carper (1978) called "personal knowledge," which refers to the knowledge of self. Personal knowledge in the sense of the knowledge of oneself is the knowledge of introspection and is a part of private knowledge. The private nursing knowledge comprises those cognitive elements that are required and used in nursing practice, including the nurse's knowledge of him/herself.

On the contrary, public knowledge refers to knowledge of the discipline that is available at large and has the characteristics of systematization

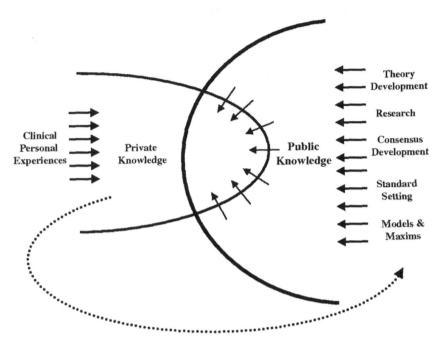

Figure 1.1. Relationship between public and private knowledge in nursing.

and generalization. However, the level of systematization and generalization may vary according to the maturity of a discipline and the degree with which a discipline is able to integrate new knowledge into a coherent system, which encompasses epistemological questions. When nursing scholars discuss nursing knowledge in general, they are referring to the public nursing knowledge that exists in various forms, such as empirical, theoretical, descriptive, ideological, or philosophical. Nursing knowledge development is oriented toward enriching the public knowledge, as it is the source and foundation of the discipline's performance at both individual and aggregate levels. The theory–practice gap we often talk about refers to the apparent lack of alignment between what is available in the public sector and what is being used in individual practice (Kim, 1993b).

Figure 1.1 shows the interrelatedness between the knowledge in the private and public spheres in the development of nursing knowledge. Hence, in practice disciplines public knowledge is not only gained and developed through scientists' work but also by accessing what becomes accumulated and refined in practicing nurses' private knowledge.

My exposition in this book, therefore, deals with how we may systematize nursing knowledge in the public sphere, although the private knowledge held by practicing nurses is a rich source of such systematization.

Nursing knowledge in general may refer to any epistemic aspects of nursing. However, nursing knowledge considered in this book focuses only on the core of nursing related to nursing practice, and ignores those aspects of nursing knowledge considered in a broader sense, such as knowledge about nursing history or its professional organizations. The focus here is on epistemological issues rather than on professional issues. I address specifically the knowledge that is directly related to understanding, explaining, and sometimes predicting nursing practice and its relationship to clients and to outcomes of practice.

Nursing certainly has made a great deal of progress in accumulating the scientific and theoretical basis for its practice as depicted in the description of the development, yet a systematic view of that knowledge gives a fuzzy picture. Confusion still exists regarding what classes of phenomena should be included in a system of theoretical understanding and explanations in nursing. However, one must remember that the boundaries of subject matter for scientific fields, even for the well-established ones such as physics, chemistry, or economics, become revised through an evolutionary process.

A scientific field goes through stages of boundary redifinitions that are based partly on the kinds of major phenomena or subject matter it deals with (e.g., money flow in economics, energy and matter in physics, or personality development in psychology) and partly on what is happening in the scientific fields in general. This idea agrees with Shapere's position (1977) regarding formation and reformation of a scientific domain as constituting a unified subject matter. Well-established associations between phenomena in a scientific field are exposed to scientific scrutiny by a variety of methodologies and from entirely different perspectives. Eventually, the propriety of categorizing scientific problems into a field of scientific knowledge may be questioned, and reformulation of the boundary may occur.

The criteria for deciding boundaries of fields may also be considered superfluous or ambiguous. Thus, subject matter may be reclassified or redescribed in different fields, especially with the emergence of new scientific fields. This happened in the 19th century in sociology when it became differentiated from economics. On this evolutionary basis, nursing as a scientific field became differentiated from medicine and has been going through the process of claiming certain classes of phenomena as its proper subject matter, and subsequently abandoning and reclaiming other subject matter as the field became clearer in its definition of what major scientific problems it seeks to answer. In addition, it appears that the monistic claim of a theory to be completely general and universally relevant is neither fruitful nor appropriate for nursing. Since a diversity of phenomena can be claimed as nursing's subject matter, and since the field has yet to be organized in such a way as to lay definite claim to a body of specific knowledge, multiple theories are not only useful but also necessary.

With these ideas as background, and in the same spirit espoused by Berger (1963) and by Berger and Kellner (1981) for sociology, I propose a framework to be used to delineate theoretical elements for the field of nursing. My main attempt is to show how one can examine relevant phenomena systematically with a nursing perspective using this framework. This framework is offered as the *metaparadigm framework for nursing* that draws out the boundaries for nursing's subject matter. I propose a backtracking, for I believe we are ready for a thoughtful reconsideration of what we have said about nursing in theoretical terms. We are now at a crossroads, after fervent discussions concerning what kinds of theories nursing should be developing and from what philosophical perspectives we must address nursing's subject matter. During the past 10 years, the field of nursing knowledge has progressed in a truly multifaceted, pluralistic manner. That situation has resulted from the development of multiple theories with various scopes, the adoption of pluralistic philosophical orientations in developing nursing knowledge, and the application in nursing studies of various scientific methods. We are at a point in our scientific development that requires a careful examination of and reflection upon the construction of the theoretical foundation of nursing based on a unifying framework.

One of the major reasons for the apparent lack of a systematic view of nursing knowledge, I believe, is the continued use of the so-called four metaparadigm concepts—*health, person, environment,* and *nursing*—in discussing nursing theories and nursing's conceptual issues. These concepts served as the starting points in thinking about nursing's emphasis when they were introduced by Yura and Torres (1975) and reinforced by Fawcett (1984). However, these are merely key concepts that nursing may need, so as to formulate meanings from which various ontological and explanatory positions may emerge. These concepts cannot be used as four cornerstones that set up the conceptual boundary for nursing's subject matter, as some nursing scholars have been trying to do. They are empty as boundary-specifying constructions, and are only useful in asking nursing scholars to formulate specific conceptual orientations for further theoretical thinking. The proposed metaparadigm framework for nursing thus is different from these "metaparadigm concepts," as the proposed framework is a boundary-specifying guide for delineating conceptual and theoretical issues regarding nursing's subject matter.

This metaparadigm framework is a typology that includes four distinct conceptual domains: *client, client–nurse, practice,* and *environment.* This typology is an analytical tool to be used to classify and posit concepts and phenomena within specified boundaries. By doing this, conceptualizations and theoretical ideas can be derived or examined with a conscious knowledge of the empirical locality of phenomena. This will help nurse scholars to conceptualize and theorize about specific entities in the nursing world, and to derive scientific understandings and explanations from whatever philosophical or theoretical perspective they may hold. The idea is to show how phenomenal elements relevant to nursing study are translated into theoretical terms and, in turn, how theoretical concepts are specified in the real world of nursing. Therefore, inductive, deductive, and interpretive approaches are considered appropriate for expositions in nursing based on this typology. These approaches are used to illustrate theoretical thinking through which systematization of ideas, abstraction at theoretical levels, and development of theories can result. This book does not go into specific ways of using theories, however. The "use of theories" here refers to the many ways of expanding, refining, and testing that scientists do through research, critical evaluation, and theory reconstruction.

Staring with conceptualization as the first step in theory building, my intention is to present various sorts of theoretical thinking, free of any specific theoretical bias or philosophical bent. Thus, I shall not provide formal guidelines for evaluating nursing theories, nor provide synoptic discussions and summaries of "major nursing theories."[1] Specific detail of major nursing theories and conceptualizations will be analyzed and discussed in appropriate sections as examples of theoretical thinking.

In chapter 2, the terms and concepts used in concept development, theoretical expositions, and theoretical analysis are defined to the extent that they are used in this book. The coverage in this chapter regarding definitions is far from comprehensive. There are many fine writings on this subject, and readers are referred to several original sources for understanding terms in a variety of perspectives and uses.[2]

In chapter 3, a model of nursing epistemology is presented, which is based on an explication of specific cognitive needs for nursing practice. Nursing practice has to be guided by a specific set of knowledge that satisfies five distinct types of cognitive needs, namely, *inferential, referential, transformative, normative,* and *desiderative* needs. This model undergirds my position regarding philosophical and theoretical pluralism in nursing knowledge and offers ways to systematize epistemological questions that plague nursing as a human practice discipline. These five different cognitive needs, critical to nursing practice, point to the five different spheres of knowledge that need to be developed for practice. This is an overarching framework that can guide knowledge development in nursing.

In chapter 4, the general description of the typology of nursing domains is presented. The rationale for the typology of four domains for nursing as *client, client–nurse, practice,* and *environment* is presented. This typology is an organizational construct, developed for systematizing many classes of phenomena that are essential for nursing studies. This is a boundary-specifying general guide that is used to delineate aspects of the real world into coherent sets of theoretical elements. As a boundary-specifying typology, it guides in the selection and specification of nursing concepts and theories. It is used as a mapping device for the analyses that follow in chapters 5 to 8.

Chapters 5 to 8 are the main focus of the book and consider conceptualization of essential phenomena at several different theoretical levels, taking up one domain at a time. Chapter 5 deals with the domain of client; chapter 6 deals with the domain of client–nurse; chapter 7 deals with the domain of practice; and chapter 8 deals with the domain of environment. In each of these chapters, a general conceptual mapping that is specific to the given domain is delineated and discussed, and conceptualizations vis-à-vis the map are given. Applying the concept analysis method specified in chapter 2, two representative concepts for each domain are analyzed as examples of concept development in the domain. The main focus of these chapters is the delineation and development of concepts.

The focus in chapter 9 is theory development. Different type of syntax for theory development from the heuristic, descriptive, explanatory, and prescriptive orientations are presented for each domain and across domains. Theoretical statements linking phenomena within each domain and across domains are examined in order to show that relevant and critical relationships may be brought together in "theories *in* nursing" and "theories *of* nursing." For each domain, models of explanation are presented as guides that can be used to develop theoretical ideas. Theory development is also examined by overlaying the model of nursing epistemology on the typology of four domains, specifying various types of knowledge-development approaches.

The last chapter addresses the next step in theoretical thinking that follows from the exposition in this book. Some of the problem areas and issues in theoretical thinking in nursing are discussed, highlighting areas for future emphasis and concern. The issue of pluralism in nursing knowledge development is taken up in relation to systematization of knowledge.

NOTES

1. There have been several books and articles written with these purposes as the primary focuses. See, for example, Hardy, M. E. (1978). Evaluating nursing theory. In *Theory development: Why, what, how?* (pp. 75–86). New York: National League for Nursing; Barnum, B. J. S. (1994). *Nursing theory: Analysis, application, evaluation* (4th ed.). Philadelphia: J. B. Lippincott; Fawcett, J. (1994). *Analysis and evaluation of theoretical models of nursing.* Philadelphia: F. A. Davis; and Meleis, A. I. (1997). *Theoretical nursing: Development and progress* (3rd ed.). Philadelphia: J. B. Lippincott.

2. Among the many published works for this subject area, the following classics may be of help to serious students of theory development: Hempel, C. G. (1952). *Fundamentals of concept formation in empirical sciences.* Chicago: The University of Chicago Press; Popper, K. R. (1959). *The logic of scientific discovery.* New York: Harper & Row; Kaplan, A. (1964). *The conduct of inquiry.* San

Francisco: Chandler Publishing; Reynolds, P. D. (1971). *A primer in theory construction.* Indianapolis: Bobbs-Merrill; Dubin, R. (1978). *Theory building* (rev. ed.). New York: Free Press; Blalock, H. M., Jr. (1969). *Theory construction: From verbal to mathematical formulations.* Englewood Cliffs, NJ: Prentice-Hall; and Suppe, F. (Ed.). (1977). *The structure of scientific theories* (2nd ed.). Urbana, IL: University of Illinois Press.

Terminology in Theoretical Thinking

OVERVIEW

This chapter presents the definitions and meanings of the terms and concepts used in theory construction and theoretical analysis. Its intention is to clarify the meanings of the theoretical terms and to provide the reader with clear definitions of these terms as they are used throughout this book. The meanings presented in this chapter have been taken freely from several scholars and indicate ideas and understandings of the terms that are in accordance with the accepted usage in the scientific field. The terms discussed in this chapter are: phenomenon, concept, theory, theory type, theoretical statement (i.e., proposition and hypothesis), measurement of concept, level of conceptual description and analysis according to holistic and particularistic modes, and method of conceptual analysis. Additionally, the terms *metaparadigm*, *metatheory*, and *paradigm* are defined according to the meanings attributed to them in this book.[1]

PHENOMENON

The term *phenomenon* is used to designate reality, that is, what exists in the real world.[2] A girl's love for a certain boy is as good an example of a phenomenon as an apple ripening on a tree or a patient's grimace at seeing his wound. However, this term in the scientific usage refers to the aspects of reality that are relatively regular and enduring rather than fleeting or rare occurrences. Because phenomena exist even when they are not recognized to exist by any humans or named by scientists, it is the role of science to discover, identify, and delineate general features of phenomena and thus gain systematic descriptions and explanations of them. This view, that phenomena exist regardless of human perception or recognition, is counter to the tenets of absolute constructivism, which holds that all elements exist only as humans register them to be represented by attributed entities mostly expressed in linguistic terms. Because this is a critical debate that cannot be handled adequately in this book, we take the aforementioned view, specifically, forging an alliance with scientific pragmatism to guide our exposition of this book.

Woodward suggests that phenomena are "relatively stable and general features of the world which are potential objects of explanation and prediction" and that data "play the role of evidence for claims about phenomena" (1989, p. 393). In scientific considerations of reality, we are often—in fact almost always—exposed to multiple phenomena having similar or different meanings and characteristics. Throughout human history we have used various means of communication, especially language, to form ideas about phenomena we encounter and share such ideas with each other for intersubjective understanding. We take for granted the meanings and labels we attach to various phenomena we encounter in our ordinary lives. However, phenomena of interest for scientific study are established through specific scientific language so as to be understood and used in a more strict and rigorous sense.

As the first step in looking at reality in such a restricted sense, scientists must adopt a classification system by which each phenomenon is considered a member of a kind or class. Both the exactness of a class definition and the scope of a class depend on the person who is categorizing as well as on the historical conventions that have become accepted in the scientific world. By using a classification system, we are able to categorize many aspects of reality broadly or narrowly, depending on the context in which phenomena are studied. For example, general systems theorists will categorize many different types of phenomena, such as the ecological environment on earth, the life cycle of a butterfly, or the circuit of a computer, into system/nonsystem categories. On the other hand, biologists will categorize such life forms as jellyfish, salamander, and whale into the classification system of coelenterates/arachnids/amphibians/mammals.

This "naming of phenomena" into the same kinds gives order to the perceiver of reality. In fact, the phenomenon of jellyfish refers to the exact same thing as the phenomenon of coelenterates. The only difference is that the phenomenon of jellyfish is a class within the phenomenon of coelenterates. This means that as a phenomenon is thought of as having certain entities, that phenomenon is expressed as a concept, that is, through language. Hence, this "naming of phenomena" is, de facto, concept formation. Gillett states that "in grasping a concept we are mastering the use of a term in the interactions and practices of those with whom we have to do" (1987, p. 103); hence, through concepts referring to specific classes of phenomena, we are able to share the meanings and identity of those phenomena.

A major issue regarding phenomena is demarcation, that is, determining the boundaries for inclusion of phenomenal elements as sets. Although many phenomena (for instance, physical and biological phenomena such as dogs, humans, trees, viruses, birthing, and singing) exist within natural boundaries in relation to space and time, many others (such as human experiences, behaviors, feelings, or social conditions) exist in an undifferentiated, intermingled, and/or interpenetrated manner. Thus, naming a phenomenon or an aspect of a cluster of phenomena via conceptualization is a way to specify boundaries and to extract specific identities with labels. Although the major aim of conceptualizing a phenomenon or a set of phenomena is to assign specific linguistic labels to the selected phenomena, often two or more concepts can share some phenomenal elements within their boundaries. For example, the concepts of anxiety and depression refer to human experiences and states, some of which are unique to each concept while others partake of both concepts. A high body temperature is a central phenomenal element for the concept of fever, but it can also be considered a phenomenal element for the concept of inflammation. Thus, the specificity in identifying boundaries and demarcations in phenomena is a key to conceptualization, and this is dealt with in identifying descriptive features of concepts.

CONCEPT

The term *concept* is adopted as a procedure of labeling and naming things, events, ideas, and other realities we perceive and think about. In our ordinary lives, we know numerous concepts through our language and use them in communicating with others and in thinking about reality and ideas. Hence, humans are born into the linguistic culture that has evolved through the history of our existence. Humans' linguistic culture is based on established conceptual systems used in our ordinary lives. However, concept and conceptual thinking are important aspects of science at another level, as scientists use them to formulate and understand phenomena of interest for scientific investigation.[3]

A concept is a symbolic statement, describing a phenomenon or a class of phenomena, expressed by a definition. Gillett (1987) suggests that "a *concept* is a semantic and cognitive tool that unifies a set of experiences...and allows one to repeat acts of judgment within and across situations." Also, concepts embed specific meanings. Whereas a phenomenon exists in the real world, a concept of that phenomenon is articulated in a symbolic construct, having a semantic value, formulated through the workings of the scientist's mind. Because concepts are derived from conscious efforts to name aspects of the world, a concept may refer to a single, unique case or to a class of phenomena having the same properties that are specified in definitions or according to what Wittgenstein (1968) called "family resemblances."

There are several different theories of concepts, such as: the classical view that a concept refers to a category of phenomena that share a set of properties necessary and sufficient for membership; the prototype view, that aligns with the Wittgenstein's "family resemblances" idea; and the exemplar view, that uses an exemplar as the key referent for a concept (Margolis, 1994; Medin & Smith, 1984; Rodgers, 2000a). The concept of Christianity, for example, refers to a single, unique entity, which however can be a member within a concept of religion. Categorizing phenomena into *a class of phenomena* allows a concept to be narrow (i.e., limited) or broad (i.e., all-encompassing). Hence, *pain*, as a concept, is broader than *headache*, in that pain is inclusive of the phenomenon known as headache.

A concept may refer to a class of abstract phenomena or a class of concrete phenomena. Abstract concepts are ideas of reality and have no specific spatiotemporal referents, such as the concept of *number*, which only has symbolic meanings without specific empirical contents and was the central object of analysis as an abstract concept offered by Frege (1884/1980); or *illness*, which has empirical contents and refers to general cases. They encompass symbolic meanings or general cases. In contrast, concrete concepts refer to phenomena having exact references to time and space. Thus, a concept of *disability*, as an example of an abstract concept, may be defined as "a state in which a person is unable to carry out human actions that are normally expected," whereas a concept of *quadriplegia of Korean War veterans* is a concrete concept, as it refers to a class of phenomena that exist in certain people in the world.

Both abstract and concrete concepts may also take on varying levels of specificity. For example, *health* is a more general abstract concept than the concept of mental health, whereas *fetal death in a hospital* is more general than *Ann Smith's miscarriage* as a concrete concept. The level of generality of viewing a given set of reality is thus a matter of choice. A conceptual ladder of abstraction from the class–subclass perspective suggested by Blalock (1969) is a way of increasing abstractness. One can link mental images about a class of phenomena from very concrete to most general. Blalock (1969) suggests that the class–subclass perspective specifies a mode by which a generalization about a class of phenomena is made, linking more concrete subclasses to a general, highly inclusive class.

Concepts are used in theoretical statements to refer to phenomena of concern. Thus, *dream* is a concept in Freud's psychoanalytic theory (1955a, 1955b), as are the *unconscious*, the *id*, and *sleep-preservation*. Rogers (1990) proposes *unitary humans, energy fields, homeodynamics, helicy, resonancy,* and *complementarity* as the major concepts in her theoretical model. Roy and Andrews (1991), on the other hand, identify *adaptation level, adaptive mode, focal stimuli, contextual stimuli, residual stimuli, cognator,* and *regulator* as the major concepts in Roy's adaptation model.

Because scientific concepts are linguistic constructions with specific usage, they result from a process called *conceptualization*. Conceptualization refers to an intellectual act of delineating aspects of reality into like categories so as to give them specific "names" (i.e., labels or terms). Hence, this is a work of classification. Because such delineation depends on the range of focus that is used in the intellectual act, objects of conceptualization vary in different scientific disciplines. However, scientific concepts are not necessarily "constructed," as many are extensions of natural, ordinary language. Thus conceptualization also includes how such extensions are specified for scientific uses.

For our purposes, the frame of reference is always nursing. This means that our interests in the real world and conceptualization of those interests are limited to what happens to people in need of nursing care or receiving nursing care, and how whatever happens in such situations occurs in particular ways. Thus, the phenomena of interest and the concepts that describe them for theoretical, scientific studies in nursing are those aspects of reality that are critical to influencing nursing practice.

Although there are many different ways of categorizing concepts according to their characteristics, for the exposition of this book I have adopted a classification scheme of "*property*" and "*process*" concepts. Nursing is basically concerned with two kinds of reality: (a) *the state of things*, such as whether or not the patient has abdominal pain, what the anxiety level is, or what the patient knows about the emergency care of bleeding, all of which refer to the characteristics of property; and (b) *the way things happen*, such as how a person learns to take blood pressure, what a patient is experiencing when he says "I don't care" or what becomes of the digitoxin a patient takes, all of which are concerned with the nature of occurrence. The first kinds of phenomena are labeled as "property" concepts, the latter as "process" concepts. In this way, some phenomena may be conceptualized in both ways, as *both* property *and* process concepts, depending on the analytical perspective taken in conceptualization of the phenomena.

For example, many scientists have used the concept of stress as a property concept that is expressed according to amount, extent, or type of stress. In contrast, others also have used it as a process concept by which the phenomenon is identified as action. The course of events associated with the impingement of noxious stimuli on objects—including humans—is inclusively described in such a definition. Similarly, "thought" is a property concept, "thinking" a process concept. As is true of any classification schema, this is also an arbitrary, analytical construct that appears to meet the test of mutual exclusiveness and exhaustiveness as criteria of typology formulation.

This system of classification of concepts into property and process types is useful in an analytic sense. By questioning the essence of a conceptual definition as either property or process, we are also questioning the focus with which conceptualization is carried out. This is theoretically important, for concepts are the main building blocks of theory. Explanations of relationships between two concepts differ according to the definitions of the concepts. This, then, brings us back to the issues in defining concepts.

Definitions of concepts are statements that explicate meanings embedded in those concepts and cannot be synthetic (Gupta, 2008). Definitions of scientific concepts need to be precise in articulating meanings, using clarifying methods such as description, explication, and stipulation, and should go beyond the commonsense definitions of nominal and dictionary types. Because scientific concepts refer to general cases (although at varying degrees of abstraction), definitions require precision in language use and in meaning. This is especially critical for concepts in human sciences in which terms in ordinary language are often brought into the scientific context, because terms in ordinary discourse tend to be inexact, change over time, and have different meanings and different uses depending on users and contexts of their uses. Because definitions of concepts are the primary ways of specifying the relationships of those concepts to referred phenomena, the meanings explicated in the definitions specify the nature and scope of such relationships.

DESCRIPTIVE FEATURES OF CONCEPT

In sciences, concepts and their definitions need to be expressed further according to their descriptive characteristics and features. This is necessary because definitions alone cannot impart the full meanings embedded in concepts, and concepts are used in theories and research to develop knowledge rather than just in ordinary discourses as in natural language. Therefore, it is essential for concepts to take some descriptive designations that will guide their identifications. This is so especially because most concepts are "cluster" concepts rather than "single-character" concepts. Descriptive characterizations of concepts begin with the definitions of concepts. The prevailing position accepted by scientists regarding concepts aligns with Wittgenstein's (1968) idea of "family resemblances" in general, especially with respect to how concepts are explicated for their descriptive characteristics. This is because the classical view of concepts, which requires specifying a set of properties necessary and sufficient for membership, has been found to be untenable by many philosophers.

In general then, concepts are described by the identification of threads of common features that are typical in phenomena referred to by specific concepts. Descriptive features of a concept may refer to appearance, structure, quality, pattern, variability, and activity as key aspects of it. For example, the descriptive features of *pain* as a concept would include how it exists (a sensation of hurt felt in many different ways, locally or holistically), how it affects the person (elevated pulse, activity variation, emotions, etc.), how it varies (intensity, quality, and duration), and how it is experienced physically, emotionally, socially, and politically, etc. The details and characterizations used in concept descriptions tend to differ according to philosophical orientations of scientists.

Whereas concepts are described according to given sets of guidelines when their conceptualizations are grounded in specific theories, they are often described without formal guidelines. Concepts developed from interpretive perspectives such as phenomenology are described by "themes." However, disciplinary perspectives determine all concept descriptions, because disciplinary perspectives determine the fields of vision and the foci for attention applied in conceptualizations. Whether or not concepts and their definitions and descriptions are theory-dependent is a philosophical debate that has been going on through the era of positivism and the post-received-view era. At the most general level, scientific concepts are theoretically determined because disciplinary perspectives, which are established by philosophical and theoretical orientations of disciplines, are applied to frame them. A large sector of scholars and philosophers goes further, with the notion that scientific concepts are determined within specific theories, which can be very broad or very specific. For example, Hempel (1966) distinguishes "descriptive" (or "analytic") definitions from "stipulative" ones, noting that scientific concepts are of the stipulative type, as stipulative definitions "serve to introduce an expression that is to be used in some specific sense in the context of a discussion, or a theory, or the like" (p. 86). This debate is philosophical, and scientists must determine their own positions according to their ontological and epistemological perspectives.

The relationship of concept definitions and descriptions with regards to the reality and empirical world has raised an additional debate in philosophy. Abell (1971) declares that theoretical concepts must ultimately be expressible as observational concepts. The necessity for a distinction between theoretical concepts and observational concepts was one of the major tenets of positivism, and was articulated by Hempel (1965) in his distinction of theoretical concepts from observational concepts for which the rules of correspondence (bridge principles or auxiliary theories) are used to make logically sound linkages between these two sorts of concepts. This position allows a variety of observational concepts that can be linked logically to theoretical terms. This is a departure from Bridgman's initial proposal (1927) for operationalization, which called for definite testing (observational) procedures to determine specific features of scientific terms, a notion that dominated many sciences, including the social sciences, for several decades. Although the concept of operationalization has remained a way of specifying theoretical concepts in observational terms, the strict sense advanced by Bridgman has been abandoned in most sciences.

A set of descriptive features of a theoretical concept, then, is the base from which empirical contents for the concept are logically derived. The process by which scientists make such derivations is through deduction, following a hierarchy of conceptualization. This process, known as operationalization of concepts, then, means designations of observational concepts having immediate referents in the real world as sense impressions and as the counterparts to the theoretical concepts. The concept of operationalization is directly associated with positivism, and has been viewed as suspect by many scientists during the past three decades. This is especially due to the questioning of what constitutes "observations" and how the unobservable may be operationalized in sciences. It also has been argued against by interpretivists and postmodernists on the ground that pure objectivity is neither possible nor necessary in sciences. However, a somewhat loose notion of the concept of operationalization has been generally accepted in response to the need to translate theoretical concepts in research in this postpositivist era. In the social sciences, for example, development of measurement tools for theoretical concepts has been applied through the identification of "essential" descriptive features as the first step.

Scientific concepts in theories are variable concepts, meaning that members (that is, clusters of phenomena) belonging to a given concept can occupy qualitatively different positions with respect to the descriptive features of that concept, both theoretically and empirically. This means that although they are members of the same class (i.e., the same concept) by definition, there are intrinsic variations that put one member in a relative position to others. For example, for the concept of gender, two distinct member-types are possible—male and female; and for the concept of pain the variations may be determined according to quality, such as dull versus sharp pain, or according to quantity, such as high versus low pain. In the positivist tradition this variability in concepts is handled through operationalization and measurement.

The value or character of a concept can be one of several different types: *qualitative* concepts can be specified as nominal or descriptive types, and *quantitative* concepts can be specified as ordinal, interval, or ratio types. These characterizations are commonly used for operationalization and measurement. As scientists uphold intersubjectivity in dealing with the variable nature of concepts that are critical in sciences, quantification becomes an issue. There are debates regarding the points that (a) all concepts must be operationalized in quantitative terms, (b) some concepts are quantifiable whereas others are not quantifiable because of the nature of the phenomena to which they refer, or (c) quantification is an artifact of human construction and has no connection to the genuine nature of phenomena. Quantification is viewed as increasing generalizability, assuring objectivity, and decreasing bias in scientific work, even as it is viewed as inauthentic and artificial, increasing the loss of critical information embedded in concepts, and failing to capture the real properties of concepts. These are philosophical questions deeply related to the nature of theories and the role of scientific understanding. In human sciences, this debate is much more complex because of the subjective nature of many human phenomena, as well as because of the interpretive nature of human experiences according to language, context, and history.

LEVEL OF CONCEPTUAL DESCRIPTION: HOLISTIC AND PARTICULARISTIC MODES

The most fundamental difficulty a serious scientific thinker encounters in conceptualizing certain "happenings" of interest is deciding the level or the limit to which such happenings (i.e., phenomena) should be considered. The level of description one selects influences the kinds of theoretical questions and outcomes that are generated in the analysis of phenomena. Hofstadter (1979) treats this issue as one of "holism" versus "reductionism." Holism is an analytical approach that looks at the object as a whole, without regard to its parts. In the holistic mode, one's focus is on the generic property of object as a totality. In contrast, Hofstadter's reductionism is a mode of analysis by which the meanings of an object's parts are brought into focus. In describing these modes in the context of listening to a Bach fugue, Hofstadter states that "the modes are these: either to follow one individual voice at a time [reductionist mode], or to listen to the total effects of all of them together, without trying to disentangle one from another [holistic mode]."[4]

The issue is this: A set of phenomena can be viewed either as a global happening or as a collection of several discrete happenings. These two approaches to viewing a set of phenomena will direct and differentiate what follows with respect to description, explanation, and measurement. For example, scientists may study humans as a whole composed of many integrated parts, or humans as a collection of different parts. It is necessary to have a global concept of humans if one is interested in understanding humans as a totality, a unified entity. A holistic view of humans is concerned with human operations as involving the totality of the person and having meanings with respect to the total being. On the other hand, it is quite possible and sometimes desirable for scientists to study many aspects of human affairs separated out as singular or discrete occurrences without explicitly making a global reference to the wholeness of humans. Again, this is a matter not of right or wrong, but of *perspective*. For the exposition of and analysis in this book, the terms *holistic* and *particularistic* have been adopted as two levels of description and analysis applicable to theoretical thinking in the nursing framework.

The *holistic* view of a situation, a happening, or an object is directed to perceiving and conceptualizing the characteristics presented by the situation, the happening, or the object with respect to its meaning as a totality. In contrast, the *particularistic* view of a situation, a happening, or an object disaggregates the situation, the happening, or the object and selects out the aspects that are of particular interest for description and analysis. In a particularistic mode, the scientist takes as given those aspects of the situation or object that exist outside of the conceptual realm of particular interest.

CONCEPT DEVELOPMENT

For any scientific discipline there is a set of essential, key concepts that are the objects of knowledge development in that field. Such concepts for a given discipline are predetermined as the discipline coalesces around the sheer nature of what the discipline considers its proper subject matter, or are advanced by theoretical specification and concept development in a progressive manner. Often these two processes are combined. In nursing, concept development as a process has come to occupy an important position in knowledge development since the 1970s, as the nature of nursing's subject matter took shape not only within nursing itself but also in the sciences, most particularly in the health sciences. As stated in chapter 1, development of concepts was the focus of knowledge development during the third phase of nursing knowledge development. Many nursing scholars proposed various approaches for concept development during this phase. However, in nursing, the terms *concept development* and *concept analysis* were used somewhat interchangeably, as many scholars considered concept analysis to be the major strategy for concept development in nursing.

Concepts as the basic units of scientific theories have specific meanings and features. Concept development refers to approaches used to advance concepts for theory development, and is aimed at clarifying existing concepts or explicating new ones. Rodgers (2000a) suggests that approaches in concept development vary according to what sorts of conceptual problems—Laudan's "internal" or "external" problems (1977)—the scientist is trying to address, and that the choice of approach may depend upon "the concept of interest and the purpose of the inquiry." Walker and Avant (2000) also recommend concept analysis as a method of choice when there are concepts already in the literature that are unclear, outmoded, or unhelpful; the strategies of concept derivation and synthesis are more appropriate when new concepts are needed in the discipline.

On the other hand, Penrod and Hupcey (2005) regard concept analysis as purely analytical of the existing literature, its outcome a summative description rather than a synthesis for clarification, and propose a method for concept advancement or refinement, starting with concept analysis as the first step. Rodgers (2000b) proposes an evolutionary approach to concept analysis, based on the assumption that concepts change over time, historically and contextually, in their uses, and that concept development is based on understanding such changes over time through their various uses. A hybrid model of concept development (Schwartz-Barcott & Kim, 2000) was proposed as an approach to developing concepts in nursing through theoretical, fieldwork, and analytical phases in which prior understanding, clinical confirmation, and analytical rigor are the bases for concept development.

Most of the concept development approaches proposed during the 1980s and 1990s in nursing are undergirded by the philosophy of realism or pragmatism, in which concepts developed through such approaches would either be viewed as representing the truth of their existence or be treated as satisfying the approximation of the truth until better conceptualizations can emerge. This philosophical grounding has been questioned by relativists and postmodernists with a view that, in the sciences, concepts can neither be universally determined nor applied acontextually.

Among nursing scholars who have voiced such concerns is Paley (1996a), who argues that concept analysis is a futile endeavor, as concepts do not get clarified through analysis. Concepts, to him, are not *a priori* to theories, as the adherents of the Walker and Avant method (2000) seem to believe, but acquire meanings only within theories. To relativists a concept has specific meanings determined by the theory or theoretical framework of which that concept is a part. In a similar position, Parse proposes, "concept inventing" as an approach to creating "unitary" concepts within a simultaneity perspective (1997b, p. 63).

Concept inventing is akin to concept formulation methods applied in deductive theory building in which concepts are formulated specifically within a theory, their meanings determined by the assumptions of the theory. From a different perspective, Wuest (2000) proposes "concept critique" as a method of concept development in critical paradigms as a dialogic process through which heightened understanding of meanings and transformations could be achieved ultimately. These are controversies that require continuing debate and conscious attitudes in the scientific community. It is necessary for each scholar to articulate the philosophical perspective on which her/his conceptual, theoretical, and empirical work is founded.

For the exposition of this book, my views on concepts are that: (a) a concept has meaning within given perspectives, where perspectives could be singular or layered, and could be at the most general level a disciplinary principle, and at the most specific level a theoretical statement; (b) a concept has to be defined and its critical features identified to clarify the definition; and (c) a concept has to refer to a class of or set of phenomena.

METHOD OF CONCEPT ANALYSIS

The first analytical technique scientists use in theoretical thinking is concept analysis. Whereas conceptualization refers to the act of arriving at an abstract understanding of a phenomenon, concept analysis refers to critical evaluation of the conceptualization that has been arrived at. Thus, conceptualization is a form of active theoretical thinking, whereas concept analysis is a form of reflexive theoretical thinking. Concept analysis is a critical evaluation of the product of conceptualization vis-à-vis scientific criteria of sound conceptual characteristics. In this book, concept analysis is used as a method of evaluating the stage and rigor of conceptualization that has taken place regarding selected concepts.[5]

Criteria for concept analysis are guidelines for examining the characteristics of a concept. Reynolds (1971) proposes three desirable characteristics of scientific concepts: (a) *abstractness*, indicative of independence from time and space, allowing concepts to have more universal and general meaning complexes that make them nontrivial and essentially important for scientific pursuits; (b) *intersubjectivity of meaning*, specifying definitional clarity and agreement among scientists with regard to phenomenal references; and (c) *descriptive clarification and intersubjectivity of descriptives*, including measurements, indicating congruity between theoretical definitions and descriptive characterizations, and agreement in the methods selected to express the meanings of theoretical concepts in empirical terms. Definition of concept serves as the basic tool to indicate and reduce the meanings of abstract concepts symbolically. Kaplan (1964) also suggests that one may use either indicative and reductive strategies or both in defining conceptual terms.

The method of concept analysis adopted in this book uses Reynolds' criteria for scientific concepts, with modifications. I have adapted Reynolds' criteria regarding operationalization and measurement by broadening them into "descriptive features." This is done by embracing the notion that the characteristics of concepts can be expressed not only through measurements but also in various descriptive terms. The specific components of concept analysis involve (a) definitional clarification of the concept selected for analysis, (b) differentiation of the concept from related concepts, (c) descriptive features of the concept, and (d) relationship of the concept to other concepts. All of these steps are carried out through a comprehensive review of the literature and with insight gained through clinical experiences or other related scientific work.

Concept analysis can be done either within a specific theoretical system or without a specific orientation to a particular theoretical system. Concept analysis carried out within a theory is less complex, because the theoretical orientation directs conceptualization toward a specific predisposition in selecting out characteristics of phenomena. Analysis of a concept without specific reference to a theory is thus far more complex, because the concept has to be analyzed for its meaning and descriptive features according to various theoretical orientations. Nevertheless, a comprehensive concept analysis allows progression toward theory construction as well as consequent theory analysis.

THEORY AND THEORETICAL STATEMENTS

Scientists use theories and theoretical statements as the basic tools for explaining problems of concern. Conceptualization of reality is linked to theories and theoretical statements for scientific descriptions and explanations. At this point, it might be useful to clarify what is meant by theory and how it is used differently from such related terms as theoretical statement, proposition, and hypothesis.

Theory is defined as a set of theoretical statements that specify the nature of phenomena or relationships between two or more classes of phenomena (and, therefore, concepts) so as to understand a problem or the nature of things. In general, a well-formed theory contains at least three components (*assumptions*, *concepts*, and *theoretical statements*) that are integrated together to provide a specific type of scientific understanding. A set of assumptions of a theory (which are also referred to as premises, presuppositions, and suppositions by some authors) comprises foundational, general belief statements about: (a) the worldviews that undergird the theory; (b) the theoretical perspectives and rationale by which the theory's perspectives are formulated; (c) the scope of the proposed theory; and (d) the style or form of scientific understanding adopted in the theory. A set of concepts identified and defined in a given theory specifies the phenomenal boundary with which the theory is formulating scientific statements. And a set of theoretical statements provides the exact nature of scientific understanding proposed in a given theory.

The purposes of theory are multifaceted. Theory is an intellectual tool used to understand and explain the world in which we live. The ultimate motivation, though, is in our desire to "control" the world to our benefit. Theory provides a systematic basis for sorting out regularities from irregularities. By knowing what is happening (i.e., having descriptive knowledge) and then finding out how something occurs (i.e., having descriptive or explanatory knowledge), we are able to move toward knowing the kinds of changes we must make for some things to occur. Whereas conceptualization is mainly directed toward descriptive knowledge, theory is oriented to understanding, explanation, and prediction. As we become able to explain and predict certain phenomena, both control and prescription become possible for us. Certain phenomena can be produced by manipulating components (e.g., elements, factors, or variables) of theoretical formulations in research. However, the idea that theory should be oriented only toward explanation and prediction leading to control and prescriptions has been challenged and rejected by many philosophers and scientists in recent years. Scientists are increasingly considering theories rich in scientific value even when they are oriented basically toward description and understanding.

In practice sciences, the role of theory extends beyond simple description, explanation, and control of phenomena. Practice sciences need prescriptions for action and intervention. Prescriptive theories (situation-producing theories, as designated by Dickoff, James, & Wiedenbach, 1968a, 1968b) are used to develop intervention strategies. Approaches to solving practical problems are "prescribed" according to theoretical knowledge. In nursing, Dickoff and James' classification of theories (Dickoff, James, & Widenbach, 1968a, 1968b) into (a) factor-isolating, (b) factor-relating, (c) situation-relating, and (d) situation-producing types has been subjected to much debate. There is general agreement, thus far, on the need for prescriptive theories, which can be applied to "regulate" nursing therapies, as the highest level of theoretical formulation in nursing. However, nursing theories may be considered as belonging to one or more of three types: *descriptive, explanatory*, and *prescriptive* theories, each type serving different sorts of scientific understanding.

The focus of theory is usually on unexplained phenomena considered to be problematic or important. A problem exists for a given phenomenon when its nature is puzzling, its variation is not obvious, or it affects other phenomena profoundly. These are instances that require understanding, explanation, or solution. For this reason, many theories are not simply drawn out of the "thin air," but are derived from other theories. Theory is a systematic way of designating orderliness between or among elements of reality. Theory is always tentative to a certain degree, because it is based on logically derived conjectures.

At the most elementary level a theory consists of *concepts* and *theoretical statements*. Theoretical statements in a theory are merely notations that illustrate behaviors (or states) of the concepts and designate relationships among concepts. Theoretical statements may be descriptive or explanatory. Descriptive statements express the nature of things and characteristics of phenomena. In contrast, explanatory theoretical statements specify relationships in a causal or an associational manner among two or more concepts. Theoretical statements are either propositions or hypotheses. A *proposition* is a theoretical statement that specifies the nature of concepts, or relationships among concepts. A theoretical proposition can be descriptive, specifying characteristics, patterns, or regularities of concepts. It also can be explanatory, specifying systematic ways regularities and irregularities occur among two or more concepts. A *hypothesis*, in comparison, is a theoretical statement that is to be tested in a specific empirical situation for verification.[6] Thus, a hypothesis has a referent proposition from which it is drawn. Whereas a proposition deals with more general classes of the phenomena in question, a hypothesis is concerned with subsets of the same classes of the phenomena. All theoretical statements have to be able to be tested or verified and should have empirical referents implied in the statements. A logical deduction is the method used to derive empirical statements from many levels of abstract theoretical statements. This indicates that concepts in propositions tend to be broader and more general than concepts in hypothesis.

An example of a theoretical statement in nursing theory would be Roy's "adaptation level" proposition: "The greater the adaptation level, the greater the independence in activities of daily living" (Roy & Andrews, 1991). The concept of adaptation level, expressed as a quantitatively varying concept, is related to another concept, independence in activities of daily living, which is also expressed as a quantitatively varying concept. This statement by itself contains very little information, and a reader would not be able to understand the full meanings of the proposition. This is because the statement is derived from a theoretical system in which a special language has been developed for terms such as "adaptation level." In this statement, whereas the concept of adaptation level is quite abstract and holistic, the concept of independence in daily living is not. The abstract and holistic concept of "independence" has been somewhat reduced to refer to certain aspects of an individual's functioning freedom, that is, activities of daily living. By defining the exact meanings of the two concepts in the statement and specifying empirical referents of the concepts, it is possible to deduce a hypothesis of the proposition so as to test it in the empirical world.

The scope of theory is determined by the nature of the phenomena it is intended to explain and the complexity of theoretical statements. Thus, subject matter for a theory may be very broad and all-inclusive or very narrow and limited. For nursing, four levels are identified: *grand theory*, *mesotheory*, *middle-range theory*, and *microtheory*.

The term *grand theory* is usually used to refer to a theory that tries to handle phenomena in a general area of a scientific field, such as Parsons' general theory of action (1951), Einstein's theory of relativity (1961), Freud's theory of psychoanalysis (1955a, 1955b), or Rogers' theory of unitary humans (1994). In most instances, grand theories require further specification and partitioning of theoretical statements for them to be empirically tested and theoretically verified. Grand theorists start their theoretical formulations at the most general level of abstraction, and it is often difficult to link these formulations to reality. The early theoretical efforts for "theories of nursing," such as the works of Rogers, Roy, and Johnson, seem to have focused on developing grand theories in nursing.

The term *mesotheory* is proposed to designate nursing theories that are less general than grand theories, but more general than middle-range theories in their scope. This term is proposed because nursing deals with phenomena that are located empirically in four different domains, as discussed in this book. Because grand theories refer to those dealing with the subject matter of nursing in an all-encompassing way, it seems necessary to have a term that refers to theories that deal with a broad spectrum of phenomena in a specific domain. Such theories are not middle-range in the sense the term is used by Merton (1968) and accepted in nursing, and are more abstract and deal with broader classes of phenomena. King's theory of goal-attainment (1981), Watson's theory of human care (1988), and Newman's theory of health as expanding consciousness (1994) may be considered mesotheories of nursing. The nursing phenomenon of interest for King's theory is "transaction," referring to phenomena between client and nurse. Transaction is used to explain the nature of goal attainment in the client. King's theory deals with phenomena of goal attainment generally applicable in all nursing practice situations, whereas Watson's theory (1988) deals with general features of the client–nurse relationship. Newman (1994) particularly addresses human health from the notion of expanding consciousness.

A more realistic and testable level of theory is what was proposed as the theories of middle range (Merton, 1968). *Middle-range theories* in sociology, such as the theory of reference group, theory of social exchange, and theory of power have been developed and tested rather successfully during the past 20 years, although many of these theories have not been integrated to form a grand theory that explains the social reality in a comprehensive manner. In nursing, very few middle-range theories were developed and tested in the early years of the profession's theoretical development. During the past 10 years, however, there has been an increasing level of interest among nursing scholars for the development of middle-range theories. Although a specific definition of middle-range theory has been firmly established neither in social science literature nor in nursing literature, it is generally accepted that middle-range theories refer to theories that are "testable and intermediate in scope" (Suppe, 1996). Many middle-range theories have been developed in nursing, as evidenced in several recent books that discuss such theories (for example, Smith & Liehr, 2003, 2008). Middle-range theories are developed by applying various analytic and research methods, and include among many, the theory of self-transcendence (Reed, 1991), the theory of uncertainty in illness (Mishel, 1988, 1990, 1997), the middle-range theory of unpleasant symptoms (Lenz, Pugh, Milligan, Gift, & Suppe, 1995, 1997), and the theory of women's caring (Wuest, 2001).

Microtheory is a term used by some scientists to refer to a set of theoretical statements, usually hypotheses, which deal with narrowly defined phenomena. There is a great deal of debate as to whether this should be called a "theory," as it tends to be rather limited in its explanatory power and is composed of mere postulations of hypothetical thinking. In nursing, Im and Meleis (1999) and Im (2005) proposed situation-specific theories as a special type of practice theories, and termed them as microtheories. Situation-specific theories are those that focus on specific nursing phenomena, reflecting clinical practice issues, and circumscribed by specific populations or particular fields of practice (Im, 2005). This does not mean that situation-specific theories are the only type of microtheories available; as microtheories are generally referred to as those composed of a set of testable hypotheses or with a narrowly defined scope. Theories developed by applying the grounded theory approach, which have not been formulated into what Glaser and Strauss called formal theories (1967), may be included here as a type of microtheory.

The difference among the levels of theory just noted is not only at the level of abstraction with which concepts are delineated, but also with respect to the range of explanation the theory seeks to attain. Thus, a theory can be characterized both according to the level of sophistication of its explanation and in view of its scope.

Theory development as the central focus of scientific work can be pursued by *inductive, deductive,* or an *interpretive* approach. An inductive approach refers to developing or constructing theories beginning with empirical data or phenomena as they exist in actual situations. An inductive approach discerns regularities, both descriptive and explanatory, that exist in reality, with generalizations about the discovered regularities formulated into theoretical statements. On the other hand, a deductive approach begins with generalized ideas about phenomena. The deductive approach is based on a set of foundational notions about the nature of explanation, and proceeds using a system of deductive logic to come up with a theory moving from general ideas about phenomena to more specific theoretical relationships. In recent years, scientists are increasingly combining both approaches to develop theories aligned with what Hanson (1958) called *retroduction.* A retroductive approach is oriented to reconstruction and revision of theories. Theories are viewed as emerging mostly from existing theories; with the need for theory reconstruction originating from anomalies and deviations observed in reality. Such observations present ideas inductively about what other ways a given theory may be revised and reconstructed. This inductively derived understanding thus becomes the basis for deductive reconstruction of a given theory.

More recently, an *interpretive* approach has been proposed and applied by scientists within the interpretive tradition for theory development, especially in the human sciences. Taylor (1985) suggests interpretation as the basis for the development of "the science of man." He believes that the traditional empirical scientific mode of studying the human sciences is inadequate because the empirical sciences base knowledge development on brute data only, neglecting the meanings embedded in human affairs. Thus, a hermeneutical science of humans studies "the intersubjective and common meanings embedded in social reality" through interpretation. Theories developed through interpretation provide "*ex post* understanding," an explanation different from predictive explanations of empiricism. Interpretation as an approach to theory development then uses texts (or text-analogues) for the readings of meanings, which "are for a subject in a field or fields,...are partially constituted by self-definitions, and...can thus be reexpressed or made explicit by a science" (Taylor, 1985, p. 52). Theories developed through the interpretive approach are of a different character than those developed in the traditional empirical sciences, because such theories are not for verification but for intuitive explanation. As Gadamer (1976) states, in the human sciences theories provide ways of understanding through a fusion of horizons.

During the past decades, we have been struggling with and debating about not only what classes of phenomena should be included in a system of theoretical explanations in nursing science, but also what approaches may be most fruitful and appropriate for developing that knowledge. We also have been engaged in debates about the differences between "theories *of* nursing" and "theories *in* nursing" and their respective propriety, legitimacy, and relevance in the scientific study of nursing. Scientific knowledge in nursing can be expanded and enriched by studying, developing, testing, and refining *both* types of theories. This should not be viewed as a disadvantage but as an advantage for nursing.

By definition, *theories in nursing* develop through the process of borrowing. Nursing as an applied scientific field has the responsibility to apply theories and knowledge developed in other fields. Such "borrowed" theories can be used to describe, explain, and predict specific phenomena that we confront in our work. This involves translating and using the theories for nursing-relevant phenomena, treating them as subclasses of those for which the original theories were developed. For example, the motivation theory of learning can be applied to study patients' difficulties in learning to carry out specific self-care procedures. A modification of the theory through repeated empirical specifications in nursing situations will thus result in the motivation theory of patients' learning. The responsibility for the selection of relevant and important ideas from such theories and for the codification into "theories *in* nursing" rests with nurse scientists. These individuals make theoretical connections between original theories and phenomena of importance to nursing, and specify the linkages, both theoretical and empirical, between them. Because nursing is concerned with several different aspects of human life, many theories from biological, social, psychological, and other behavioral sciences can be refined and reconstructed as theories in nursing.

In contrast, *theories of nursing* are those developed to describe, explain, and predict "nursing" as a class of phenomena proper. For such theories, it is necessary to define and differentiate nursing phenomena from the subject matter of other fields. It involves identifying the conceptual properties of selected phenomena in a specific way—that of nursing. There have been many attempts at this by such nursing theorists as Rogers, Roy, Orem, Neuman, and Parse at the grand theory level, others such as King, Watson, and Newman at the mesotheory level, and many more at the middle-range level. We are progressing steadfastly in developing theories of nursing, as we are gaining headway in "naming" and "describing" distinct classes of phenomena as specific to nursing. It is necessary to incorporate both kinds of theories into the discipline of nursing if we are to aim for comprehensive understanding within the field.

PARADIGM, METAPARADIGM, AND METATHEORY

The term *paradigm*, made fashionable by Kuhn (1970), is used in this book to refer simply to a scientific perspective that encompasses specific orientations and approaches adopted for a given subject matter. It includes perspectives about the nature and form of explanation and the dominant methods of scientific work. From this usage, it is possible to identify several different paradigms actively pursued in nursing, such as holistic paradigm, systems paradigm, behavioral paradigm, phenomenological paradigm, interpretive paradigm, and critical paradigm. This usage is a very much simplified version of the original proposal by Kuhn (1970), who emphasized two specific meanings of paradigm, one denoting "the entire constellations of beliefs, values, techniques, and so on shared by the members of a given community" (p.175) and the other referring to the specific models of puzzle-solutions adopted for solving scientific problems.

The term *metaparadigm* has gained usage in the nursing literature to refer to generic features of nursing science. Here, *metaparadigm* refers to the epistemological considerations at a higher and more general philosophical level. The "meta" in this word is adopted to mean "beyond" and "transcending" paradigms to a higher and broader epistemological level. Metaparadigm is concerned with general issues of the subject matter of a discipline with respect to what the general contents are, to how such contents are organized, and to what a discipline is concerned with as a knowledge structure. In nursing, metaparadigm is commonly used in talking about metaparadigm concepts. Health, client, nursing, and environment as the metaparadigm concepts for nursing have been used as the key concepts nursing must define and incorporate into theoretical work. This is one usage of the term, but it is a limited usage. In this book, the term *metaparadigm* is used not in conjunction with concepts but as an adjective in referring to epistemological, disciplinary concerns that transcend paradigms, theories, and methods.

Although the term *metatheory* is not in vogue in nursing, this term is being discussed fervently in other social and behavioral sciences. *Metatheory* is most commonly defined as the analytical work regarding issues associated with theory development and knowledge generation germane to a given discipline, such as a systematic study of the underlying structure of theory in a given discipline (Ritzer, 1992; Ritzer, Zhao, & Murphy, 2006). Ritzer (1988) proposes a typology of metatheories. Fuhrman and Snizek (1990) identified cogent areas of metasociological work in sociology (metasociology, including metatheory) as mapping of sociology's cognitive structure, debates on sociology's core-concepts, discussions on various assumptions about human nature and their implications on the study of society, and ideological investigations that link sociology to other disciplines and philosophy. Turner (1990), on the other hand, insists that metatheorizing should be limited to directing the development of better theories. In nursing, metatheorizing has been active during the past 20 years, as evidenced by the articles assembled in books edited by Nicoll (1997) and by Reed and Shearer (2009) and numerous books published in analyzing theoretical works in nursing such as Meleis (2004) and Barnum (1994). Nursing knowledge will be developed most richly through both metatheorizing and substantive theorizing, with metatheorizing providing the necessary critiques of, reflections on, and formulations of what the discipline's knowledge should be about, and substantive theorizing advancing specific contents of that knowledge.

In summary, I have mainly presented my usage and understandings, omitting comprehensive discussions of various semantic, disciplinary, and scientific usages of the terms. The terms also take on somewhat different analytic meanings in the field of philosophy of science. In addition, there are many more terms and concepts used in theory-development literature.

A comprehensive discussion on the subject requires another kind of passion. Thus, they are not pursued here, not for a lack of passion for such a pursuit, but for the consideration of "propriety" of the context in which this book is written.

NOTES

1. See also: Kim, H. S. (1997). Terminology in structuring and developing nursing knowledge. In King, I. M., & Fawcett, J. (Eds.), *The language of nursing theory and metatheory* (pp. 27–36). Indianapolis, IN: Sigma Theta Tau International Center Nursing Press.
2. One comment about the debate that is going on over a differentiation between "absolute" reality and "conscious" reality may be in order. Many philosophers of science have debated the definition of reality. The history of scientific discovery tells us that we are ever encountering phenomena that we were unaware of in our past. This suggests that there exists an "absolute" reality to be discovered, to become aware of. A contrasting view to this is the argument that what we cannot perceive to exist is not reality, and that reality is bounded by the consciousness and perceptiveness of humankind at a given time, for what we cannot fathom to exist cannot be real to us. Such arguments are interesting and paradoxical. But for now, let me ask for the readers' indulgence to accept my position, for purposes of this book, that a reality needs to be conceptualized in the human mind for it to be problematic.
3. Concept formation refers to three different senses. The first sense is the formation of concepts for a linguistic culture, that is, how concepts within a linguistic cultural system become formulated and transmitted through its history. The second sense is the formation of concepts in individuals as we learn language; that is, how an individual comes to establish and make connections between what is perceived and thought of and terms that refer to them. This second sense refers to the process of linguistic learning in humans. The third sense is concerned with how terms are established within scientific disciplines and how terms come to have specific intersubjective meanings for scientific understanding. This third sense of concept formation is of interest in this book.
4. This Hofstadter story labeled as "prelude" should be of interest to readers who want to follow the arguments for holism and reductionism. See Hofstadter, D. R. (1979). *Goedel, Escher, Bach: An eternal golden braid* (p. 282). New York: Vintage Books.
5. See for other approaches to concept analysis and concept development in nursing: Rodgers, B. I., & Knafl, K. A. (2000). *Concept development in nursing: Foundations, techniques, and applications* (2nd ed.). Philadelphia: W.B. Saunders.
6. I do not believe it fruitful to debate over what the proper meanings and definitions of these two terms are. Although there are many different ways and different levels of specificity with which these terms are used in the scientific community as well as in nursing, the distinction proposed here seems the most accepted use.

3 Nursing Epistemology

OVERVIEW: THE NATURE OF NURSING KNOWLEDGE

Nursing's efforts to define itself as a legitimate knowledge system began in the 1950s with its movement to detach from medicine as a distinct discipline and a profession. Nursing knowledge as a system of knowledge for its disciplinary base has been termed "nursing science," mostly to locate the discipline within the legitimate world of the modern knowledge system from this early period.

On one hand, there has been a continuing effort to establish nursing as a specific science, for instance, by Rogers (1970, 1992), who proposed that nursing is a basic science whose phenomenon of concern is unitary human beings in mutual process with their environments, and by Barrett (2002) and Parse (1998, 1999), who also claim nursing science as a basic science encompassing "the substantive discipline-specific knowledge that focuses on the human-universe-health process articulated in the nursing frameworks and theories" (Parse et al., 2000, p. 177). On the other hand, the fervent development of nursing knowledge during the past 3 decades with the adoption of empirical methods and research and with an alignment with positivism has fostered a sense of nursing discipline developing as an empirical science.

At the same time, in response to the discordance and the feeling of discomfort with the notion that nursing knowledge was becoming aligned solely with science, nursing scholars began to specify different types of knowledge for nursing. This has to be understood in the context of that period during which the concept of science was basically tied to empiricism, with the natural sciences as its models. As one of the first suggestions in this regard, Donaldson and Crowley (1978) proposed a syntax of nursing composed of two sets of value systems, that is, that of science and that of professional ethics, as criteria for acceptance of true statements for the discipline of nursing. Thus, in this view, nursing knowledge is composed of two sets of statements syntactically organized as either the science or the ethics. This proposal specifies two different sets of knowledge for nursing—one scientific, and the other ethical—which are then developed and systematized according to different modes of knowledge development.

Carper's seminal article (1978) proposing four patterns of knowing raised the consciousness of nursing scholars regarding the ways nursing can develop its knowledge. It has led theoretical thinking to move beyond the scientific/empirical modes of knowledge generation in nursing. However, Carper (1978, 1988) has not been clear as to whether the patterns of knowing refer to the processes of gaining knowledge or to four types of knowing in nursing practice inherent in individual practitioners. This is especially true as Carper designates empirics as a science of nursing having a set of systematic explanatory structures, while positing the other three types of knowing as processes rather than as systems of knowledge. She thus specifies aesthetics (or "esthetics"), equated with the *art* of nursing, to encompass knowing of particulars in individual experiences, and identifies empathy as the mode of an aesthetic pattern of knowing. She then attributes personal knowledge in practice to be a "subjective, concrete and existential" knowing of the self (i.e., the nurse) that is critical in clinical encounters; she identifies ethics as the moral component and refers to the ethical pattern of knowing as the knowing and understanding of different philosophies of morality, of different ethical frameworks for moral judgments, and of different orientations vis-à-vis obligations. These statements suggest that Carper's four patterns of knowing refer to one system of knowledge (empirics) and three processes of knowing inherent in practice.

Thus, although she seems to propose a knowledge system of the empirics, Carper does not specify parallel, organized systems of knowledge for ethical, aesthetic, and personal knowing. This has created misconceptions in the literature. Some have considered the fundamental patterns as the modes with which individual nurses arrive at their own knowledge, whereas others have thought of these patterns as four specific types of nursing knowledge. Chinn and Kramer (2003) adopted Carper's four patterns of knowing to identify four types of knowledge for nursing practice as science (empirics), ethics, aesthetics, and personal knowledge.

Thus, they set apart empiric science as having specific methods for developing knowledge from three other types of knowledge, which are developed by modes other than the scientific. On the other hand, Paley and colleagues (2007) argue that Carper's four patterns of knowing in nursing have elevated four types of knowing to the same level of authority in influencing practice, a situation which, if taken seriously in practice, is likely to produce practice that is entrenched with errors in judgment and misuse of information. Therefore, for Paley the issue is not the nature of knowledge itself but how different ways of knowing actually influence practice.

Although many other critiques on Carper's patterns of knowing in nursing have appeared in the literature (see, for example, Schultz & Meleis, 1998; White, 1995), Carper's paper contributed to the realization and acceptance of diverse types of knowing or knowledge for nursing, stimulating scholars to examine different ways of knowing and different modes by which nursing knowledge may be developed (Benner, 1984; De Raeve, 1998; Edwards, 1998; Fawcett et al., 2001; Kirkham, Baumbusch, Schultz & Anderson, 2007; Moch, 1990; Munhall, 1993; Rycroft-Malone et al., 2004; Van der Zahm & Bergum, 2000).

Along with this dialogue on Carper, nursing's realization that scientism, or positivistic inquiry, is limiting in its capacity to address its subject matter satisfactorily stems from the 1980s (among many discussions, see Allen, Benner, & Diekelmann, 1983; Thompson, 1985; Watson, 1985). This view has prompted much debate, which remains with us as a deeply felt chasm between "tough-minded" and "tender-minded" scholars. To date, the discourse remains contentious, locked in an "either/or" position concerning an exclusive epistemology for nursing.[1]

Here, nursing science is pitted against nursing art (which sometimes has been equated with the humanities) as two different, separate, or parallel aspects of nursing. Darbyshire (1999) has suggested that nursing has become embroiled in a cultural battle between two opposing sides—the humanities against the natural sciences—with nursing weighted heavily toward the natural sciences by way of its adopting natural scientific methods. Yet, even as a sector of nursing scholarship continues its pursuit of knowledge through natural science, another sector has distanced itself from this mode and begun to align with the philosophy and modes of the human sciences, especially in terms of interpretive philosophy and methodology. In addition, still another sector has entirely moved away from the notion of science, declaring nursing to be a humanistic discipline—in short, an art.

On this issue, there are thus three positions, which have not been reconciled by the profession:

1. The nursing discipline is to be identified solely as nursing science (Giuliano, Tyer-Viola, & Lopez, 2005; Meleis, 2004; Rolfe, 2006; Roy, 2007, among many others), as one of the human sciences (Holmes, 1990; Playle, 1995; Van der Zalm & Bergum, 2000, among others), or as unique (Mitchell & Cody, 2002; Newman, 2002; Parse, 1999; Rogers, 1994).
2. The nursing discipline is an art, one of the humanities, which distinguishes its unique nature of practice (Appleton, 1994; Baumann, 1999: Watson, 1994, among others).
3. The nursing discipline consists of two dimensions, that is, nursing science and nursing art, nursing science being its knowledge base and nursing art being the base for practice (Darbyshire, 1999, for example).

Even a cursory look at the nursing literature reveals the fact that nursing scholars have adopted not only diverse theoretical orientations (unitary models originally developed in nursing, systems models, cognitive models such as the self-efficacy framework, biobehavioral models, self-care and functional models, symbolic interactionism, psychodynamic models, and psychosocial models) and different modes of inquiry (including empirical, interpretive, and critical modes), but also different ontological and epistemological philosophies in their theoretical advances.

Omery, Kasper, and Page (1995) present nine different philosophical orientations viewed as having relevance to nursing knowledge development; these range from empiricism, pragmatism, paradigmatic historicism, and science as problem solving, to feminism, phenomenology, hermeneutics, critical philosophy, and poststructuralism. It is certain that we are grappling with philosophical pluralism as well as theoretical pluralism in nursing. In viewing pluralism, especially relative to the various worldviews represented in nursing, as creating diversity and fragmentation, Reed (1995) offers a "neomodernist" worldview (defined as the "developmental–contextual" worldview) as the unifying perspective for nursing's knowledge development. Her position advocates adopting a singular paradigm as a desirable and necessary step in dealing with the pluralism.

However, as Emden (1991) suggests, there apparently is an increasing cross-camps discourse that may bring about a deeper understanding of what kinds of contributions the different types of inquiry make for the development of nursing knowledge. Several voices urge the acceptance and necessity of multiparadigm epistemology for nursing that embraces multiplicity of theories, perspectives, and philosophies (Booth, Kenrick, & Woods, 1997; Engebretson, 1997; Fawcett, 2000; Geanellos, 1997; Schultz & Meleis, 1998; Tarlier, 2005). In the same spirit, Omery, Kasper, and Page propose that "a plurality of philosophies may be necessary to reflect the many facets of nursing science; that is, no one view may be sufficient to embrace or drive nursing knowledge in its totality" (1995, p. x). Proposals for reconciliation between nursing science and nursing art are attempts to view nursing as a two-dimensional discipline, having two components requiring integration at the level of practice.

Pluralism is certainly evident in nursing (see Allen, Benner, & Diekelman, 1983; Gortner, 1993; Kim, 1996; Reed, 1995), but it is also evident in most other scientific disciplines. What is not clear is why pluralism is appropriate for nursing. Staats (1989) talks of psychology as having developed into fields of study identified as separate entities holding oppositional positions such as "nature versus nurture, situationism versus personality, scientific versus humanistic psychology," with little or no planning with respect to their relationships to the rest of psychology. Good (1994) also identified four different approaches to the anthropological study of illness and health as "the rationalistic–empiricist" tradition, the cognitive orientation, the "meaning-centered" tradition, and the critical medical anthropology. Ritzer, Zhao, and Murphy (2006) specify four metatheories, identified as positivism, hermeneutic, critical theory, and postmodernism in sociology, each of which addresses how sociological theories must be developed and is mostly posed as an oppositional and competitive perspective against others regarding sociological knowledge. Bhaskar (1986) suggests it is inevitable that "on the new, integrative-pluralistic worldview which emerges, both nature and the sciences (and the sciences in the nature) appear as stratified and differentiated, interconnected and developing" (p. 101).

What remains open and vague regarding nursing knowledge at present is the indeterminate character of nursing knowledge as generally accepted by the discipline as well as the haphazard ways knowledge is being developed without concern for how each piece of knowledge contributes to the total system of nursing knowledge. In view of this state of nursing science and the rampant pluralism in nursing knowledge development with respect to perspectives, theoretical frameworks, theories, and methods of inquiry, it is critical to have a unifying framework for epistemological discussions about nursing knowledge. This is because nursing is a practice discipline in which knowledge is developed to be applied in practice. By discerning the philosophies, intellectual commitments, and theoretical orientations, we may be able to gain an insight for a unifying framework that brings together multiple—sometimes rival, sometimes complementary—knowledge in nursing. The essential purpose in this proposal for nursing epistemology is to find a way to systematize nursing knowledge and offer a coherent way for the users of nursing knowledge, that is, the nursing practitioners, to examine and use the knowledge effectively in practice.

NURSING EPISTEMOLOGY

From this background, then, I propose a *nursing epistemology* as a way of critically comprehending our knowledge both for knowledge development and for practice. I have proposed my perspective for this epistemology as a *critical normative epistemology* (Kim 1997, 2007). This philosophy is an integrated view coming from epistemological realism, emancipatory pragmatism, and normative perspective of human practice. This is based on the sentiments expressed by Good (1994) for anthropology, and Bhaskar (1986, 1991) for the social sciences. Byron Good stated for medical anthropology that "[d]isease and human suffering cannot be comprehended from a single perspective. Science and its objects, the demands of therapeutic practice, and personal and social threats of illness cannot be comprehended from a unified or singular perspective. A multiplicity of tongues are [sic] needed to engage the objects of our discipline and to fashion an anthropological—scientific, political, moral, aesthetic, or philosophical—response" (Good, 1994, p. 62). The position Bhaskar takes is that "any social science must incorporate a historically situated hermeneutics; while the condition that the social sciences are part of their own field of enquiry means that they must be self-reflexive, critical and totalising in a way in which the natural sciences typically are not. But there is neither antinomy nor unbridgeable chasm nor the possibility of mutual exclusion between the sciences of nature and of (wo)man" (Bhaskar, 1986, p. 101).

A *nursing epistemology* is offered as the base from which the types of knowledge necessary for nursing practice can be delineated and organized. My view of nursing epistemology is, to begin with, based on the belief that the reality or the essence of reality must be considered to exist *a priori* to any science, but is "obtained" for knowledge development by contextually (historically and socially) situated specific human agents who engage in producing knowledge within given hermeneutically constrained horizons. This preunderstanding must motivate us to view knowledge as relativistic, but at the same time to strive toward self-critique that can bring our knowledge closer to what truly exists. In addition, the fact of knowing as well as the experience of our lives must be viewed as constrained by our own language and language use, history, and contexts, and that knowledge development needs to be framed within continuous reflection and self-critique.

It is furthermore based on the notion that nursing is a human practice discipline, and that nursing knowledge must be that which provides the foundation from which the practice is shaped for the discipline and for individual practitioners. Nursing knowledge for a human practice discipline with a specific focus on people's health must be for the understanding and explanation of human phenomena of interest to nursing, both those of clients and those of nursing practice itself. In addition, I base this epistemological position on several assumptions.

- Human beings, ontologically, are complex in that humans are natural, physical beings existing concretely as individuals, in concert with others, and contextually engaged in their environment. But, at the same time, humans are also symbolic entities constructed by selves and others, and constrained by history and circumstance, capable of free will, intentions, and self-propelled activities. Hence, there are aspects of humans that are among nursing's epistemic concerns which are knowable objectively and are based on generalizable features, and which are only knowable by experiencing selves and through interpretations as contextually embedded phenomena.
- It is not possible for one to know (i.e., understand and explain about) human beings all at once in a unified, comprehensive fashion. We must tease out aspects of humans based on different ontological foci for proper understanding. This requires specific nursing ontology of humans that can direct us to adopt appropriately different epistemological modes of knowledge generation.
- Nursing practice as a form of human practice requires mutuality that upholds emancipation of involved human agents. Human agents engaged in practice (both clients and nurses) must coordinate their freedom, meanings, and desires as a means of gaining emancipation, mutuality, and goal-attainment.
- Nursing practice is founded upon a normative, moral, and aesthetic grounding that is formulated through historical, social, and personal processes that go beyond the way scientific knowledge is produced.
- Although knowledge needs to be developed partially and selectively within the given ontological and epistemological foci appropriate for nursing, such knowledge must be considered complementary and inclusive rather than competitive and exclusive.
- The ultimate endpoint for any systematized nursing knowledge is the knowledge of synthesis as it is used in actual practice, and can be revealed and known only by accessing the practice.

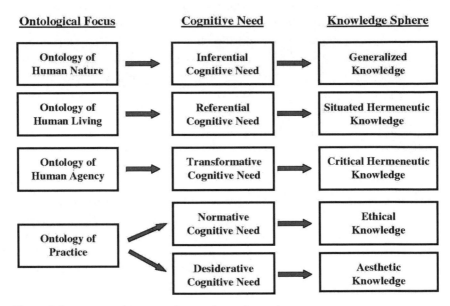

Figure 3.1. Structural elements for nursing epistemology.

These premises for the critical normative epistemology of nursing help us to view our knowledge development from four ontological commitments that point to five different types of cognitive needs, which in turn delineate five spheres of nursing knowledge as shown in Figure 3.1.

The premises expressed previously make it necessary to espouse four separate but integrated ontological commitments regarding nature, humans, and practice that must undergird nursing knowledge. Ontological commitments refer to the necessary attitudes regarding the nature of subject matter with which the discipline is concerned. Ontological commitments are based on what the discipline's functions are perceived to be in relation to its practice. Thus, these ontological commitments emanate from the definition of nursing practice. There are variations in the definitions of nursing practice offered in the literature, but there are essential characteristics that are fundamental to that practice. I offer the following as a generic definition of nursing practice (originally given in the second edition of this book), in which I identify the four ontological commitments for nursing epistemology:

> Nursing practice is a goal-directed, deliberative, action-oriented, and coordinated work for and with people for enhancing healthful living or peaceful dying, in which both patients and nurses embody the ontological realities

of human features and life, and of human agency. Nursing practice is an intentionally coordinated process consisting of scientific, technological problem solving, human-to-human engagement, and services to people with specific needs. It occurs in social situations of health care in which nurses assume particular sorts of responsibilities.

This definition specifies four ontological commitments: ontology *of human nature,* ontology *of human living,* ontology *of human agency,* and ontology *of practice.* The ontology of human nature bespeaks a commitment to the assumption that human nature encompasses humans' species-specific and group-specific features, characteristics, and conditions that exist and are possible as patterns and systematic differences influenced by innate and contextual as well as experiential forces. For example, both human genetics and human socialization play important roles in determining conditions, behaviors, and trajectories of experiences in humans. The ontology of human living, on the other hand, points to a commitment to the understanding of human living as experienced, interpreted, and managed from the totality of the living self, the individual that is conscious, meaning making, historically and contextually embedded, and reflexive all at once. This means that human living is both individually unique and at the same time contextually connected to the culture (that is, history, language, customs, habits, etc.) in which the living takes place.

The ontology of human agency commits to the assumption that humans are agents who are engaged in both independent and coordinated actions in search of certain goals. Human agents thus are both free and constrained in seeking and moving toward their goals. The paradox of freedom and constraints is the essential feature of human agency, and thus points to the need for coordination regarding means, meanings, and goals. The ontology of practice is based on the assumption that human practice is a service of one human person (the provider or the professional) to another (the patient, the client, the service user) in which the goal is specified for the recipient (the patient), thus requiring ethical, moral, and aesthetic guidelines for practice. This ontology also commits to the notion that practice is not simply scientific, technological problem solving, but is guided by *a priori* and overarching principles and desiderata.

These four ontological commitments suggest that there are different types of knowledge that align with these ontological commitments and address the specific features of the ontologies. These ontological commitments also mean that the phenomena of interest to nursing are centrally located in humans both as clients and nurses, which will need to be understood, examined, and explained from four different angles if we are to get comprehensive knowledge in nursing. The reason why these ontological commitments connote distinct types of knowledge is that fundamental features of human phenomena have to be abstracted differently from the perspectives of these four ontological commitments. The different types of knowledge for nursing, then, means the complementary nature of knowledge developed from the different ontological perspectives. The specification of these different types of knowledge for nursing associated with four ontological commitments was carried out thinking through what sorts of cognitive needs are to be met to satisfy these ontological commitments.

My contemplation and development of this nursing epistemology thus has been stimulated and influenced by Habermas's ideas on human cognitive interests. Habermas (1986) laid out three forms of cognitive interests as "establishing specific viewpoints from which we can apprehend reality as such in any way whatsoever" and the basis for thinking about social science knowledge: (a) *empirical-analytical sciences,* as governed by a "technical" interest in the prediction and control of objectified processes—"the facts relevant to the empirical sciences are first constituted through an *a priori* organization of experience in the behavioural system of instrumental action"; (b) the *historical-hermeneutic sciences,* as governed by a "practical" interest in intersubjective understanding, that is, toward mutual understanding in the conduct of life; and (c) *critical sciences,* as oriented to emancipation from "ideologically frozen relations of dependence that can in principle be transformed," that is, toward emancipation from seemingly natural constraint (1986, pp. 308–311).

This conceptualization, of course, was intended and used as a set of exhaustive categories by many social scientists (both for and against Habermas's philosophy), as well as by Habermas himself, to differentiate sciences into tripartite groups as natural (empirical), interpretive, and critical sciences. In criticizing Habarmas's philosophy of pragmatism, Bhaskar (1991) specifies five forms of reason and (as a corollary) seven levels of rationality for the human sciences from the perspective of critical naturalism. He bases his ideas on the nature of knowledge for the human sciences on three basic tenets: (a) the ontology of the world as "structured, differentiated and changing" by which closed systems are not possible, which means all theories must be exclusively explanatory and nonpredictive; (b) the epistemology for "a rational account of scientific activity, which is conceived as engaged in the continual process of the empirically controlled retroduction of explanatory structures from the manifest phenomena which are produced by them"; and (c) the metacritical dimension that calls for "an examination of the metaphysical and social bases of accounts of science" (1991, pp. 146–147). For this position, Bhaskar identifies instrumental reason with technical rationality at Level I and contextually situated instrumental rationality at Level II, critical reason with practical rationality (i.e., criticism) at Level III, and explanatory critical rationality (i.e., critique) at Level IV, emancipatory reason with depth-explanatory critical rationality at Level V, depth-rationality at Level VI, and historical reason at Level VII. These are to him hierarchically specified levels of rationality that can make it possible for knowledge in the human sciences to move toward true emancipation for humans as individuals and species. This epistemological structuring is also based on integrating theories with practice and values with facts, and shows the limits of knowledge that are apparent in the knowledge developed at lower levels of rationality.

Building on the proposals by Habermas and Bhaskar, I propose a structuring of nursing epistemology considered within a specific notion that human practice sciences differ from the human and social sciences (sociology, psychology [excluding clinical psychology], anthropology, politics, and economics). The knowledge orientation of human practice sciences is in "practice" with other humans for some form of "good" involving interactive, intersubjective processes that involve knowledge beyond understanding and emancipation. Nursing as a human practice science furthermore is grounded in a focus on specific empirical contents (such as health, illness, functioning, recovery, and health care). What I believe is that nursing knowledge has an integrative, synthesizing cognitive interest that must embrace four ontological commitments for knowledge content, and that this integrative, synthesizing cognitive interest encompassing five sets of cognitive needs must be identified as the central aspect of nursing epistemology. I also deviate from Carper's four patterns of knowing in nursing by focusing on the *cognitive needs* for nursing practice that are specified by a set of ontological commitments necessary for nursing.

I propose five different types of cognitive needs based on these four different ontological commitments regarding human nature, human living, human agency, and nursing practice as shown in Figure 3.1.[2] They are: *inferential* cognitive need, *referential* cognitive need, *transformative* cognitive need, *normative* cognitive need, and *desiderative* cognitive need. These five cognitive needs point to the types of knowledge necessary for nursing practice.

The *inferential cognitive need* is grounded in the ontology of human nature. It is based on the assumptions that (a) some aspects of reality for humans exist in patterned ways (i.e., regularities and systematic differences), (b) it is possible to develop theories that explain how such patterns exist, and (c) it is possible to understand, explain, or predict (not factually but theoretically) individual occurrences by drawing inferences from theories. Patterns and regularities may be universal or circumscribed, or broad or narrow. Theories of regularity specifying different levels of generalization make it possible to draw inferences about particular instances. This need asserts a way to understand and explain particular instances based on our knowledge of general cases from which inferences are drawn, both for a simple phenomenon such as bleeding on a knee upon scraping on asphalt (inferred from the theory of tissue damage) and for a complex phenomenon such as a patient experiencing severe pain from cancer (inferred from the juxtapositioning of several different pain theories). Whereas, as Gadamer (1996) states, sciences are never able to provide complete answers to problems, the knowledge that satisfies the inferential cognitive needs provides a beginning understanding of specific events, instances, or experiences. Such knowledge in a mature state establishes an initial foundation for understanding specific instances that can be built up and supplemented by knowledge developed to fulfill different cognitive needs. Although there are vast disagreements in philosophy regarding how inferences are made or how one achieves a best explanation through inference with given knowledge, this cognitive need is a critical way humans historically have been able to understand, explain, and sometimes predict nature. The inferential cognitive need allows a short-cut way of understanding the nature.

For the inferential cognitive need, I designate the *generalized knowledge sphere* as one type of nursing knowledge. The knowledge in the generalized sphere focuses on regularities (patterns) in human conditions, processes, mechanisms, changes, and experiences relevant to nursing. The emphasis is on developing knowledge that provides general understandings, systematic explanations, and predictions through objective validation. This does not mean that theories and knowledge developed in this sphere must be global in their generalizations. Generalizations may be limited to specific population groups or contexts. Knowledge in this sphere encompasses descriptive theories that identify patterns, regularities, and tendencies that can be used to frame human problems, situations, and experiences for understanding, and theories of explanation and elaboration that can be used to gain in-depth understandings of how human phenomena occur, might occur, or are possible. The knowledge in this sphere is developed from the empirical basis and through the logical scientific modes. The knowledge in this sphere is oriented to the need for an inferential knowledge base in nursing.

The *referential cognitive need* is based on the ontology of human living. Because human living is entrenched in uniqueness, situatedness, meanings, and contextuality, it is only through references that it is possible to gain deeper understanding of experiences of human living. The referential need means a way of understanding through knowing about similarities, differences, commonalities, and uniqueness in human living experiences posed against various backgrounds. Although each human experience can be viewed as unique, humans also share certain affinities that can be used for referential understanding. It is, as Taylor (1987) suggests, that understanding is never closed and is open in a hermeneutic circle for restatement and reinterpretation. Through the referential needs, the unexpected and the unique as well as similarities and commonalities can be illuminated, and one's insights into individual occurrences expanded.

For the referential cognitive need, I designate the *situated hermeneutic knowledge sphere* as one type of knowledge for nursing. This type of knowledge refers to the knowledge of enlightenment, understanding, illumination, elaboration, and appreciation regarding human experience as it is lived in a subjective, meaning-making, and situation-bound fashion. The focus is on humans' subjective, experiencing, living selves in situations and their meanings to them, which are idiographically etched and reveal private ways of being and experiencing. Knowledge developed in this sphere for nursing is *referential* rather than *inferential* in that it can give us insights, appreciation, sensibility, and depth understanding about individual clients' experiences as well as our own (i.e., nurses') experiences. Knowledge for this sphere is developed through depth-descriptive, meaning-understanding, and interpretive methods of inquiry and includes theories of uniqueness, of differences, of contexts, and of meanings. The referential cognitive need is satisfied by knowing as many different stories, various interpretations, and as much uniqueness as possible regarding human living experiences. The knowledge in this sphere can provide nursing with enriched understanding that is necessary to individualize nursing practice.

The *transformative cognitive need* is based on the ontological commitment regarding human agency that is unshakably intertwined with the socially coordinated nature of living. This ontology thus embraces human practice tied closely to human freedom but at the same time as a form of social praxis. Human agency is associated with the conditions of human engagement with other humans and in social situations framed within the concept of human freedom. This ontological commitment acknowledges that individuals engaged in coordinated living are exposed to and experience various forms of struggles, constraints, dominations, and disharmony in relation to the exercise of genuine human freedom. This cognitive need is similar to Habermas's critical cognitive rationality by which he proposes emancipation and mutual understanding as the goals of knowledge (1986). This is a need to acknowledge, understand, and transform various systematic distortions that become established for humans, circumscribing their freedom and actions. This is a postmodern awakening regarding human living by which we acknowledge limitations, hurdles, and distortions arising from and interpenetrated in social praxis produced by history, culture, language, and power. Such constraints affect (often unknowingly, sometimes consciously) all aspects of human living, such as how we determine health and illness, how we express our needs for care, or how we view others as well as ourselves regarding competence. The transformative cognitive need is therefore based on the assumption that such constraints need to be understood, corrected, and transformed to attain unconstrained, genuine living for all, including patients and nurses. This need is also based on the assumption that when people "practice" under distortions, genuine human living is not attained.

For the transformative cognitive need, I designate the *critical hermeneutic knowledge sphere* as one type of knowledge necessary for nursing. It refers to the knowledge of interpretation, critique, and emancipation that is embedded in human living in contexts and with others. Humans' lives in general and more specifically in the context of health and nursing care are intertwined with and interpenetrated in history, context, and others. The focus is on coordinated living between people, including clients and nurses. It includes knowledge about mutual understanding through interpretation, hermeneutic understanding through fusioning of horizons in an interactive sense, and emancipatory projects oriented toward "autonomy and responsibility" and the removal of distortions and domination in human living. The knowledge in this sphere is *dialogical* and *transformative* and depends on the use of language, and in nursing it gives us the base from which coordinated work of practice, of getting well, and of living together are formulated. Knowledge for this sphere is developed through hermeneutic analysis and critique, deconstruction, discourse analysis, and emancipatory projects aimed at discovering and understanding the nature of distortions, which provide self-knowledge to people and develop ways to reform and transform people for emancipation and change in ordinary living and in health care.

The *normative cognitive need* is based on the ontological commitment regarding what constitutes human practice. Ontologically, nursing practice is guided by normative ideals, ethical principles, and value orientations regarding what is right and good for recipients of nursing care (Holmes & Warelow, 2000). Nursing as a human practice discipline is firmly established with goals that are for clients (patients), and requires of its practitioners to engage in practice that ensures the maximum, the best, and the right outcomes for each client. For this to happen, nurses have to rely on the knowledge of normative expectations and ethical guidelines for conduct and decision making, and values regarding effectiveness, efficiency, and quality related to goal attainments.

For the normative cognitive need, I designate the *ethical knowledge sphere* as one type of knowledge for nursing. It refers to knowledge that is necessary for nursing to determine what is normatively expected, and aspired to in its practice. It refers to the knowledge regarding the general and specific normative standards of nursing practice, value orientations embedded in the discipline of nursing and practice, and the grounds for ethical practice. It provides the grounding for making connections between "what is known" in other spheres of knowledge in nursing practice and "what must be" in nursing practice. The focus is disciplinary. Knowledge in this sphere addresses what the nature of ethical frameworks for practice are, how they get established, generated, or changed, and their relationships to the larger culture and context.

The *desiderative cognitive need* is also based on the ontology of practice with a focus on practice as a form of self-presentation and self-expression. It emphasizes the aspect of practice that encompasses harmony, beauty, and creativity, resulting in individualized, unique caring. This sort of ontological commitment regarding practice has been expressed by Holmes (1992), who advanced the notion of nursing practice as aesthetic praxis. This separates the aesthetic ground of nursing practice from the moral ground of nursing practice and signifies the desiderative cognitive need to be oriented to the aspect of goodness associated with desirability rather than necessity. Whereas the normative cognitive need is oriented to the need to know what is expected and required, the desiderative cognitive need is oriented to the need to know what is desirable.

For the desiderative cognitive need I designate the *aesthetic knowledge sphere* as one type of knowledge for nursing. Knowledge in this sphere provides the basis for grounding nursing practice in the values of goodness, harmony, and individuation. Knowledge in this sphere addresses various modes of self-presentation and self-expression necessary to create aesthetic practice, and different aesthetic frameworks for practice in relation to events, situational context, society, and culture. It also attends to how values and value standards for aesthetic practice become established, changed, or interpreted.

These five knowledge spheres founded upon four ontological commitments and five different types of cognitive needs make up the knowledge that is necessary for nursing practice as shown in Figure 3.2. As shown

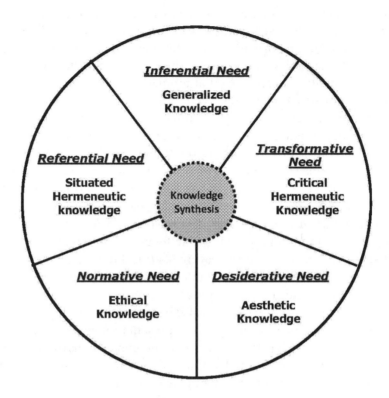

Figure 3.2. Schematic representation of nursing epistemology.

in this figure, these five spheres are coalesced together into a central sector for synthesis. Knowledge synthesis drawing from these five types of knowledge is the process through which knowledge is used in nursing practice. The bulk of presentation in this book on theoretical thinking in nursing is concerned with developing knowledge in the generalized knowledge sphere with the inferential cognitive needs. This is because developing generalized knowledge requires approaches and methods of logical and empirical rigor, as systematization is the key in this type of knowledge.

KNOWLEDGE SYNTHESIS

Nursing has been unwittingly developing knowledge in all of these five spheres, although the empirical and positivistic orientation applied to the generalized knowledge sphere is still quite dominant in our knowledge development. Knowledge in these five spheres is critical as it is the comprehensive, unifying base from which nurses must draw knowledge that is applicable and useful in singular, unique clinical situations. It means, then, that the ultimate synthesizer and knowledge generator must be the nurse in practice.

Practicing nurses must be able to come to know the critical aspects of their clients, situations, and their own practice by alternately dissecting each stratum to view through one lens and at the same time layering and knitting together the multiple strata to produce "the practice." Synthesis of knowledge in practice involves how (that is, method) nurses bring forth knowledge that exists in many different sectors (such as in the public domain, in themselves, in clients and families, and in situations) to bear relevance in specific situations, and what (that is, content specifiable in the five knowledge spheres) sorts of knowledge become incorporated into nursing work carried out in specific situations.

Knowledge synthesis is carried out by nurses in practice by eliciting nurses' personal knowledge, drawing upon situation-specific knowing, and accessing public knowledge. The five knowledge spheres therefore identify different types of knowledge to be systematized for nursing as the public knowledge. Nursing epistemology is for the systematization of the public knowledge of nursing that is developed, applying various inquiry methods, including scientific, philosophical, analytic, and dialogical ones.

NOTES

1. The terms "the tough-mined" and "the tender-minded" were coined by William James (1955) and reiterated by Phillips (1987). The descriptors identified by Phillips (1987, p. 84) for "the tender minded" are rationalistic, intellectualistic, idealistic, free-willist, anti-naturalistic, anti-realist, hermeneutic/interpretive, relativist, qualitative, and epistemologically charitable, and for "the tough-minded" are empiricist, sensationalist, materialistic, fatalistic, skeptical, naturalistic, fallibilist, epistemologically uncharitable, and proscientific rationality.
2. I have earlier proposed four cognitive needs for the nursing epistemology. I have differentiated what was termed as the desiderative cognitive need into two types of need, as there seems to be essential differences between the need to determine what is good from bad and what is right from wrong on one hand and the need to determine what is desirable.

4

Conceptual Domains in Nursing:
A Framework for Theoretical Analysis

Social facts cannot be adequately explained by psychological facts; psychological facts cannot be adequately explained by physiological facts; physiological facts cannot be adequately explained by chemical facts. The facts at any level of integration need to be explained and can only be fully explained in terms of that level.

—*William A. White*

OVERVIEW

This chapter presents a typology of theoretical domains for nursing. The typology is composed of four domains: client, client–nurse, practice, and environment. It is an organizational construct, developed for systematizing many classes of phenomena that are essential for nursing studies. The rationale for the typology and the theoretical meanings of the four domains as boundary-maintaining devices are discussed. The typology is presented as a device that can help us to make sense of reality in the frame of reference that is nursing.

The intellectual and theoretical preoccupation we have for understanding nursing phenomena forces us to view reality from a nursing angle of vision. By doing this we can bring those elements needing critical attention to the center of the field of vision, while pushing away those with less importance and little significance into the peripheral region or to the area outside of the field of vision. The typology as a metaparadigm framework is a tool and a guide that can be used to separate out the aspects of the real world we encounter into coherent sets of theoretical elements. In this book, the typology is used as the framework with which theoretical ideas are analyzed from the nursing perspective, and as the organizing guideline for the presentation of theoretical ideas in the following chapters. Whereas the structure of nursing epistemology presented in chapter 3 is a framework for the determination of the types of nursing knowledge, this typology of four domains is concerned with how we organize the contents of nursing knowledge. The typology is a device by which we can organize what "problems" nursing as a scientific discipline is trying to solve.

This typology as a metaparadigm framework for nursing's conceptual system is an analytical device proposed for systematizing phenomena and concepts of interest to nursing study—that is, content-systematizing. As Turner (1986) suggests, development of analytical schemes is an important and necessary aspect of theorizing in a discipline. A typology divides the universe of interest into an order, so that each phenomenon or concept can be located within a conceptual boundary specified within the typology. It is a classification schema by which relevant phenomena of interest to nursing are delineated, differentiated, and studied within the perspective of the discipline. In this typology, four "domains"—four specific conceptual areas of study—are proposed. The term *domain* is used to refer to an area of study that is identified by a common phenomenal boundary.[1]

A scenario is used in the first section to show how one arrives at theoretical notions from the nursing perspective as opposed to other perspectives. The scenario is used as the basis for an examination of elements in this "reality" through the process of focusing on the nursing angle of vision. The typology of four domains is then presented, focusing on the general meanings and theoretical applicability of the domains. For each domain, examples of relevant phenomena and concepts are given to show the process of conceptualization on the holistic and particularistic levels. The last section deals with the utility of the typology in conceptual development and theory construction.

Scenario

Mr. Milton Jones[2] is a 58-year-old African American patient who has been hospitalized at a university medical center for liver transplantation. Liver transplantation was done 5 days before, and he was transferred from the intensive care unit 2 days ago to this acute surgical unit for postsurgical care.

He had a reoperation for ligation of bleeding vessels on the second day after the liver transplantation due to bleeding in the hepatic bed. He is resting in a semi-Fowler's position, and is dozing on and off. His wife is at his bedside reading a book, and conversing with her husband in short spurts.

His medical history includes hemophilia A (factor VIII deficiency), diagnosed in his infancy. The hemophilia was manifested by multiple hemarthroses because of which he received left hip and left knee replacement surgeries and bilateral ulnar-nerve entrapment 13 years ago, was complicated by hepatitis C infection, and chronic hepatitis diagnosed 2 years ago. He further was diagnosed 8 months ago with hepatocellular carcinoma. This led him to be a candidate for a liver transplantation, which had been performed at this hospitalization. He had a history of essential hypertension, benign prostatic hypertrophy, and urinary tract infections.

On this day, he still has two Jackson-Pratt drains and a T-tube drain on his transplantation site. He has an IV (intravenous) line for his medications. He still has some pain in his surgical site, which is managed with non-narcotic pain medication, and has begun a physical therapy regimen. His primary nurse for the shift is Mr. James Holten, RN, who had not cared for this patient before. The nurse is aware of the critical need to monitor the patient's status change regarding bleeding in addition to providing the routine care for patients with liver transplantation. Mr. Jones's laboratory work for the previous day revealed hematocrit of 28% and aPPT (activated partial-thromboplastin time) of 23 seconds. The hematocrit level has been stable for 3 days at this level, and the aPPT has become elevated from 15 seconds of the previous day. Adequate factor VIII levels at the normal range are continuing following the surgery without the return of the inhibitor.

Ms. Linda Reynolds, RN, CCRN, is a clinical coordinator for liver transplantation patients at this hospital, and has had long discussions with Mr. Jones and his wife before the liver transplantation regarding what to expect immediately following the surgery. She believes it is time for her to discuss with the patient and his wife his posthospitalization course in greater detail, as he is expected to be discharged to home within a few days if he does not experience any other postoperative complications.

Mr. Jones is to continue with immunosuppressive therapy that includes prednisone, antithymocyte globulin, mycophenolate mofetil, and tacrolimus. He is also to continue with hydrochlorothiazide, lisonopril, and atenolol for his hypertension. There is a strong indication that factor VIII will stay at the normal range being produced by the allograft, allowing the termination of factor VIII replacement therapy.

Mr. Jones weighs 198 pounds with a height of 5 feet, 11 inches; he has mild limitations in flexion and extension of the right elbow, extension of the right hip, flexion of the left and right knees, and dorsiflexion of the right ankle, with no joint effusions revealed at the time of admission.

Mr. Jones is an assistant principal at a high school in a medium-size city where he lives with his wife, located about 80 miles from this hospital. He has two adult daughters who are both married and have children, one of whom has a diagnosis of hemophilia.

APPROPRIATENESS AS NURSING'S SUBJECT MATTER

The first question we need to address (and establish) in considering and analyzing this scenario in a nursing context is whether there are some aspects of this reality that can be claimed to have nursing "meanings" and "problems" for nursing to address scientifically. Of course, one might say that it is superfluous to pose such a question, since the reality is occurring in a hospital, to a patient, and one of nursing's important places of action is in a hospital with patients. Such obviousness notwithstanding, we shall make a formal claim upon this situation by applying the definition of nursing.

Nursing is a service to people for the promotion of individual health. Thus, a situation requiring services or interventions of health promotion is a legitimate place for nursing. Since Mr. Jones's situation requires interventions that are unique to nursing, it is justifiable for us to claim this reality as having nursing phenomena. Yet this does not mean that the situation cannot be claimed by other scientific disciplines as having unique meanings and problems that are applicable only to their fields. This possibility is the main reason for the necessity for a specific angle of vision, a selected frame of reference, in studying a given phenomenon. Although nursing is concerned with health and health care, not all aspects of health and health care constitute the proper subject matter of nursing. Adopting Berger's phrase (1963), we might state that nursing does not study phenomena that another field is unaware of, but it examines and studies the same phenomena in a different way, from the perspective of nursing.

MEANING IN NON-NURSING PERSPECTIVES

In an effort to make clear the later discussions concerning the perspective of nursing in analyzing the scenario, let us examine possible claims of phenomena in the scenario by other, non-nursing perspectives first. We will look at the perspectives of medicine, physical therapy, social services, medical science, and psychology to contrast the meanings of studying the same reality in different ways from different angles of vision.

First, let us take the perspective of medicine. The medical frame of reference in pursuing problems of health is based on a number of carefully delineated models of normal and abnormal human conditions and of modus operandi for diagnosing and handling such human conditions as diseases and pathologies. In the medical frame of reference, a physician will pose the following questions related to the scenario because these or others similar to these are important aspects of the phenomena to medicine.

1. Mr. Jones's liver transplantation has been successful so far. However, he was re-operated on for bleeding in the hepatic bed. What is the likelihood of recurrence of bleeding, and how can it be detected?
2. What is the probability of rejection of Mr. Jones's transplanted liver?
3. How can the reappearance of factor VIII inhibitor be prevented after the liver transplantation for Mr. Jones?
4. What combination of drugs would be the most effective immuno-suppressive therapy after the liver transplantation for Mr. Jones?
5. What is the likelihood of re-emergence of hepatocellular carcinoma?
6. What should be done to prevent future hepatitis?

These questions point out the medical frame of reference; the reality of the scenario presents itself in the phenomena associated with the surgical course of treatment for this patient, including current status and prognosis, and risks involved in current and future medical managements. Therefore, the medical frame of reference directs attention to studies of medical diagnosis, pathological findings, and treatment protocols necessary for removal of pathologies.

The frame of reference for physical therapy will question the problems related to the range of motion, mobility, and use of body in everyday life, including range of motion, muscle strength, neuromuscular competence, musculoskeletal intactness, and limitations in use. The focus in physical therapy then is on raising questions regarding how to assist Mr. Jones to gain a greater degree of competence or to find ways to accommodate his life with limitations, given the history of hemarthroses and hip and knee replacements.

In contrast, the social services frame of reference will view the reality of the scenario along the lines of the following questions:

1. What is the health insurance coverage for Mr. Jones?
2. What are income consequences of Mr. Jones's extended sick leave due to this hospitalization and related recovery?

3. Is the family going to need some sort of assistance with social welfare services during this episode of illness?

The frame of reference for social services is the effective and efficient utilization of private and public resources in case of crisis and disruption in individual and family life. Thus, it is appropriate for this perspective to examine the reality of the scenario with such questions as those presented above.

These examples of questions based on different frames of reference indicate to us how the same situation may be perceived in many different ways, with different and specific solutions. These questions, posed in specific clinical situations, can be raised to the level of knowledge development by converting them into problems the discipline needs to have answered. These questions, on the other hand, may be answered by drawing from theoretical knowledge established in the specific discipline.

There are various ways of linking the reality of this scenario with scientific studies. One way would be to use such questions to begin inductive studies to arrive at generalizable answers. Another is through a deductive system in which scientists identify appropriate aspects and elements of the reality as empirical counterparts to theoretical concepts they are investigating. For example, a medical scientist who is interested in relationships between a certain protocol of immunosuppressive therapy and the occurrence of organ rejection can easily include Mr. Jones as a case in such a study. Similarly, a psychologist who is interested in studying relationships between the concepts of *locus of control* and *decision making* may want to investigate Mr. Jones's postsurgical activities and behavior from that perspective.

Different definitions of a situation made in the context of scientific angles of vision allow divergent theoretical questioning and multiple empirical conceptualizations. This is, indeed, what is meant by studying the same phenomenon in different ways.

PERSPECTIVE OF NURSING

We now turn to the question of how nursing should perceive the phenomena in this scenario. We can pose many questions haphazardly, as the questions were presented with other perspectives in the above section. However, since the aim is to present a systematic view of this reality from the nursing perspective, I propose a method by which the phenomenal elements in the scenario are dissected and disentangled rather than con-

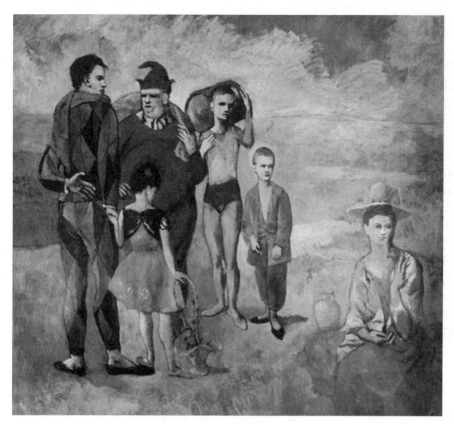

Figure 4.1. Picasso: *Les Saltimbanques.*

ceived as a conglomerated, global phenomenon. This does not mean that the scenario cannot be perceived and conceptualized as one global phenomenon, only that the theoretical usefulness of such an approach may be too complicated at this point, or meaningless for nursing explanations.

It is somewhat like viewing Picasso's *Les Saltimbanques* (*The Entertainers*; Figure 4.1). A viewer as a lover of art appreciates the total mystery and beauty of the painting as a piece of work that moves one's heart and sense of aesthetics. He or she finds a certain message in the painting, such as "solitude," "pathos," or "waiting." Whatever message the viewer perceives, he or she perceives from the totality of the painting as it is presented to him or her. This is the holistic mode of perception, as defined in chapter 2. In this mode, the viewer is totally involved in the piece of art as a whole thing, representing a specific but all-encompassing meaning.

However, another viewer may gain quite a different kind of appreciation and understanding of the painting by dissecting the painting and viewing it in one of many possible different meaning systems. These may include: (a) the physical attitudes depicted in the painting—how each person in the painting stands and looks at one another, (b) the emotional tones of the painting—how the emotions are depicted by the painter in different expressions assumed by the "entertainers," or (c) the blending of color tones—how colors are used for the persona and the background. This second viewer uses a specific guideline for viewing art (i.e., a particular mode of perception and analysis within a frame of reference that is art) to understand the meanings of the given phenomena. This second viewer's understandings would be specific to the interrelatedness of objects on canvas, the mixture of emotional tones as depicted in images with figures and colors, or the use of color itself. This viewer has thus adopted the particularistic mode of perception.

In essence, the quality of impressions gained by viewers of a painting, such as the first viewer, would depend on the extensiveness and refinement of the general knowledge the viewer has acquired about painting, art, and beauty. In contrast, the second viewer adopts an analytic posture for understanding what is presented before him or her, making it possible for this viewer to appreciate the art in the context of its selected meanings and qualities.

Thus, the proposed method here is to adopt the analytical mode of examining a phenomenon so that we may be able to understand the hidden aspects of the reality and examine various elements in a phenomenon within different frames of reference. Since this analytical method is akin to the particularistic mode of description and analysis, it is necessary to eventually consolidate it into the holistic mode of analysis. The essential distinction between holistic and particularistic analysis is in the focus of description. Holistic analysis is aimed at examining properties and forces of an object or a situation as a whole. Particularistic analysis, on the other hand, is aimed at focusing on a specific aspect or element of a situation or an object without explicit regard for the whole. Therefore, for any particularistic level, there is a related holistic level, and for any holistic level there is a more global holistic level, making the first holistic level particular.

These thoughts on analytical modes indicate that it is possible to pose questions regarding the scenario from the nursing perspective on various levels. We can thus abstract the following elements from the above scenario that are directly related to Mr. Jones, the client:

1. Mr. Jones is uncomfortable due to various drains, has some pain in the surgical incision, and is following the routine postoperative regimen for mobility.

2. He has had a life-long chronic illness that had required a continuous therapy and monitoring. He developed various complications from the chronic illness, one of which had required hip and knee replacements, resulting in minor limitations in movement.
3. He is in a course of recovery that may extend beyond discharge from hospital.
4. He felt fortunate to have been selected to receive a liver transplantation, and feels hopeful about resuming normal life after recovery. However, he is worried about the possibility of rejection.
5. He had been distressed when he was taken for a re-operation due to bleeding, and is fearful of bleeding again.
6. Bleeding has been his major concern throughout his life. The prospect of a normal factor VIII is exhilarating.
7. He feels deeply remorseful about his grandson's hemophilia.
8. He is somewhat overweight and is not very active.

These are major elements of the scenario, requiring explanations and understanding if nursing is to provide effective care to Mr. Jones.

From the interaction between Mr. Jones and the nurses (Mr. Holten and Ms. Reynolds), we can also abstract several different phenomenal elements relevant to what generally goes on between a client and a nurse:

1. Mr. Jones and Mr. Holten exchange greetings, talk about drainage, surgical incision site, etc.
2. Mr. Holten checks the drains, makes notations about various amounts of drainage, and examines the incision and the IV site.
3. Ms. Reynolds approaches both Mr. and Mrs. Jones to discuss what will happen after his discharge. Mr. Jones has asked his wife to write down their questions beforehand. So, they begin with the listed questions.
4. Ms. Reynolds shows and goes through the booklet for liver transplantation patients.

These statements refer to phenomena that exist or could be apparent when the client and the nurse are together as an interactive pair. These phenomena raise important questions for explanation and understanding from the nursing perspective, as nursing involves a service delivered to humans (i.e., clients) by other human agents (i.e., nurses). Phenomena in the client–nurse interaction belong to general categories of human-to-human contact and interaction phenomena, but are particular sorts specific to the context of nursing.

In addition to these two sets of phenomenal elements in the scenario that are important to nursing's understanding of Mr. Jones's care, the following questions must be posed with specific regard to nursing interventions and practice:

1. How did Mr. Holten organize the data on Mr. Jones?
2. What are the specific problems Mr. Holten has identified in Mr. Jones as requiring nursing approaches and interventions?
3. What are the alternative approaches the nurse has identified for the delivery of nursing care during Mr. Jones's hospitalization?
4. What are the priorities that need immediate attention from nursing staff for Mr. Jones?
5. What should the nurse do in monitoring the drains?
6. How could the nurse assist Mr. Jones to cope with the effects of immunosuppressive drugs?
7. How should Ms. Reynolds determine Mr. Jones's regimen after being discharged to home during his recovery?
8. What is the discharge plan for Mr. Jones?
9. How should the nurse assist Mr. and Mrs. Jones to handle liver transplantation on a long-term basis?

These questions are related to the kinds of nursing activities the nurse needs either to carry out or to consider carrying out for the patient. Although knowledge related to some of these questions depends on understanding obtained regarding this client and this client–nurse relationship, these questions point out the need for a specific set of knowledge that pertains to nursing practice itself.

Supplementing the phenomenal elements in the client, the client–nurse, and nursing practice, we can also abstract different elements from the environment of Mr. Jones. The following can be specified as having significant meanings to nursing:

1. Mr. Jones is on a regular ward after being in an intensive care unit for two days following his surgery.
2. His wife sits at the bedside, appearing very supportive to his needs.
3. The nurses on this unit are not familiar with Mr. Jones.
4. Mr. Jones's ordinary life is in a medium-size city, with his children living in the same town. His daughters and grandchildren live close by, making frequent visits.
5. He has a large social network, through the school where he works and the church he attends.

These are some of the elements in the environment that are relevant in gaining answers to nursing questions such as:

- Do these factors influence or explain Mr. Jones's health in any way?
- Are there any critical aspects of his environment that influence the way Mr. Jones responds to his hospitalization and recovery?
- Do any of these factors have an influence on the way nursing care is provided to Mr. Jones?

These four sets of delineation indicate that it is possible to disentangle the situation of nursing care into four areas of focus: the client, the client–nurse relationship, the nursing practice, and the environment. Furthermore, the questions posed in this nursing perspective are different from those raised from the other, non-nursing perspectives. These are nursing questions, raised for the nurse's deeper understanding and explanation of the situation. The goal is to give nursing care to Mr. Jones that is scientifically appropriate and effective. The knowledge addressing these elements will be valuable to nurses in delivering nursing care to Mr. Jones. This analysis leads us to a typology that can be used systematically to analyze elements in nursing situations, a typology of four domains: client, client–nurse relationship, nursing practice, and environment.

THE TYPOLOGY—FOUR DOMAINS

Four domains—client, client–nurse relationship, nursing practice, and environment—are proposed at this point as components of a typology for conceptualization from the nursing perspective. This classification scheme is a way of disentangling realities, phenomena, and concepts within the nursing perspective. The four domains of this framework direct identification of concepts within specific phenomenal boundaries, and are suggested for use in properly "locating" phenomena of importance to nursing studies.

This suggested utility is quite different from the purposes linked to the frameworks of theory analysis advanced by Barnum (1994), Fawcett (1994), and Hardy (1978). These domains of the typology also serve quite different purposes than those derived from metaparadigm concepts such as those by Fawcett (1978, 1984), Meleis (1997), and Yura and Torres (1975). The latter (Yura & Torres, 1975) identified four subconcepts— man, society, health, and nursing—as the most common components of theoretical formulations in nursing as articulated in baccalaureate curricula.

Also, Fawcett (1978, 1984) adopted person, environment, health, and nursing as the units comprising the phenomena of interest to nursing science and as the essential components of nursing theories. Meleis (1997) adds "transitions" to the fourfold metaparadigm concept proposed by Fawcett. Although our proposed typology of four domains is an attempt to refine such suggestions, the major purpose of the typology is different from those expressed by Torres and Yura, Fawcett, and Meleis. Their main interests were in identifying essential concepts in nursing theories. The idea is to use the typology to identify essential aspects of nursing as contained within the four domains. This typology is a conceptual tool by which nursing scientists can identify a locus of concepts and phenomena within specific domains. Although the domains may be used to test theoretical comprehensiveness, the main purpose for the typology is in its usefulness in conceptual delineation and theoretical thinking about the scientific field of nursing.

More important, this typology can be used to define the nursing angle of vision in viewing the world of health care. Any conceptual or theoretical development has to have a specific reference to nursing if it is to be of value to the scientific field of nursing. The primary concern regarding theoretical thinking in nursing is not that of comprehensiveness of nursing theories, but is in ensuring that what we develop theoretically has nursing significance. The four domains point to four spheres of the empirical world in which nursing-relevant phenomena could be located, while at the same time orienting scientists toward possible relationships among concepts within and across domains. The typology is a conceptual map upon which the discipline can plot its phenomena of interest in a systematic, organized fashion so as to develop scientific knowledge. As shown in the following introductory discussions regarding each domain, and in the more in-depth expositions offered in chapters 5 through 8, the domains are used to make sense of concepts and phenomena we study in nursing.

The Domain of Client

Clients present to us rich arrays of phenomena requiring various types of considerations, understandings, and interventions, as shown in the preceding discussions regarding Mr. Jones. The domain of client is concerned with those theoretical issues that pertain only to clients, that is, the reality that belongs entirely and solely to clients. The focus is on what is happening with, presents in, or refers directly to clients. In addition, when clients are the focus, we are also concerned only with those elements in clients relevant to nursing. Clients refer to humans, mostly as individuals

Table 4.1

AN ILLUSTRATION OF RELATIONSHIPS BETWEEN SELECTED PHENOMENA AND CONCEPTS IN THE DOMAIN OF CLIENT

PHENOMENAL ELEMENTS	CONCEPTS
Diagnoses of hemophilia at infancy; chronic hepatitis	■ Chronic illness ■ Chronicity
Liver transplantation	■ Liver reorganization ■ Rejection susceptibility ■ Meaning of liver transplantation
Discomfort; pain	■ Discomfort ■ Postoperative pain
Intravenous infusion; surgical drainage	■ Invasion of body ■ Meaning of drainage
Surgery for liver transplantation and reoperation for bleeding	■ Long-term recovery ■ Anxiety for complications
History of hemarthroses; hip and knee replacements	■ Reduced mobility ■ Recidivism
Mr. Jones as a person	■ Personhood ■ Selfhood

but also as dyads and groups, who are the recipients of nursing care. The ultimate reason for nursing to regard "client" as the focus is that, by understanding happenings (reality) in the client, nursing can: (a) attain an understanding about the nature of phenomena present in the client, (b) gain knowledge regarding the client's problems, (c) formulate generalized notions about why such problems exist, and (d) deliver the most effective and needed nursing care to the client.

The elements of the Jones scenario that pertain to the domain of client were identified earlier. Table 4.1 shows how such phenomenal elements are then made to have some meaning-relations with specific concepts in the domain of client. Concepts such as pain, discomfort, chronicity, uncertainty, etc., can thus be examined and analyzed as theoretical concepts for explanations. Some of the concepts are holistic, whereas others are particularistic on several different levels of abstraction. Thus, concepts in the domain of client can be delineated in both the holistic and particularistic modes.

For example, on a holistic level, a patient who walks into an emergency unit with a swollen and injured face is considered and described according to general features that are sui generis to the human person and that describe the person as a whole, such as healthy, sick, happy, depressed, or dying. It also involves a perception of the individual with respect to characteristics that depict the person as the basic unit of analysis. Hence the following description of the person in this holistic mode of analysis:

> Marjorie Johnson, a woman of middle years with a slight figure, who appears fearful and nervous in her posture, has gross injuries of old and fresh contusions and lacerations on her face. Her face appears distorted and her posture is agitated. She looks as though in pain yet indicates that the injuries do not hurt.

On the contrary, on a particular level, this same patient is considered and described with a particular focus, the injury. A description with a particularistic focus on the injuries of Marjorie Johnson will result in the following:

> Marjorie Johnson's facial injuries consist of a 2-degree edema on the left side of the face, with a contusion of 2-cm diameter around the left cheekbone area, and a superficial cut in the mucosa of the upper lip, which is bleeding intermittently. There are several small contusions near the forehead that are sensitive and painful to pressure.

The focus of the holistic description within the domain of client is the person as a whole, as a human person, whereas the focus of the particularistic description, in this instance, is the injury. In the theoretical arena, both levels of description and analysis are necessary, so far as each level is selected for appropriate theoretical explanations.

Phenomena and concepts in the domain of client are of three types: *essentialistic, health-care experiential*, and *problematic*. A more comprehensive discussion of this sub-categorization and a detailed exposition of concepts and phenomenal elements in the domain of clients are presented in chapter 5. In addition, major descriptive and explanatory frameworks useful in studying this domain are also presented in that chapter.

The Client–Nurse Domain

The client–nurse domain is defined as the area of study in nursing pertaining to phenomena arising out of encounters between client and nurse, as nursing involves human-to-human engagements and services. This domain points to many facets of relation between client and nurse in the process of providing nursing care. Phenomena in the client–nurse domain refer to the nurse in direct contact with the client.

Table 4.2

AN ILLUSTRATION OF RELATIONSHIPS BETWEEN SELECTED PHENOMENA AND CONCEPTS IN THE CLIENT–NURSE DOMAIN

PHENOMENAL ELEMENTS	CONCEPTS
Nurse's touch of Mr. Jones while giving care	■ Instrumental touch
Talking between the nurse and patient; caring occasion	■ Caring ■ Client–nurse transaction ■ Empathy
The nurse's presence and closeness with the patient	■ Distancing ■ Presence

The domain encompasses various modes of contact, including spatial, physical, communicative, emotional, and interactive modes. Nurses and patients in nursing care situations converse, play specific roles, exchange feelings, and make connections. Contacts between client and nurse are occasions in which transfer and/or interchange of information, energy, and affection/humanity occur. Such contacts are, from the nurse's perspective, the medium for delivering nursing care and for helping clients; and, from the client's perspective, for gaining attention and receiving care. Such concepts as touch, empathetic relationship, transaction, therapeutic communication, collaboration, and therapeutic alliance belong to this domain.

Table 4.2 shows the linkages between the phenomenal elements identified regarding Mr. Jones in the preceding section and relevant theoretical concepts pertaining to the client–nurse domain. As the examples show, some concepts (such as "instrumental touch") are particularistic, whereas others (such as "client–nurse transaction") are holistic.

Phenomena and concepts in the client–nurse domain can be categorized into three different types according to the dominant features of client–nurse interchange: *contact*, *communication*, and *interaction*. Of course, these types are oriented toward particularistic conceptualization of the interchanges, and are perhaps most useful as analytical tools in studying the specific aspects of the client–nurse interchange from particular perspectives. This subcategorization does not preempt the usefulness of a holistic conceptualization of the client–nurse interchanges. A more in-depth exposition of the client–nurse domain is presented in chapter 6.

The Domain of Practice

This domain encompasses phenomena and concepts related to what nurses do "in the name of nursing." It includes phenomena particular to the

Table 4.3

AN ILLUSTRATION OF RELATIONSHIPS BETWEEN SELECTED PHENOMENA AND CONCEPTS IN THE PRACTICE DOMAIN

PHENOMENAL ELEMENTS	CONCEPTS
Observation of the patient's problems	■ Nursing assessment
Organization of data regarding the patient	■ Clinical reasoning ■ Prioritization
Formulation of alternatives in nursing care	■ Nursing decision making
Drainage monitoring; administering medication; observing the rate of IV infusion; charting	■ Nursing description ■ Nursing enactment

---

nurse who is engaged in nursing work. The concept of practice refers to the cognitive, behavioral, and social aspects of professional actions taken by a nurse in addressing clients' needs and problems and in fulfilling the role of nurse in a given nursing care situation. It encompasses phenomena pertaining to the nurse in formulating, thinking about, and contemplating nursing actions as well as those involved in the nurse doing nursing, in carrying out the work of nursing. The phenomena of concern are located in the nurse with respect to how she/he thinks, makes decisions, transfers knowledge into action, uses available knowledge in actual practice, or takes certain actions.

For the domain of practice, the main theoretical questions involve the methods by which nurses make decisions regarding nursing care and what techniques and processes are adopted for taking nursing actions. Thus, concepts such as critical nursing judgment, prioritization of nursing care needs, clinical decision making, routinization of nursing care, personalization, and nursing rule-bending belong to this domain of practice.

Table 4.3 shows the linkages between the questions presented regarding the nursing care of Mr. Jones in the preceding section and relevant theoretical concepts. These are examples of concepts that require theoretical understanding if nursing actions are to make scientific sense. As the examples show, some concepts of nursing actions are particularistic, such as drainage monitoring, whereas others are holistic, such as nursing care planning. This, then, also suggests that phenomena and concepts in the domain of practice can also be analyzed in both modes, holistic and particularistic. Phenomena and concepts in the practice domain can be organized into two processes: the *phase of deliberation* and the *phase of enactment*. A more in-depth exposition of the domain of practice is presented in chapter 7.

The Domain of Environment

The domain of environment is an essential component in developing knowledge in nursing, as it is the common source of understanding and explaining the phenomena in the client, client–nurse, and practice domains. The environment is thought to be composed of physical, social, and symbolic components, varying in temporal and spatial contexts. Environment refers to the external world that surrounds the client and that also forms the context in which client–nurse interchanges and nursing practice take place. It is composed of both immediate and remote elements.

Table 4.4 shows the linkages between the phenomenal elements that were identified in the preceding section regarding Mr. Jones and general concepts that are thought to encompass those phenomenal elements. These phenomenal elements and concepts identified for Mr. Jones's situation have theoretical significance for nursing to the extent that (a) scientific scrutiny of such concepts will illuminate understanding and explanation of the client's problems, and (b) theoretical understandings of concepts and their relationships to other phenomena will influence nursing interventions.

Just as we examined phenomena and concepts in other domains in two analytic modes, so too can the domain of environment be subjected to both modes of analysis. Environment in a holistic mode of analysis takes the form of one's global surroundings having multiple yet coherent influence as a totality on the client, client–nurse interchanges, and practice. In contrast, environment can be analyzed in a particularistic mode as composed specifically of physical, social, and symbolic elements. A more comprehensive analysis of the domain of environment is presented in chapter 8.

In a way, the typology of four domains proposed in this section is a way of reshaping the world to fit our purpose, to identify only those critical elements for scientific and theoretical scrutiny within the nursing perspective. The four domains are not separated in any formal way, except in their boundary specifications that enable locus designations of phenomena and concepts. The ways in which the domains are conceptually divided for this purpose is summarized in Figure 4.2. The figure shows subcategories that make conceptually meaningful sense and analytical clarification in thinking about each domain, as discussed in this chapter and as also expanded upon in later chapters. This typology can only serve as a way to see things more clearly and to understand the proper contexts of conceptual and theoretical development. It is a tool that can make the development of conceptual clarification less painful and less haphazard.

Table 4.4

AN ILLUSTRATION OF RELATIONSHIPS BETWEEN SELECTED PHENOMENA AND CONCEPTS IN THE DOMAIN OF ENVIRONMENT

PHENOMENAL ELEMENTS	CONCEPTS
Hospitalized in an acute care unit	■ Sensory overload ■ Social isolation ■ Territoriality
Presence of wife	■ Affection ■ Role expectations ■ Significant other
Wife, children, grandchildren; friends and neighbors	■ Social network ■ Social support
Being in a hospital	■ Health care environment ■ Hospital rules ■ Patient role expectations ■ Temporary place

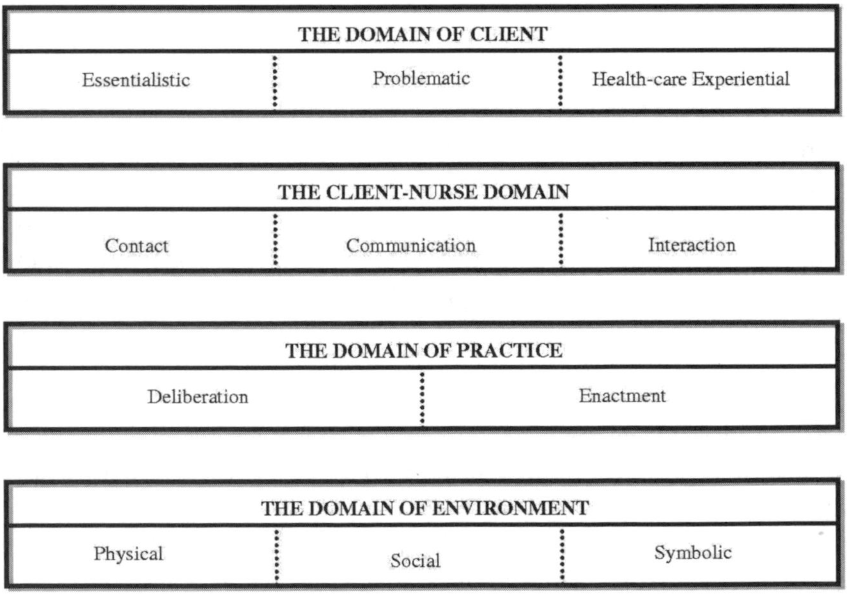

THE DOMAIN OF CLIENT		
Essentialistic	Problematic	Health-care Experiential

THE CLIENT-NURSE DOMAIN		
Contact	Communication	Interaction

THE DOMAIN OF PRACTICE	
Deliberation	Enactment

THE DOMAIN OF ENVIRONMENT		
Physical	Social	Symbolic

Figure 4.2. The four theoretical domains of nursing and their conceptual subboundaries.

UTILITY OF THE TYPOLOGY IN CONCEPT
AND THEORY DEVELOPMENT

The question, then, is how this typology aids conceptual and theoretical development in nursing. The examples of the clinical scenario and the linkages shown between the observational elements (phenomenal elements) and the theoretical concepts for the four domains as presented in Tables 4.1, 4.2, 4.3, and 4.4 refer, in fact, to the first-level, simplistic, inductive conceptualization. We have defined the boundaries for understanding the phenomenal elements in reality as having specific locus of meaning with respect to client, client–nurse interaction, nursing practice, and environment. This process enables the inferences of realities to abstract concepts and makes the understanding of aspects of reality in a general, theoretical sense, rather than as distinct, isolated, novel situations. This disentanglement of reality into many different observational concepts within the four domains also makes scientists view reality in a detached, analytic manner.

A reverse approach of deductive conceptualization for a scientist in approaching reality is also possible within the typology. For example, a scientist who is interested in the theoretical concept of fatigue will first define the concept to refer to phenomena in the domain of client. Following this definition, the scientist will formulate observational referents of the concept. The actual observation and analysis occur as the scientist selects particular situations of a client exhibiting the observational elements of fatigue. The scientist will thus focus on observing clients for the presence of fatigue since the domain of the concept is the client. The typology thus provides an easy, clear-cut way of designating units of analysis in conceptualization. For each domain, units of analysis for concepts always exist within that domain.

As the second step in theoretical thinking, concepts studied and abstracted for descriptive understanding need to be exposed for their significance in theoretical formulations. The typology is useful in theoretical formulations, for the domain identification of concepts allows scientists to define the level of comprehensiveness a given theoretical formulation will have. Theoretical development in nursing is a step beyond mere conceptualization. Theoretical development involves developing sets of interlinked propositional statements for selected concepts. Since a theoretical formulation in nursing can handle concepts within or across the domains, identification of concepts with respect to the domains can show the boundaries toward which the theoretical efforts are aimed.

The typology clarifies how encompassing a theoretical formulation is in its explanatory statements. For example, a theory of cognitive dissonance in nursing is limited to explaining the phenomena in the domain of the client, whereas a theory of social support in nursing links the phenomena in the client with those in the domain of the environment. In a more global way, a general systems theory of nursing such as that proposed by Rogers encompasses in its explanatory propositions many phenomena in all four domains.

Figure 4.3 shows many possible theoretical clusterings of concepts among and across the domains for different types of theoretical development, albeit all theoretical linkages may be appropriate for nursing. Clusterings indicate possible propositions in theoretical systems. For example, with the selection of the following concepts for each domain as shown below, we can think of many different types of theoretical formulations among these concepts (as shown in Figure 4.3):

1. The Domain of Client:
   - Pain experience
   - Non-compliance
   - Stress
   - Overweight

2. The Client–Nurse Domain:
   - Collaboration
   - Therapeutic Alliance
   - Empathy
   - Client–nurse distancing

3. The Domain of Environment:
   - Noise
   - Significant others
   - Social pressure for conformity
   - Family's eating habits

4. The Domain of Practice:
   - Priority setting
   - Discharge planning
   - Nursing assessment
   - Personalization of care

Thus, putting together these concepts can result in formulations of propositions. Possible relationships proposed in Table 4.5 serve as exam-

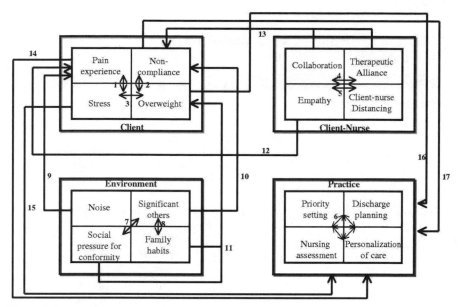

Figure 4.3. Examples of relationships among concepts within the domains and across domains.

ples of theoretical developments linking concepts within and across the domains. These formulations implicitly show that when two or more concepts are clustered together as theoretical formulations and propositions, they tend to come together as broader concepts, such as adaptation, interaction, and influence. Hence, the typology is also useful in directing the delineation of broader theoretical concepts in the process of theoretical development. These 11 examples are only some of many possible numbers of theoretical formulations linking the twelve main concepts used in this example.

As we will see in chapter 9, not all possible linkages and clusterings of concepts are theoretically meaningful in general, nor are they specifically for nursing. Therefore, although it is not difficult to make propositional connections between concepts, it is difficult to put propositions together into a coherent system of theoretical formulations. The burden is on nursing scientists to make decisions about the nature of critical concepts and phenomena that are essential for theoretical explanations of nursing phenomena. Once essential concepts are selected, the complexity of theory evolves around the main attitudes regarding the comprehensiveness of theoretical development.

The main question for theoretical development is to ask what needs to be explained and why such explanations might be important to nursing.

Table 4.5

EXAMPLES OF THEORETICAL FORMULATIONS LINKING CONCEPTS IN FOUR DOMAINS OF NURSING

DOMAIN LEVEL	PROPOSED THEORETICAL RELATIONSHIPS
Within Domains	
a. The domain of client	1. Pain experience and level of stress (Theory of stress and coping) 2. Overweight and noncompliance (Theory of balance or Theory of motivation) 3. Level of stress and overweight (Theory of stress)
b. The client–nurse domain	4. Collaboration and therapeutic alliance (Theory of collaboration) 5. Empathy and distancing (Theory of empathy)
c. The practice domain	6. Nursing assessment, priority setting, personalization of care, and discharge planning (Theory of nursing practice)
d. The environment domain	7. Social pressure for conformity and significant others (Social integration theory) 8. Family eating habits and significant others
Across Domains	
a. The domains of client and environment	9. Pain and noise (Theory of stress) 10. Noncompliance and significant others (Social support theory) 11. Overweight, family eating habits, and social pressure for conformity (Reference group theory)
b. The domains of client and client–nurse interaction	12. Pain experience and empathy (Theory of empathy) 13. Noncompliance, collaboration, and therapeutic alliance (Theory of compliance)
c. The domain of client and practice	14. Pain experience and nursing practice 15. Stress and nursing practice 16. Overweight and nursing practice 17. Noncompliance and nursing practice

The ultimate inference in any theoretical development in nursing needs to address phenomena in the domains of client and nursing action either directly or indirectly.

Holistic and Particularistic Modes— Conceptualization Within the Typology

For theoretical formulations in nursing, five levels of holistic conceptualization are possible and relevant, based on the four domains of the typology. These five levels of holistic theoretical systems in nursing are: (a) client; (b) client–nurse; (c) practice; (d) the environment; and (e) the holistic level, which includes the other four domains of client, client–nurse relationship, nursing practice, and environment. In addition, within each of these five levels of theoretical formulation, innumerable levels and types of a particularistic level of theoretical formulations are also possible. Table 4.6 lists selected concepts as "examples" of holistic and particularistic descriptions for the five levels. Scientists select and define proper levels of description for concepts chosen for specific studies within the theoretical contexts that are applied for the studies.

In many instances, the relationship between holistic and particularistic concepts for a given set of phenomena, as formulated into a proposition, takes the form of what Blalock (1969) calls "the element-class abstraction" in which a major difference in the conceptualization is in units of analysis. Such relationships and other similar relationships among different types of concepts, such as those alluded to in Figure 4.3, are discussed in greater detail in chapter 9.

A word of caution is in order at this point: There is a difference between the two modes of analysis applied to description and to explanation. Conceptual description refers to the specification of characteristics, entities, elements, or nature of a class of phenomena through conceptualization. In contrast, theoretical description and explanation focus on how and why a concept, as defined and described, occurs, often bringing in other concepts. Thus, the holistic explanation aims at comprehensive understanding of changes or characteristics of the whole, whereas particularistic explanation is oriented toward understanding particular elements of the whole. Propositions in a holistic explanatory system tend to be global, whereas propositions in a particularistic explanatory system are narrower in their conceptual focus. Holistic explanations, indeed, may be aimed at grand theories and mesotheories. Middle-range and microtheories are aimed at particularistic explanations. This suggests that explanations within each domain are mainly particularistic explanations,

Table 4.6

EXAMPLES OF CONCEPTS FOR NURSING STUDY ACCORDING TO LEVEL OF CONCEPT DESCRIPTION AND THE DOMAIN

DOMAIN LEVEL	LEVEL OF CONCEPT DESCRIPTION	
	HOLISTIC	PARTICULARISTIC
Client	■ Adaptation ■ Chronicity ■ Disability ■ Health ■ Illness ■ Personhood ■ Recidivism	■ Anemia ■ Depression ■ Edema ■ Immobility ■ Infection ■ Injury ■ Pain ■ Respiratory distress
Client–Nurse	■ Client–nurse exchange ■ Client–nurse interaction ■ Client–nurse transaction ■ Therapeutic relationship	■ Client–nurse collaboration ■ Distancing ■ Gift giving ■ Therapeutic alliance ■ Touch
Practice	■ Clinical expertise ■ Ethical practice ■ Nursing practice ■ Nursing process	■ Clinical diagnosing ■ Nursing assessment ■ Rule bending ■ Surveilling ■ Technical skill
Environment	■ Biosphere ■ Ecosystem ■ Field ■ Territory	■ Ethical standards ■ Noise ■ Pollution ■ Social support

whereas explanations across domains and in the system of all four domains tend to be holistic explanations.

SUMMARY

The typology of four domains in this chapter and the analytic modes of holism and particularism are tools by which conceptual clarity is attained in theoretical thinking. The domain typology aids nursing scientists in locating concepts. As presented in the following chapters, each domain poses somewhat distinct conceptual and theoretical problems and issues in nursing.

Holistic and particularistic modes of analysis as applied to the domain typology allow theoretical thinking in nursing to be confined to certain levels of abstraction, depending upon the need for scientific explanation and investigation. If we consider nursing as inclusive of all four domains, nursing as a general concept is at the most inclusive holistic level, whereas each domain is in a particularistic mode. Thus it is a matter of scope in analysis and observation. This methodology is important for theoretical thinking. Conceptualization and related conceptual analysis require scientists to take "confined" views of the object world, but the level of confinement depends upon whether one opts for a holistic mode or a particularistic one. These two frameworks are used repeatedly and consistently in analyzing concepts and examining theoretical statements throughout the book.

NOTES

1. Shapere (1977) defines a scientific domain as being composed of "related items for scientific investigation," constituting a unified subject matter that poses important problem(s) for scientific investigation and having the quality of "readiness" in a scientific sense to deal with the problem the subject matter presents (pp. 518–527). Although this definition can be thought of as referring to a discipline, it is possible to apply this definition to specify subareas of study within a discipline that is concerned with a complex array of phenomena. Thus, domains in this typology refer to subareas of nursing study, specifying locality of phenomena that need to be studied in nursing. Although this differentiation of nursing's subject matter into four separate domains is appropriate, since each domain contains concepts that are related to each other and poses a unified problem specific to each domain, the separate domains may still need to be combined into a larger "domain" if the larger domain poses a distinct problem that cannot be independently addressed by the subdomain solutions for the domain-based problems.

2. This scenario has been constructed based on the facts and details provided in Case 38-2008 recorded in the case records of Massachusetts General Hospital published in the *New England Journal of Medicine*. Although most of the clinical data have not been altered, other details have been added. Thus, the total scenario does not depict an actual case. See: Dzik, W. H., Laposata, M., Hertl, M., Sandberg, W. C., Chatterji, M., & Misdraji, J. (2008). Case 38-2008: A 58-year-old man with hemophilia, hepatocellular carcinoma, and intractable bleeding. *New England Journal of Medicine, 359,* 2587–2597.

5

Theoretical Analysis of Phenomena in the Client Domain

[M]an, you see, is to be both the knower and the object of known; the difficulty is that of a knower having to objectify itself and having then to form a just concept of what the object is.

—*Cassius J. Keyser*

OVERVIEW

The primary aim of this chapter is to outline and discuss how nursing scientists might go about their search for theoretical concepts within the domain of client. The main focus is on concepts of interest to nursing that exist in this domain. This is done in three stages of discussion.

Discussions in the first section attempt to clarify the essential character-istics of theoretical concepts that describe phenomena in the domain of client from the nursing perspective. The boundaries of the nursing perspective in theoretical thinking with respect to the client as the focus of attention are defined. The idea is to suggest that, as Blau puts it, "the nature of the patterns and shapes one can recognize in the welter of human experience depends on one's perspective" (1975, p. 3).

In the second section, an attempt is made to show several different ways of abstracting the phenomena of human living and of health in the domain of client. The concepts of human living and health are treated here because these have been the main focal points of theoretical thinking for many nursing theorists. This section offers discussions on the approaches that are used and useful in delineating concepts from a different intellectual scope. Approaches of delineation and abstraction are considered important in theoretical development, since it is neither necessary nor possible to observe and abstract all elements characterizing the real world in all instances. Different approaches permit abstracting selectively within proper frameworks of observation and delineation. Several non-nursing and nursing theorists' approaches in conceptualizing human personhood and health are brought into discussion in this section to compare and contrast the postures that emerge from different directions.

The third section provides expositions on how to analyze theoretical concepts for phenomena in the domain of client through two examples: restlessness and compliance. The purpose is to illustrate important strategies of theoretical analysis of concepts. These analyses are offered as preludes to the development of theoretical propositions in nursing that can be used in explanations and empirical analyses. What is not dealt with in this and in the following three chapters is the advancement of specific theoretical statements of relationships among concepts in a theoretical system. The central focus in chapters 5–8 is in abstracting, delineating, and describing phenomena of significance in theoretical terms. This step is considered a prerequisite to thinking about relationships among two or more concepts and is a necessary step for developing a theory.

THE CLIENT DOMAIN IN THE NURSING PERSPECTIVE

One of the essential skills that a nurse scientist needs if he/she is to contribute to theoretical development in nursing is the capacity to conceptualize phenomena in the client from the nursing perspective. There are a vast number of concepts that describe phenomena in the client that are not significant to nursing. The nursing perspective for this domain is specifically that of "health"—health not viewed in the context of two million streptococci invading the lung tissues or of a ruptured cerebral artery, but considered with respect to human living and behaviors of health. Concepts and relevant phenomena in the domain of client from the nursing perspective are important to the extent that the client, the human person, is the main focus of nursing. For nursing to demonstrate its credibility and relevancy in society, it is necessary for nurses to understand, explain, and predict certain happenings in clients. These "certain happenings" and definitions of them are central to this section's theoretical thinking.

The main idea is to concentrate on and direct our intellectual energy toward the study of more critical and essentially nursing-oriented concepts, selected from a vast array of possible ones. Defining a boundary is difficult because it involves a critical ability, a sense of relevance, and definite ideas about propriety for nursing. Current literature indicates that nursing scientists are approaching this boundary-definition issue in two different ways: (a) from a holistic point of view that is global and all-encompassing, and (b) from a particularistic point of view that is discrete and focused on selected aspects of the human condition.

The domain of client offers a vast array of human phenomena from which selections should be made for the study of appropriate and essential phenomena from the nursing perspective. As suggested in chapter 4, the main difference between the holistic and particularistic conceptualizations of phenomena in the domain of client is in units of analysis. Holistic conceptualization in this domain necessarily has to take in the whole person as the basic unit of analysis. Particularistic conceptualization, on the other hand, takes only parts or certain elements of the human person as the basic units of analysis.

Because it is somewhat arbitrary and difficult to select concepts of importance within the domain of client from the nursing perspective, I propose a scheme for categorization by which certain characteristics of human phenomena are classified for theoretical analysis in nursing. This classification scheme for the domain of client refers to types of concepts in a generic sense, and includes: (1) essentialistic concepts, (2) problematic concepts, and (3) health care experiential concepts.

Essentialistic concepts refer to those phenomena present in the client as essential characteristics and processes of human nature and living that are important to nursing and to human health in general. Examples of essentialistic concepts are negative feedback, homeostasis, structural integrity, coping, and self-image. Concepts referring to phenomena in human development and growth are also thought to be essentialistic. Maturation, bonding, socialization, ego-development, aging, and so on, are a few examples representing developmental concepts. Essentialistic concepts refer to normal and fundamental characteristics and processes that human beings experience in ordinary states of living and growing. The term *ordinary* refers to what is generally expected as "usual" and "normal." An understanding of these phenomena will certainly aid in understanding the human person and health from the nursing perspective, and also can be applied to understanding and explaining problems of clients.

Problematic concepts refer to phenomena that are present in human beings as deviations from normal patternings of healthy living. These concepts represent phenomena that require some kind of nursing solutions and interventions. Such concepts as pain, infection, anxiety, depression, and respiratory distress are of the *problematic* type. Problematic concepts have been the major focus of study by nursing scientists, especially those who have put effort into the development of nursing diagnosis terminologies. For this category, the term *problematic* is used to mean problematic to nursing, requiring nursing intervention. Thus, concepts such as appendicitis or bankruptcy, although these represent problematic human conditions, are not problematic concepts from the nursing perspective. Here also, the term *problematic* refers to the nature of phenomena, and does not refer to "problems" as used in epistemology. In epistemology, problems refer to puzzles requiring explanations and are the bases for knowledge-seeking activities. From the epistemological perspective, *all* concepts can be problems. On the other hand, in this exposition, problematic concepts in the client domain specifically refer only to phenomena that threaten a real person's health and healthful living.

As the last group of concepts, *health care experiential concepts* refer to phenomena that arise from people's experiences in the health care system. This category includes such concepts as recidivism, compliance, health-belief, hospitalization, recovery, etc. This type of concept is relevant for nursing studies because it refers to specific human experiences that affect either the process of health or the contents of nursing.

Table 5.1 lists examples of concepts categorized according to this classification scheme and in the holistic/particularistic modes. These examples have been drawn from the current nursing literature, unsystematically and in a casual manner, and are listed here only as typical concepts in each category according to the definitions given earlier.

This way of classifying concepts in the domain of client focuses on general meanings of phenomena. Current development in work on nursing diagnosis classification suggests that at present the discipline of nursing is interested more in the conceptualization of problematic and health care experiential phenomena than in essentialistic concepts. My belief, however, is that the discipline needs to clarify conceptualization of those essentialistic concepts that are necessary to understand many of the problematic and health care experiential concepts.

This classification scheme is one way of organizing human phenomena into appropriate categories for scientific examination from the nursing perspective. Nursing is concerned with clients' behaviors, responses, experiences, and constituents in human living to the extent that these have some bearing on their health, health-maintaining behaviors, and nursing requirements. While this scheme is useful for categorical thinking, and

Table 5.1

EXAMPLES OF CONCEPTS IN THE DOMAIN OF CLIENT FOR STUDY IN THE NURSING PERSPECTIVE

CONCEPT TYPE	LEVEL OF CONCEPT DESCRIPTION	
	HOLISTIC	PARTICULARISTIC
Essentialistic	Aging	Biologic rhythm
	Health	Dexterity
	Hope	Ego
	Independence	Hardiness
	Lifestyle behavior	Intelligence
	Maturation	Mobility
	Normality	Respiratory compliance
	Personhood	Self-image
Problematic	Chronicity	Anorexia
	Helplessness	Chronic sorrow
	Illness	Incontinence
	Maladaptation	Infection
	Stress	Irritability
	Suffering	Obesity
	Trauma	Pain
		Respiratory distress
Health care experiential	Institutionalization	Decubitus ulcers
	Isolation	Dependence
	Noncompliance	Nosocomial infection
	Recidivism	Technology-dependence

has shown that commonly studied concepts in nursing can be classified accordingly, the discipline of nursing has long been preoccupied with the idea that the conceptualizations of *human person* and *health* as two fundamental, essential concepts are necessary to structure nursing theories. Thus, major nursing theorists have put their efforts into developing some refined ideas about these two broad concepts in their presentation of nursing theories and conceptual models. Some scholars even consider it a requirement in theory development to advance the frame-specific conceptualizations of human person and health. Conceptualizations of humans and health are the foundations from which many other concepts in the domain of client are understood in frame-specifying ways. Hence, conceptualizations of humans and health are ontological in nature. Accordingly, conceptual notions about humans and health are usually the first and basic ideas requiring identification in the development of nursing curricula, nursing service philosophies, and professional standards. Of all concepts relevant for inclusion within the nursing framework, the concepts of *humans* and *health* are the most essential holistic concepts for theoretical thinking.

CONCEPTUALIZATION OF HUMANS AND HEALTH

In a holistic posture, phenomena in the domain of client are conceptualized as systems of interlinked elements, with respect either to the nature of human beings or to that of health. Although there are other concepts in the holistic mode that are important to nursing, concepts of humans and health stand out as the most important and essential ones for nursing. An understanding of what humans are all about and how things happen in humans is central to nursing, because the recipients of nursing actions as well as the performers of those actions *are* human beings. In addition, health, pertaining to life and death and states in between, is an *essential property* of humans. Health is also the main purpose of nursing work.

Thus, the nursing perspective is to conceptualize a person not just as a complex biological entity but also as a much more complexly integrated being that is psychologically, socially, and culturally embedded in existence. However, since nursing's focus is health, we cannot disregard the biological nature of humans in our conceptualizations. The nursing perspective also is to conceptualize health as a variable state in which a person assumes certain characteristics of human living associated with biological, psychological, and social functioning and responses. Nursing is concerned with certain types of human affairs and human well-being, that is, health and illness. Hence, it is natural for nursing scientists to struggle for clear conceptualizations of humans and human affairs of a particular kind, namely, healthy humans and healthy human affairs. Concepts of humans and health take on their proper meanings in the nursing perspective insofar as such conceptualizations lead to developing effective and scientifically valid nursing strategies.

In nursing, there has been a long history of preoccupation with a grand understanding of the human person philosophically and theoretically. One obvious reason for this preoccupation is, in a way, rooted in the profession's insistence on having philosophical stands on life, humans, health, and nursing. This value has been most clearly expressed in the accreditation criteria for nursing curricula throughout the years. Additionally, the profession has maintained a long-standing posture that views a human being as a whole rather than as discrete details within a maze of physio-psycho-social-spiritual components. Consequently, nearly all nursing theorists have supplied us with their specific visions of what humans are and how one should understand human affairs under the latent or sometimes manifest claim of viewing humans as wholistic beings. Likewise, we are also supplied with various conceptualizations of health by nursing theorists, motivated apparently by similar reasons.

A person is usually conceptualized in a global sense and is described in a synthesized fashion, indicating what a person is all about. Thus, nursing conceptualizations of humans are generally founded on philosophical (i.e., ontological) views of human existence, and are directed toward unified views of people that are useful and valued for nursing practice. This approach of aligning the conceptualization of humans with the basic tenets of the profession permits development of "models of humans" that are the foundations for a scientific growth of knowledge in the field. Such an approach has been used in psychology, sociology, economics, political science, and medicine. For example, Simon's model of man (1957) has been used in administrative science and the social sciences as the basis for the field's theoretical and empirical work. Likewise, Comte's (2009) positivistic conceptualization of the human being has influenced the early theoretical development in sociology in Europe. Models of human beings provide scientists with the basic attitudes and abstract tools to make detailed propositions in the development of specific theories of human beings.

In contrast to the ways models of humans are developed and used in scientific fields, conceptualization of health in nursing is a movement to a somewhat particularistic level of thinking. In this sense, models of health are less global than models of humans and may develop from the main philosophical ideas of humanity, but are specifically oriented to describing the nature of health, which is only one aspect of human affairs. Conceptualization of health is similar to those used for the development of conceptual models of "wealth," "knowledge," or "power" in the sense that the focus of conceptualization is on certain characteristics of human life, not in human life itself.

These considerations point up analytical differences in the approaches for "models of humans" and "models of health," although both concepts are holistic concepts for nursing. In general, models of humans are ontological and address the basic existential questions regarding body/mind and the nature of human life, whereas models of health are conceptual, focusing on identifying specific phenomenal elements that define health. Irrespective of the approaches adopted by theorists, the focus of attention for theoretical consideration remains on those phenomena in humans related to health insofar as a model is developed from the nursing perspective.

Although health as a concept is implicitly inferred more often in models of humans, it is explicitly defined and developed in models of health. The difference in the approaches for developing models of humans and health seems to be the placement of focus: The first approach for a model of humans focuses on "human person" from a philosophical orientation, whereas the second approach for a model of health focuses specifically on "health" as the major phenomenon of interest. Thus, the two approaches pose different problems in specifying descriptive features of health, in that the first approach requires conceptual descriptions of humans, specifically addressing how health is encompassed with such descriptions, whereas the second approach needs to specify descriptive features of health only with respect to its conceptual constituents. Regardless of the approaches adopted for explaining human phenomena in a holistic mode, models of humans and health developed from the nursing perspective ultimately must be brought to bear on nursing questions. In addition, models of humans and health are the basic frameworks for development of theories in nursing on various levels and within a wide range of scope. Theoretical development for nursing thus has to be viewed to have some connections to particular models of humans and health that provide the basic tenets and premises for specific delineations of theoretical statements and definitions within a theory.

These two approaches as conceptual models and theoretical systems in nursing are currently the main efforts that are being fervently pursued in nursing, especially in the continuing refinements of the so-called grand theories of nursing. The desire seems to be to develop a general nursing theory of a grand type through a model of humans or a model of health. However, models of humans and health are conceptual models that can be the baselines not only for theories of grand type but also for meso-level, middle-range, and microlevel theories.

Although several serious attempts to develop models of humans and health are currently being made in nursing, the next section examines several other models of humans and health that have been developed by theorists in other disciplines prior to presenting the nursing models. This is done to provide a generalized baseline to compare and contrast how models of humans and health have been developed in the scientific community (including nursing), and to consider the relationships of nursing models of humans and health to other approaches. This approach of presentation is used to show that nursing models of humans and health should be examined within the broader context of the "idea systems" present in the scientific community in general.

MODELS OF HUMANS

It is difficult to be comprehensive in discussing models of humans. Since our conceptualization of *homo sapiens* has been and will continue to be closely tied to prevailing philosophical attitudes about life, humans, and the universe, the history of dominant philosophies provides an important base for a basic understanding of how several different models of man have emerged in the recent past. For our discussion in this section, first I present only briefly several different models of humans that are being debated in the scientific world and that are considered relevant to nursing. This is done mainly to provide a background for the discussion of and comparison with nursing models of humans. A more comprehensive discussion follows regarding several models of humans developed within the conceptual models of nursing. Philosophical and conceptual linkages between models of humans developed in other relevant scientific disciplines and those developed in nursing indicate that scientific ideas in general do not arise out of a vacuum but have connections with the prevailing general paradigm of the scientific world.

Early scientific attempts at developing unified models of humans can be traced back to 19th-century positivism. Scientific thinkers such as Huxley, Darwin, Spencer, Moleschott, and Engels influenced the creation of a concept of humanity in which a person is mainly thought of as a member of a species having animalistic instincts and wants. Models of humans prior to the 19th century were so closely tied to the dominant religious beliefs and philosophies, backed by scant biological and physical understanding of human life, that the influence of those models on the conduct of human practice was profound, yet arbitrary. The arrival of positivism encouraged many scientists to try to explain human behaviors by reference to animalistic patterns. Twentieth-century logical positivism also influenced the conceptualization of humanity in many fields, such as psychology, biology, and sociology. In addition, Husserl's phenomenology and various philosophical ideals of existentialism complicated theoretical thinking concerning the concepts of humanity that emerged in many directions during the 20th century.

Models of Humans in General

As an archetype of empiricism and physicalism, the Skinnerian model of humans was developed with the main focus on human behaviors. Skinnerian conceptualization is based on behaviorism, which has enlarged upon the basic ideas about the stimulus–response proposition of human behaviors. Both psychological and social versions of the behavioral model of humans are based on the premise that human behavior is learned, maintained, extinguished, and modified by means of reward and punishment.[1] In a behavioral model, a person emits activities in a present situation based upon the experiences he or she attained either directly or vicariously as the consequences of previous activities; the consequences either reinforce or extinguish learning and repeating of activities. Behaviors are evaluated according to need/disposition or deprivation/satiation principles. Such behavioral models of humans resulted from the late nineteenth and early twentieth centuries' preoccupation with a value-free, positivistic approach to the generation of scientific knowledge.

In a somewhat different orientation, Bernard (1957), Cannon (1932), and Selye (1956, 1976) developed a physiological conceptualization of humans. A person is viewed as striving to adapt in the most efficient manner possible to demands or stresses that are put upon the person, either as a total organism or in parts, but always striving to maintain stability within the self. Theirs was an attempt to unify a person into a whole being, opposing the scientific advances and efforts that dissected a person into organs, cells, and different functional attributes. The method of studying humans through the use of autopsy and surgical techniques in the early 1900s influenced many scientists to view humans in a dissected form. Medical and pathological atomists' conceptions of humanity have their roots in such development. Although there still exist scientists whose work is based on the atomistic view of humanity, the most dominant concepts of humanity in biomedical fields are stress-adaptation models. Much of the current work in stress-adaptation models is based on the conceptual premises of the original ideas postulated by Cannon, Bernard, and Selye.[2] This stress-adaptation model was extended in the recent decades with the model of psychoneuroimmunology (Ader & Cohen, 1975; Ader, Felten, & Cohen, 2006; Goodkin & Visser, 2000), introduced to explain health and illness by linking stress, psychological processes, and neuro-biochemical processes. Recent advances in biochemistry and brain physiology have further developed the conceptualization of health and illness on this model.

René Dubos's model of humans (1965) is an extension of this view of adaptation and describes all aspects of the human environment as providing ephemeral conditions. A person is thought to exercise adaptive abilities by selecting among alternatives to achieve a self-directed end, given the external conditions that are encountered at a given moment. Dubos's human, furthermore, is a product of the lasting and universal characteristics of human nature, inscribed in being, and yet is capable of establishing a personal history; thus, the person possesses both phylogenic and ontogenic adaptability. A person is seen as an organism responding to stimuli of environmental challenge in a manner that is based on rationality, that is, that although some responses are based on the direct effects of the stimuli on the organism, most of a person's responses are usually determined not by such direct effects but by the symbolic interpretations he or she attaches to the stimuli.

Thus, Dubos's human treats and responds to actual environmental stimuli in a chained sequence of direct reactions, indirect reactions that occur as ripple effects of the direct reactions, and responses to personalized symbols that are generated by the impinging stimuli. This human trait, according to Dubos, makes the individual's responses to any environmental factors extremely personal.

Alfred Korzybski's theory of humans (1921), emerging from the engineering and mathematical orientation in the wake of Russell's mathematical logic and Einstein's theory of relativity, is concerned with somewhat different aspects of human nature. This model views humans as having the characteristics of time-binding power beyond the space-binding capacity of animals and the matter–energy binding property of plants. Although the language used in the description of a person in this model is highly oriented to the physical sciences, it describes a person as a life form different from animals and plants, having another dimension of orientation, that of time. It is a departure from both the theological and the biological conceptions of humans. A person and his or her capacity are conceptualized as: (a) bound to past achievements, (b) the user of ever-increasing, inherited wisdom, and (c) the trustee of posterity. This model of humans is rooted in Descartes's idea of universe as comprising space, matter, and time, and was developed against the backdrop of Einstein's proposition that links human movement in time and space to other objects in a relativistic fashion. It views humanity's basic *modus operandi* as "creative competition," by which new ideas and more goods are produced in a rational manner. By juxtaposing Korzybski's theory of humans with Einstein's theory of relativity, Polakov suggested that "man measures an event from the standpoint of his own system regarded as at rest" and that a person is a relativist having a unique personal system of reference in space–time contexts (1925). An illuminating aspect of this model having a physical perspective is its conceptual likeness to Dubos's model, in which personally accumulated history is stressed.

In addition to the behavioral model discussed earlier, there are several different concepts of the psychological model of humans. Three views stand out distinctively, indicating different orientations. The psychoanalytic models of humans advanced by Freud and reformulated by many scientists[3] are based on the ideas of organizational and dominational relationships among different psychological elements in humanity. The id (or the instinct), the ego (the consciousness), and the superego (the controller) are the main human elements that determine self-generated actions and a person's relations to the outside world. Ego as consciousness plays an important role in attaining, maintaining, and controlling human responses in the psychoanalytic models of man. A person's actions are the extensions of suppressions of the id's wants and the superego's controls by the consciousness, and yet expressed by the dominations obtained by different aspects of the personality for pleasure and power.

On the other hand, Maslow (1967, 1973) attempts to generate an idea of humanity by interfacing human needs that are basically psychological in nature with the biological make-up of the human organism. Maslow's concept of a person as an organism that is oriented to self-regulation, self-government, and self-choice is akin to the rationalist view of humanity. However, it is based on the notion that human needs are fundamentally biological. He classifies human needs into two types: (a) the basic needs, including safety and protection, belongingness, love, respect, self-esteem, identity, and self-actualization; and (b) the metaneeds, including truth, goodness, beauty, justice, order, law, unity, etc. These needs are seen as tied to the structure of the human organism itself. He conceptualizes variations in human conditions according to satisfaction and deprivation of need, and views deprivation as the cause for disease or illness.

Gestalt psychologists' view of a person as a personalistic, holistic being is a more recent concept of humanity in psychology. This concept of unitary human being suggests that human activities are produced by integrated efforts of a person to express what he or she knows and how he or she deals with this knowledge within the context of given biological conditions. The Gestalt view of a person is understood not in his or her componental characteristics but as the whole depicted in his or her experience and behaviors.

Psychological models of humans also have limiting explanatory use for human phenomena in the nursing perspective. Only selected phenomena in the client can be studied within theoretical systems that are based on psychological models of humans for nursing.

Another conceptualization of humans to emerge, rooted in Cartesian philosophy, Kantian rationalism and Russell's system of mathematical logic, is economic models that view a person as being able to maximize preferences based on rational behaviors. The major premise of the economic model is global rationality, implying a perfect fit between a human choice and a preference, as in the game–theoretical model of von Neumann–Morgenstern. However, Simon (1957) suggests a model that emphasizes "striving for rationality" rather than the "rationality" itself as the basis of human behavior. Simon's human strives for rationality and yet is basically oriented to a goal-satisfying rather than a goal-maximizing mode of decision-making behaviors. Simon's human makes decisions and selects choices among alternatives through a satisfying mode, a mode through which a person finds "a path that will permit satisfaction at some specified level of all of its needs" (Simon, 1957, p. 271). A satisfying mode is defined by an individual's aspirational level at the point of choice. Simon further advances his thinking on the concept of bounded rationality and its relationship to human behavior in his conceptualization of "thinking man." He recapitulates "satisficing" and "bounded rationality" as the basis of human behavior in the following way:

> …a picture of Thinking Man, a creature of bounded rationality who copes with the complexity that confronts him by highly selective serial search of the environment, guided and interrupted by the demands of his motivational system, and regulated, in particular, by dynamically adjusting, multidimensional levels of aspiration.[4]

What is projected as central to human existence and human affairs in economic and administrative models of humans is rationality. These models are conceptually concerned with circumscribed aspects of humans, decision making, and choice behavior. These conceptualizations are not concerned with the total organismic person as physical–biological being. For them, such biological natures are only important to the extent that they influence preferences, needs, and evaluations of utilities. Therefore, human aspects other than rationality are only contextual to studying the processes through which a person handles himself and the external factors. If we were to apply these models of humans directly to viewing the client in the nursing perspective, the theoretical explanations of human phenomena would be limited to "choice behaviors." Thus, such a model is useful only in studying particularistic phenomena in the domain of client.

Of course, there are many more models of humans that have been proposed by scientists in different disciplinary orientations. For example, Parsons' model of social humanity is composed of personality and organism, acting and interacting with objects and other human beings in the social world (Parsons, 1951). A person acts and interacts within given cognitive, cathectic, and evaluative motivations. The Parsonian individual is a product of integration of cultural values and social norms. Furthermore, human deviant behaviors are viewed in the context of functionality to the social systems rather than to the individual's motivations or needs. A social person thus is a constrained being, acting within the limits of individual, social, and cultural standards and expectations.

From the perspective of social action, Hollis (1977) distinguishes two models of "man," as Plastic Man and Autonomous Man. Hollis's Plastic Man is a being constituted by adaptive responses stemming from the interplay between nature and nurture. On the other hand, Hollis' Autonomous Man is a being with a subjective self whose basic apparatus for social actions is rationality.

Another example is a biomedical model. In addition to the dissected view of human system as a biological being, there has been a growing interest in medical fields for a development of conceptualization of humanity that encompasses bioethical issues that have raised many moral questions in the practice of health care in recent years. In an attempt to view humanity in the context of biomedical ethics, Fletcher (1979) proposes a composite human model. He specifies the necessary characteristics of a human person as follows: (a) minimum intelligence, (b) self-awareness, (c) self-control, (d) a sense of time, (e) a sense of futurity, (f) a sense of the past, (g) the capacity to relate to others, (h) concern for others, (i) communicability, (j) control of existence and freedom, (k) curiosity, (l) change and changeability, (m) balance of rationality and feeling, (n) idiosyncrasy and individuality, (o) neocortical function, (p) not non- or antiartificial, (q) not essentially parental, (r) not essentially sexual, (s) not a bundle of rights, and (t) not a worshipper. This model raises several moral and ethical questions regarding the values of life and existence. Although such a model can create a great deal of controversy and discussion, it can serve scientists to view human life and human existence from quite different perspectives. More importantly, when such a model is applied to human services, there are many practice implications. In any event, such a model at least provides a framework upon which evaluation of human nature may begin and questions related to human interventions are addressed.

Focusing on intervening in human problems in a general way, Stevenson, in his exposition in *Seven Theories of Human Nature* (1987), selected theories of human nature, which are based on the combination of a theory of the nature of the universe, a basic idea about human nature, a specification of determinants for what is wrong with human affairs, and a proposal for a way to correct the wrongs (p. 9). Based on these premises, Stevenson offers seven models of humans: (a) the Platonic theory of human nature, embracing dualism of body and spirit, by which major problems of humans are identified in a context of harmony and justice, to be corrected by the supremacy of reason; (b) the human model of Christianity; (c) the Marxist model of humans, which focuses on economic conditions of human life; (d) the Freudian psychoanalytic theory of humans, in which the deterministic nature of the human condition and human development is emphasized; (e) the existential model of humans, which is grounded in human existence and freedom; (f) the behaviorist model of humans, within which environment is the major force for explanation of human behaviors; and (g) the Lorenzian model of humans, in which humans are viewed as a sort of animal.

An emerging view of human activities includes cyberspace, referring to a concept of the human person that encompasses both the "real" and the "virtual." For example, Pollock (2008) offers a concept of the human person as "supervenient"; that is, as interacting with virtual cognition that then influences bodily functions. This conceptualization embraces that of the human mind as a "virtual machine" akin to Peirce's (cited in Hartshorne, Weiss, & Burks, 1935/1958) notion of states of mind being "virtual." On the other hand, as virtuality disembodies the concreteness of things, such as the human body, humans in a virtual reality exist with respect to time only, without occupying space.

These theories of human nature from various philosophical positions point to different conceptualizations of human ills (or problems) and how problems that are inherent in the nature of humans can be corrected or remedied.

These are but some of the eclectic examples of models of humans in a variety of scientific fields that suggest varied viewpoints and different angles of vision. As this cursory review of such models suggests, our conceptions of humanity are closely related to philosophical ideas about meanings attached to differentiating the subjective from the objective and about a person's relations to the world and herself or himself. Scientific advancement and technology, as well as the dominant modes of scientific investigation, also influence our ideas about human nature, capacities, and variabilities. Disclosures briefly discussed in these pages indicate that a person may appear differently when objectified with the tinted glasses of the biologist, the psychologist, the sociologist, the mathematician, the physician—even the philosopher—with different ideological commitments. Yet a person may also be perceived in the same manner even among scientists of different disciplinary orientations and of varying perspectives. It is also obvious that scientists use their conceptual models of humans for different purposes—for development of a theory of humans, an ethical basis of scientific inquiry, a framework for human intervention, or as a starting point for philosophical discourse.

These examples also indicate that models of humans conceptualized in other disciplines have limited theoretical utility for nursing if they are applied directly to nursing without expansion or modification. This enlightens our thinking and directs us toward developing nursing models of humans. For nursing explanations, it is necessary to have nursing models of humans, notwithstanding the contributions to the discipline of nursing of models of humans derived from theoretical developments in other fields. The specific nature of essential phenomena in nursing within the domain of client requires a conceptualization of humanity that addresses such a specific nature.

Nursing Models of Humans

In nursing, then, what should a model of humans describe? Nursing models of humans generally describe humanity with respect to placement in and operations related to health and well-being. Conceptual models proposed by several nursing theorists of the 1970s and 1980s such as Rogers, Roy, Orem, and Johnson have attempted to do this. I shall attempt at this point to summarize the mental images that these nursing theorists have projected in their models of humans. This exposition is presented to show examples of the models, not as exemplary models for nursing. Of course, it needs to be made clear that these theorists describe their ideas in an implicit manner and do not refer to their conceptualizations of humanity by the term "models." Health is usually the major theme handled in nursing models of humans as the essential descriptive characteristics of humanity. The current conceptualization of humanity in nursing models can be categorized into six major types, according to their respective views of health as an essential human condition:

1. "Balance" as the essential human characteristic for human existence and health
2. "Process" as the mode through which humans' existence and living are actualized
3. "Configuration" as an integrative basis of human existence and health
4. "Aggregation" of parts as a way to express the human condition
5. "Experiencing" as the basic characteristic of human existence and health
6. "Meaning making" as the essential feature of human living

This idea of differentiating conceptual approaches to formulating models of humans—balance, process, configuration, aggregation, experiencing, and meaning making—is proposed here so as to attain a clear mental picture of the variety of human phenomena proposed by different thinkers in the field of nursing. By introducing this classification, we are also able to compare nursing's human models with those discussed earlier. The balance model, for instance, is a conceptualization in which human phenomena are considered in relation to integration and stability, and Selye's "stress" model of humans is simply a balance model in which human phenomena are mainly considered with respect to equilibrium.

The process model is a conceptualization in which human phenomena are explained as ever-changing, continuing activities. Dubos's adaptive model of humans is of this kind, in which a person is depicted as an ever-adapting, growing entity.

The configuration model refers to a conceptualization of human phenomena in which integration among different elements and subsystems is taken to be the major characteristic. Gestalt human models and systems models are of this type.

The aggregation model is a conceptualization in which a person is viewed as an entity composed of different elements. Human phenomena are expressed as the additiveness of different elements that make up a person. The biological and medical models of humans tend to take this form of conceptualization of humanity.

The experiencing model takes humans' experiencing at present in a given context as the primary focus for understanding human living and existence. Models based on existentialism and Husserlian phenomenology, with their emphasis on the "life world" of individual, subjective persons, are of this type.

On the other hand, the meaning-making model emphasizes humans' reflexivity and hermeneuticity as the basis for human life and health. Taylor's human science model of "man" takes this form of conceptualization of humanity (1985).

Johnson's behavioral system is an example of the balance model. Johnson (1980) refers to humanity as a behavioral system comprised of patterned, repetitive, and purposeful ways of behaving. Human behaviors are formed into an organized and integrated functional unit. Human health is implicitly expressed as the state of behavioral system balance and dynamic stability. According to Johnson, it is not the nature of properties or state of a person that is central to his or her health and existence, but rather the system of behaviors as parts of an organized and integrated whole. Thus, although labeled as a "behavioral" model, its premises are quite variant from the classical behavioral models of reinforcement and extinction. This concept of balance as the expression of health is akin to the systems theorists' view of humanity that considers a person as striving to attain the maximum balance and homeostasis. From the latter's perspective, a system's adaptiveness with respect to stability is the central process for an explanation of variants in system-states, whether referred to as behaviors or as states.

Although Johnson identifies subsystems within the human behavioral system, it is ultimately the behavior as a whole that is the phenomenon of interest to her. Johnson states that this conceptualization is not intended to provide a framework for marking the boundary of what aspects of the behavioral system are appropriate from the perspective of nursing. An implicit inference in Johnson's model is that any possible or actual imbalance or deviation from the dynamic stability of the behavioral system is a potential target for nursing intervention. However, the specific types of behaviors or imbalances that are the main targets for nursing intervention are neither clearly indicated nor implicitly stated.

The conceptual ideas projected in Rogers's model of "unitary man" are related to process. Rogers (1970, 1989, 1992) conceptualizes an individual as a human energy field that is an irreducible, indivisible whole, continually engaged in a mutual process with the environmental energy field for the pattern of life that moves toward increasing diversity and negentropy. For Rogers, a person is an emergent energy field characterized by a pattern whose identity is specified as a single wave. This pattern of human energy field is an abstraction representing the unitary character of humans, but is not a reality. Its character is also abstracted to be continuously changing, unique, and integral with its environmental energy field. Human energy field pattern manifests through a person's mutual, simultaneous process with her/his environment through the homeodynamics of integrality, helicy, and resonancy in one's personal evolution in pandimensional reality.

Rogers depicts a person as not having specific goals in his or her evolutionary journey through the life process, except for an increasing diversity in accordance with the law of change process. Furthermore, a person's goals in the life process are unpredictable rather than deterministic. This means that a person's goals in the life process change with the progression of the process itself, and that goals are revised and formulated according to changes in personal evolution. What is most explicit in this model is the irreducible unity of a person as a mutually processing being, having personal identity and existence defined by his or her pattern. Thus, it is not possible to understand Rogers' human evolutionary identity or process without having the knowledge of the characteristics of the environmental field or the person's mutual processing within it. Rogers also postulates mutual field process as the dynamics of change that bring about relative and increasingly diverse patterns in both the human and environmental energy fields.

Thus, Rogers's human is an ever-changing unitary entity whose characteristics are not determined by genetics, destiny, or predetermined patterns of growth, but are expressed by changes in its field pattern through the processes involving three homeodynamic principles. Goals of life are never fixed, nor are the patterns of change that are possible for an individual's life. As an abstraction, Rogers's human is an indivisible, irreducible unity identifiable by its single-wave pattern, which is relative, changing, and integral with one's environment.

Rogers implies that health is expressed as the process of life in its unity. She postulates that nursing seeks human betterment by guiding people to design ways to fulfill their different rhythmic patterns, uses the knowledge of the science of unitary humans creatively to support changes in clients' energy field patterns that are relative and diverse, and is responsible to individualize care for individuals that fits with their uniquely diverse field patterns of change (1992). The pattern of life process that an individual attains expresses whether or not he or she has realized his or her health potential. What is not specified in the model is an explicit definition of "health potential." Rogers' implicit notion of health is that of a person in a state of continuing, relative diversities, not defined by any standardized expectations, but expressed only as evolutionary, sequential pattern changes. To Rogers, the human–environment field is a mutually processing unity that generates field pattern changes; it is treated as though it has a consciousness or goal-directedness for changes that are relative and increasingly diverse, occurring unpredictably and with creativity. The model gives the impression that the human–environment integrity is as critical for human existence as a person's integrity itself.

In the Roy Adaptation Model (Roy, 1976; Roy & Andrews, 1991; Roy & Roberts, 1981), a person is perceived as an adaptive system receiving "inputs" (identified as stimuli from the external environment, or generated by the self), processing them by internal and feedback processes inherent in an individual's ever-changing abilities, and producing "outputs" as either adaptive or ineffective responses.

Roy expands this view of adaptation by a model of humans that views persons as coextensive and having mutual relationships with their environment and with a God figure, and that persons mediate their actions through thinking, feeling, and creative abilities. With this expansion Roy reformulates the definition of adaptation as "the process and outcome whereby the thinking and feeling person uses conscious awareness and choice to create human and environmental integration" (2007, p. 158). To Roy, adaptation has a positive connotation, a state of "all systems go," a "green light" in specific relation to what is happening to the person at a given moment in a given environment. Roy's human responds to stimuli in four basic adaptive modes: (a) physiological needs, (b) self-concept, (c) role-function, and (d) interdependence. Adaptive or ineffective responses result from the functioning of two basic mechanisms of controlling and responding: regulator and cognator.

Because Roy conceptualizes a person as having four distinct modes for adapting to stimuli, the concept of humanity according to this model is that of configuration, although there is an element of balance suggested in the model. A person is depicted as a configuration of responses in four adaptive modes. Thus, human responses are the major phenomena of interest in Roy's model and are analyzed for their adaptiveness in relation to four sub-sectors in an individual. Health, then, is relative to the person's responses to stimuli that promote the person's general goals of survival, growth, reproduction, and mastery, manifested within each adaptive mode. A person who responds ineffectively to stimuli is seen as capturing and spending energy for the particular set of stimuli, exhibiting behaviors that are incongruent with the valued goals. Roy's human is a reactive entity whose basic mechanisms become activated in response to impinging stimuli. The characteristics of creativity and self-determination are not emphasized in this model.

These three nursing models of humans are contrasted here to provide concepts of humanity that are quite different from one another, yet have a shared, significant identification within the nursing perspective. These nursing theorists' ideas suggest that in the nursing perspective a person may be described according to the nature of his or her behaviors (Johnson), the level of diversity in patterns exhibited in the person's mutual processes with the environment (Rogers), or the characteristics of responses to stimuli impinging on the person depicted either as adaptive or ineffective (Roy). As shown here, the concepts of balance, process, configuration, aggregation, experiencing, and meaning making as the distinguishing characteristics of human models can only be used to identify the dominant features of models rather than to confine them to specific types.

As indicated in these discussions, it is possible, then, to imagine a room with nursing scientists perceiving the client in many different ways and analyzing health problems with different conceptual orientations. Rogers will wonder about the rhythm and diversity in the client's energy field patterns and the nature of integral changes in the patterns emerging within the pandimensional universe with its current nature. Johnson's posture will be that of analyzing the client's behaviors in the context of the integration as a whole person-system. In contrast, Roy will evaluate the client's responses to the situation as adaptive or ineffective and identify the focal, contextual, and residual stimuli that cause deficits in the adaptive responses.

As Barrett (1978) suggested, a person becomes Janus, and each scientist or theorist or philosopher is imprisoned in his or her seat for a view of particular features. The question is whether a scientist should get up from his or her seat and walk around to obtain views of all the features from different angles, or should remain in one position so as to attain an in-depth understanding of features from that one particular perspective. It is certainly a paradox for scientists, who wish to be comprehensive in the understanding of a phenomenon and at the same time desire to gain a detailed knowledge of a single aspect of that phenomenon.

The crux of the matter is in the complexities: A person eats, plays, and fights; laughs and cries; does good for others and commits sins; falls in love and falls out of love; makes friends and seeks solitude; is happy, sad, and plainly content; makes decisions and follows the decisions of others blindly; and is healthy, ill, disabled, and dying. All these and more make the conceptualization of a person difficult. Nursing models of humans, therefore, can at least confine our theoretical interests to selected human features.

Conceptualization of Humans in the Nursing Perspective

As the discussion in the preceding section shows and the literature reveals, there is no unified perspective within nursing as to the *conceptualization of humans*. While some scholars may argue that it is both acceptable and necessary to have multiple conceptualizations of humans in the nursing perspective, we need to consider what are the essential features of humans that should be accounted for in the conceptualization of humans in the nursing perspective. Nursing is a practice discipline that is concerned with providing services to humans directly regarding their health. Therefore, conceptualization of humans in the nursing perspective has significance in considering what the recipient of nursing care (i.e., the client) is like as well as what the practitioner of nursing is about.

Mrs. Dorothy Kingsley, a 73-year-old widow, has been discharged from the hospital after a hip replacement. She lives alone in an apartment in an elderly housing complex and manages to do most of the things that need to be done. She sometimes uses a wheelchair to move around, although she is able to walk slowly and hesitantly with a walker, and has put on a nice housedress that hangs loosely when moving about. She is slight in her stature, and has a very modest stoop. She has lost some of her hearing ability, especially in her right ear, but is not keen on using a hearing aid although she has one. Her voice is round, and she speaks with large gestures with both hands. As she walks with her walker, her grips are tight and her closed mouth slants downward as though in some strain. Small lines around her eyes, however, reveal good-naturedness and a quick smile. She feels lucky for having had the surgery, and is confident that she will be able to go about in a few weeks to the malls for lunch or visit friends. She is on medication for hypertension, and feels well in general except for some pain and immobility associated with the surgery at present.

How do we see Mrs. Kingsley as a human being and as a client? What should nursing's ontological gaze be in seeing this patient? A nurse's conceptualization of Mrs. Kingsley would be: She is an elderly woman living independently with some limitations in her mobility and discomfort requiring temporary support, with hopefulness for recovery that will allow her to resume her patterns of living, with a chronic illness under control, and having a generally positive outlook on life. As a client of nursing, Mrs. Kingsley requires nursing attention regarding support needs, recovery, prevention of reoccurrence of fractures, maintenance of hypertension control, and continuation of independent living. This picture emerges from a general nursing gaze that is understood to represent the nurse's general perspective regarding humans as nursing clients. However, such general pictures may be further refined or detailed according to specific theoretical perspectives in nursing.

With the focus on clients, then, I refer back to the ontological commitments regarding human nature and human living presented in chapter 3. The ontologies of human nature and human living as the foundational guideposts for nursing knowledge development are also the elementary foundations for conceptualizations of humans in the nursing perspective. As far as nursing is concerned with health, and health is tied to humans with bodies and selves, nursing's conceptualizations of humans need to refer to how humans experience and live with their bodies and selves as independent individuals as well as with others and in situations.

This ontological position suggests that humans are bodies and selves intertwined to carry on "living" in the totality of experiences through sensing, realizing, thinking, knowing, and responding to occurrences and changes that are internal and external to them. Although historically nursing has been concerned with the human body and care of the body, there has been a gradual silence about the human body in the nursing discourse (Harder, 1992), as nursing began to separate itself from medicine and align with the human sciences in recent decades. This moving away from the focus on humans' physicalness to the emphasis on experiences, feelings, and meanings has created some confusion in viewing humans in the nursing perspective.

Nursing continues to be engaged in "body work" that involves caring for and treating parts of the body or the body as a whole, since we cannot deny the intrinsic relationship between our bodies and health. But at the same time nursing is also concerned with helping people with their emotional, social, existential, and spiritual aspects of life. To overcome this paradoxical contradiction apparent in the nursing views of humans, three human features need to be captured in an integrated fashion in conceptualizing humans in the nursing perspective: *human body, personhood and self,* and *human living.* This way of thinking, that is, viewing humans to encompass three features, is in no way to suggest that unitary views of humans that reject compartmentalization of these features are not valid. It is necessary to accept these features as valid, even if they cannot be considered to exist as separate entities as in unitary or holistic conceptualizations.

The human body, with its appearance, make-up, concreteness, and boundedness, begins with the biological but is existential in that it exists as an entity as it is experienced in time and space. Benoist and Cathebras (1993) suggest that the Cartesian conception of the human body as an object led the way to the modern biomedical concept of the human body as an entity separate from or devoid of spirit or soul. Furthermore, the representation of the human body according to its biological and physical features has been objected to by many scholars as delimiting the body's humanness and not expressing the "true" qualities of humans. Biopsychosocial models both in medicine (Engel, 1977) and nursing are examples of attempts to overcome this biological reductionism.

Phenomenological and existential ways of thinking have led us to the notion of personhood and self in connection to embodiment. Lawler (1991) states that "our understanding of the body is firmly interwoven with the nature of personhood and with the meaning of being human, and our notion of human existence requires a bodily form that is recognisable as human" (p. 56). Gadow (1980) also suggests that humanness and human experiences may be conceptualized as phenomenological relations between the self and the body. Personhood and self signify the subjectivity that is possible only through reflexivity, consciousness, and meaning making. Ontologically, how the body and the self are connected to reveal humanness and human existence is problematic, as evidenced in various theories of human nature. The notions of "mindful body" and "bodily mind" reflect the continuing debate and confusion regarding the nature of integration between the body and the mind (either as consciousness or spirit). The mind as constituted in personhood and self transcends the conceptualization of it in a psychological or neuropsychological sense, and refers to the ability to construct one's being as an existential idea.

The human body also is a vehicle with which we are social beings, capable of symbolizing and interacting as well as being controlled and controlling. The human body is no longer a simple configuration of physical, materialistic elements, but constitutes both the physical/material and the symbolic and cultural. The human body exists and has meanings for its capacity to have relations with space and time, and to perform both mechanistic and expressive activities, but also for its ability to project messages and identity in cultural context (Benoist & Cathebras, 1993). Human existence and living is concretized through the body, and the body mediates living in its many particular forms, such as eating, talking with friends, or loving, and in its entirety in a holistic sense, such as being a mother, a nurse, a worshiper, etc.

The human body cannot just be understood from the biological perspective, but has to be viewed as a synthesis incorporating the biological nature and the results of social and cultural processes (Guarnaccia, 2001). Scheper-Hughes and Lock (1987) present three "bodies" of humans as analytically separate but overlapping conceptualizations: the first as the *individual body* or the lived experience of the body-self; the second as the *social body* that is used with symbolic representations for understanding nature, society, and culture; and the third as the *body politic* that is used for regulations, surveillance, and control in relations with others. Lupton (2003) also illustrates meanings of different conceptualizations of body—the gendered body, the sexual body, the clean body, the disciplined body, the sporting body, the commoditified body, and the dead body—which may lead to different ways of conceptualizing health.

With the advent of technology, the human body is increasingly constituted by nonhuman entities such as the artificial heart, prosthetics, and

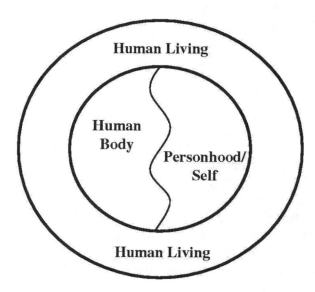

Figure 5.1. Connections among human body, personhood/self, and human living.

transplanted organs, which then can be seen to comprise a "virtual body." In another sense, the virtual body refers to the human body as configured in virtual reality by way of various representations of self (in cyberspace). The virtual body represented with virtual structures has also been used to understand health and disease (Colwell, 1996; Nissan, 2008).

Be that as it may, human bodies are labeled as deviant or normal, hygienic or unhygienic, controlled or needful of control by the institutionalized power of medicine (Foucault, 1973). The human body, then, gets intimately tied to human living not as a strict biophysical entity, but as one encased within a complex meaning structure.

However, human living is carried on meaningfully in a form that is more than the composition of biological and mechanistic responses and activities, and is mediated by personhood/self. Hence, human living includes both: (a) animalistic, biological activities and behaviors that come to have specifically human meanings, such as eating, which is not simply an act of getting food but is an act having meanings in personal, social, and cultural contexts; and (b) those purely human, beyond-animalistic activities, such as worshiping, creating poetry, or simply reading a newspaper. As illustrated in Figure 5.1, the human body, personhood/self, and living may be seen as connected in an embedded, interpenetrating fashion to project humanness.

Nursing's ontological concern with humanity lies in these three features as they impact on health individually and in concert. Specific conceptualizations of humans in the nursing perspective thus need to be developed with philosophical assumptions regarding the human body, personhood/self, and human living, as well as the relations among them with respect to health. Any version of biological, phenomenological, or behavioral reductionism is inadequate to address the theoretical and practical issues confronting nursing, as nursing is work for human health that is grounded in the human body, personhood/self, and human living. From this, we can postulate human living from the perspective of health and illness in four integrative dimensions: (a) living of one's body, (b) living of oneself (personhood), (c) living with others, and (d) living in situations. Human experiences of living are through these four dimensions that are always integrated and interconnected. Living of one's body refers to how the body gets engaged in the living through the body's capacities, limitations, sensations, boundaries, and constituents, whereas living of oneself (personhood) means living with one's history and genealogy, desires and wants, dreams and hopes, ideas and opinions, choices, habits, and knowing.

On the other hand, living with others is based on the sociality of humans and refers to communality of human existence involving coexisting, communicating, coordinating, exchanging, and interacting. Living in situations is based on the fact that all living instances occur in situations and contexts, and refers to situational embeddedness of human living (Kim, 2000). This dimension refers to the understanding that human living has to be understood in the context of situations that offer both the condition of possibility and that of limitation. These four dimensions of living establish the characteristics of human living. Human living in these four dimensions is modified by and influences various states of health and illness, suggesting such a four-dimensional schema as the pivotal focus for nursing, as shown in Figure 5.2.

I am proposing therefore a model of humans that embraces the notion of human living as the primary focus, with human body and personhood/self as integrating elements that characterize human living that is expressed in four dimensions.

MODELS OF HEALTH

Another holistic approach to conceptualizing phenomena in the client domain has been specified earlier as models of health. The theoretical

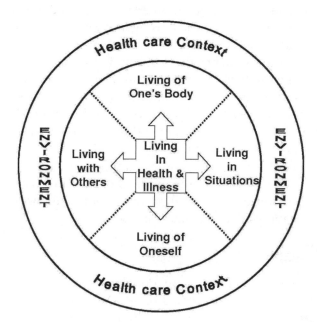

Figure 5.2. Human living in health and illness.

focus of this approach in nursing is to view health as having particular meanings for nursing actions. Thus, in this approach, health would be defined with respect to nursing care needs and nursing interventions. Although health as a concept is rather global, as with the concept of person, it encompasses rather selected sorts of phenomena in humans. Because of this, many models of humans contain the basic notions about the phenomena of health, as indicated in the discussions presented in the preceding section. Health represents a circumscribed aspect of human phenomena and can be conceptualized in more particularistic modes. Taking the medical–anthropological perspective, Lupton (2003) discusses various approaches to the conceptualization of health, ranging from the functionalist's approach in the tradition of Talcott Parsons; to the political–economic approach, in which health is viewed as a resource; to the social constructionist approach, in which health is viewed to be formulated through social, historical conventions and belief systems; to an approach that views health as lived experiences; to the critical approach from poststructuralism, in which health is viewed as something to be structured through language and power.

The literature in general indicates that the traditional models of health may be differentiated into two distinct types: structural models and functional models. *Structural* models of health are oriented to looking at human structures and properties as the major indicators of the phenomena of health. In contrast, *functional* models of health view health as intrinsically tied to human functioning. In addition, health is conceptualized according to *integrative* models, in which holistic conceptualizations of humans are the starting points. In this section, models are examined according to these three types. Models of health proposed by scientists of other disciplines as well as by nursing theorists are examined together in this section according to the types by which the models are classified. However, there are many other ways of classifying health conceptualizations, and these three types certainly do not encompass all the various different models of health. This section, thus, introduces how various models direct conceptualizations of health to have different meanings and characterizations.

Structural Models of Health

The structural, property-oriented approaches are rooted in the long history of considering "health" as opposite to sickness, disease, and illness, beginning with the ancient ideas (i.e., Egyptian and Greek) about the relationship between the way one feels and the nature of bodily constituents. Structural models of health are oriented to distinguishing the "normal" nature and constitution of elements in a human person, especially in the body—the physical being—and the deviations that exist that influence the way a person feels, performs duties, and behaves. In general, these models are clinically and/or medically oriented models, in which causes for change and deviations are the main epistemological interests.

Thus, for the conceptualization of health in such approaches, it is essential to know what causes deviations, hence the development of a string of theories seeking to explain pathophysiological phenomena, starting with early demonic theories of disease. Historically, many of the medically oriented theories of disease belong to this type of approach. Examples are Galen's theory of humoral imbalance as the basis of diseased states; the miasmic theory of illness of the 18th century, by which the production of disease is attributed to invasion of the body by earthly, noxious miasma; the germ theory of the 19th and early 20th centuries; the general adaptation syndrome as the basis of stress/adaptation; and the current biochemical theories of pathology.

Health in a structural model is indicated by signs and symptoms (that is, conditions) a person experiences or exhibits. These are considered changes and deviations from the normal in the human elements and structures. Currently, there are two general structural models of health: the clinical model and the adaptation model.

Clinical models, generally having a historical linkage to earlier conceptualizations of "disease" in medicine, are oriented to explaining health in pathological terms. Clinical models view health as a state in which there is an absence of abnormal signs and symptoms and as an opposite state of "diseased." In a diseased state, a person is in acquisition of an undesirable, abnormal, or deviant entity or property in human structures, with specific known or unknown etiologies.

The terms, signs, and symptoms in this context have negative, undesirable connotations. While current clinical models in general have been reconciled with the unified view of a human as a free-flowing integration of mind and body, there is a tendency in clinical models to have a deterministic view of what might go wrong with human nature in given situations. The earlier conceptualizations of health in clinical models were implicitly based on the dualism of the "psyche" (the mind) and the "soma" (the body). Incorporation of the ideas on psychosomatic interdependence is a more recent development in clinical models. Yet the recent interest in psychopharmacological research indicates persisting adherence of clinical models to physicalism as the major philosophical orientation.

The deterministic view in clinical models is evident in the continuing search for causal factors for diseases. Clinical models usually assume the scientific posture that seeks to identify and understand characteristics of diseased states as primary for correcting those diseased states.

Adaptation models are of more recent development. The concept of general adaptation syndrome (Selye, 1956, 1976) popularized the view of health in relation to an individual's responses and behaviors to stresses and noxious stimuli. Health in these models is conceptualized as a state of coping and adapting within a continuously changing environment. Health indicates that a person maintains his or her integrity of structures and yet changes his or her nature and behaviors to respond effectively to situational demands. Engel (1970) suggests that health and disease are phases that result as the human organism strives to master and handle stresses that are continually posed by environments on multiple levels, that is, cellular, chemical, physiological, and behavioral levels. He views a state of health as one in which an organism functions effectively as a whole, fulfilling needs, successfully responding to the requirements of the environment, and pursuing its biological destiny, including growth and reproduction (Engel, 1975). This state of health is specifically tied to the adaptation that occurs in the human organism.

Adolf Meyer's work on stressful life events, the framework of Howard and Scott (1965), and the work of Hinkle (1961) and Wolff (1962) propose ecologically oriented adaptation models of health, in which health is viewed as adjustments to one's social environment and occurrences in life situations. Such ecologically oriented adaptation models consider the ecological influences as structurally demanding and causing changes in the structures of adaptation.

Fabrega (1974) proposes a somewhat different adaptation model, which he calls a "phenomenologic" view of health and disease. The basic assumption is that disease needs to be understood in the context of an individual's subjective experiences. Such subjective experiences are thought to be shaped by social and cultural patterns. Characteristics of disease in the phenomenologic model encompass changes in the state of being, such as in the state of feeling, thought, self-definition, impulses, and so on. These changes are seen as discontinuous with everyday affairs and are believed to be caused by socioculturally defined agents and circumstances. The main "change" of structure of interest to Fabrega is an altered concept of self-identity. In a phenomenologic sense, an altered self-identity is defined as disturbed feelings, bodily sensations, beliefs about how the body functions, self-derogatory convictions, imputations of moral guilt, etc. As the major form of disease state, it is inclusive of discomfort, disability, discreditation, and danger, according to Fabrega (1974).

Among nursing models in which health is considered as a concept, Roy's adaptation model treats health as a state of structural characteristics in adaptive processes (Roy & Andrews, 1991; Roy & Roberts, 1981). Roy suggests that a state of health is possible for a person who is adaptive. A person is healthy when he or she is able to direct energies to respond to multiple stimuli of life rather than expanding and concentrating on one set of stimuli. In essence, Roy's model views health as having certain property and structural characteristics in an individual organism. A state of health is attained when an individual receives an appropriate type and amount of stimuli and has structural integrity in adaptive modes and mechanisms.

Health in structural models is operationalized and measured most appropriately as feeling-states, perceptions, and sign/symptom complexes. State-characteristics that are considered the indicators of health in these models are: (a) measured objectively and compared to the established norms as the expression of "healthy" state, as in the clinical measurements of blood pressure, body weight, level of hemoglobin, size of liver, etc.; (b) expressed as experiences and perceptions, as in feelings of pain, headache, depression, fatigue, discomfort, or respiratory distress; or (c) assessed as behaviors of adaptation, as in adaptive versus maladaptive behaviors, negative versus positive responses, or enhancing versus destroying behaviors.

Instruments developed with this approach in the conceptualization of health are found in works by Given, Simoni, and Gallin (1977); Kennedy, Northcott, and Kinzel (1978); and Wan (1976), among many others. In the same tradition, Turnbull (1976) treats health for nursing from a strictly structural perspective. Measurement of wellness and health is expressed as intactness, symmetry, nourishment, or productivity. Structural models of health are thus oriented to describing health on the basis of changes that are present in human structures, producing variations in feeling states, behaviors, and appearances of the structures.

Functional Models of Health

Functional models begin with a premise that health is a state of variability in human functioning. The functionalists' approaches view dimensions of health and variations in the state of health vis-à-vis human ability to perform required functions. Optimum health refers to the normative reference point of desired capacity and functioning.

Naegel (1970) perceives health as "a condition necessary for the realization of two of our regnant values: mastery of the world and fun." Health as a "state" allows one to do what one wants to do and to be what one wants to be. As an opposite "state," illness is seen to impede activity and to limit one's autonomy, and it is a state of frustration and deprivation. In addition, Naegel sees health as a moral good that is desired by all but vaguely defined: health is part of the condition of participation in social life as a valued state. In this view, health is globally described in social, functional terms. Health is a state in which a person is able to participate in the affairs of the world and the affairs of self with the freedom of the individual. To Naegel, autonomy is the basic functional requirement for an individual's freedom of pursuit, and health is the end-state in which the individual's autonomy can be enjoyed.

If we are to designate Naegel's concept of health as a functionalist's orientation in an individualistic sense, then Parsons' concept of health is a functionalist's approach in a social sense. Parsons (1951 and 1958) conceptualizes health as a socially desirable and normative state that is functionally important to the social system. To Parsons, health is a functional requirement for maintaining integration in the social system in an aggregated form. From this assumption, an individual's health is defined as his or her capacity to assume roles and perform essential social tasks satisfactorily. Twaddle (1974) consolidates both the biological and the sociological meanings of functioning into a more inclusive conceptualization of health. In addition, health is a state "labeled" by self and others, according to Twaddle.

Twaddle proposes the following postulates as the essential ideas about health and illness:

- Health and illness are defined normatively and refer to "standards of adequacy relative to capacities, feeling states, and biological functioning needed for the performance of those activities expected of members of a society," and yet deviations from the norms are rather ambiguously defined by that society.
- Health and illness are designated according to the norms of functioning in the biological context, in that parameters of biological functioning are used as the criteria designating the health status.
- The norms for differential labeling and designation of health status are not consistently applied to social groups, in that the norms tend to be differently interpreted among different social groups, social situations, and times, and differently applied by different individuals.[5]

Correspondingly, health is a designated state in which adequacy in one's capacities for role and task performance is judged by self and others against normative and socially held standards. What is most essential for these functional approaches, then, is the definition of "normal" or "expected" human functioning and capacity for functioning. Insofar as a person is capable of functioning as expected and adequately, an enlarged heart, an absence of a kidney, or the presence of discomfort and pain is not essential to this conceptualization of health. Engelhardt (1976) also notes that the conceptions of health and illness are tied to our ideologies and expectations concerning the world, in that we identify and judge certain states as illnesses according to what we consider as dysfunctional, deformed, or violating the norms of a reasonable expectation with regard to freedom of action on our part as humans. He considers this an instance of "*hubris*." Many recent studies indicating different evaluative standards of health applied to the general adult population and those applied to the aged suggest that differential criteria for evaluation of health status do exist for subpopulation categories.

The functional approaches have been used quite frequently in health services research. Efforts to develop indicators of health that depart from the classical, clinical measurements of abnormalities have evolved into several indices of health that are based on functioning. For example, as a most comprehensive approach, the Rand Health Insurance Study (Brook et al., 1979) has used physical, social, and psychological functioning as the basis for the development of health status indicators. Kaplan, Bush, and Berry (1976) also carried out a survey study in which normative designations of functioning capacities were assessed so as to use them as a reference guide for health-status designations. The long-standing use of activities of daily living (ADL) scales in rehabilitation and gerontology is an example of application of the functional approaches for health assessment.

In nursing, Orem's self-care model is a version of a functional model of health. Orem conceptualizes health in relation to self-care deficits, which are expressed as deficiencies in any one of the self-care foci identified in three categories (universal, developmental, and health-deviation) of self-care types (1991). Orem states that "health includes that which makes a person human (form of mental life), operating in conjunction with physiological and psychophysiological mechanisms, and a material structure (a biologic life), and in relation to and interaction with other human beings (interpersonal and social life)."[6]

Health is a state of wholeness or integrity of the person vis-à-vis his or her capacity to provide self-care. Since Orem views a human being as a unity functioning biologically, symbolically, and socially, one has to be able to perform deliberate actions to be functional and healthy. Health is thus attained by sufficient and satisfactory self-care actions responding to varying demands for attention to self. Effectively performed self-care action contributes to human integrity, human functioning, and human development. Orem further proposes that the client's health, in the nursing perspective, should be considered according to three types of self-care requisites (1980 and 1991).

Universal self-care requisites are considered to have six foci: (a) air, water, and food; (b) elimination; (c) activity and rest; (d) solitude and interaction; (e) hazards to life and well-being; and (f) normalcy. Developmental self-care requisites encompass two categories: (a) conditions that support life processes and promote the process of development, and (b) provisions for preventing exposure to deleterious conditions or for developing strategies to deal with harmful conditions. Health care deviation self-care requisites are related to six categories: (a) preventive and proactive health-seeking, (b) therapeutic, (c) compliance with medical measures, (d) awareness of adverse effects of health care, (e) self-concept generating, and (f) accepting and adjusting to health deviation consequences. Thus, self-care is the functional capacity to handle such requirements and is considered as deliberate action, either routine or programmed. Usually, self-care actions performed in daily living become routine, while new self-care actions have to be learned in response to given, specific demands.

Although Orem attempts to conceptualize health in a nursing frame of reference, moving away from medical, psychological, and sociological orientations, the self-care model suffers from its implicit assumptions of "unbounded rationality" as the basis for choice of actions and of "deliberateness" in choices as well as in actions. What is not handled adequately in the conceptualization of the model is the role of unconscious, reflexive, and autonomic human responses that define a person's functional capacities that are responsible for many types of self-care activities.

Integrative Models of Health

As shown in these discussions of various models of health, a purely structural or functional conceptualization of health appears to be inadequate and incomplete in abstracting the complex phenomena of health. Recent interests in applying the general systems or holistic approaches for a conceptualization of health are attempts to overcome such inadequacies.

Departing from the conventional perspectives and approaches presented in the preceding section, Newman (Newman, 1979, 1994; Newman & Jones, 2007) proposes a theory of health based on Rogers's model of unitary humans. Newman's basic assumptions regarding health, which is viewed as the spectrum of disease at one end and nondisease on the other, are six-fold:

- Health encompasses conditions of illness or pathology that are accompanied by varying degrees of incapacitation.
- Conditions of illness or pathology are manifestations of the total pattern of the individual.
- The manifested patterns of the individual precede structural or functional changes.
- The manifested patterns of the individual are not pathology itself, and thus removal of pathology in itself will not change the patterns of the individual.
- Being ill is healthful when it is the only way an individual's patterns can become manifest in a given life-process situation.
- Health is the expansion of consciousness and is the totality of the life process.

To Newman, the phenomena of health comprise the concepts of movement, time, space, and consciousness. Newman poses five general propositions, considering the expansion of consciousness as the expression of health. Hence, the processes that specify how an individual expands consciousness will explain how an individual progresses in life with respect to health.

Newman considers time and space as the basis of life processes, having a complementary relationship. Time and space are postulated to be in a complementary elasticity by which an individual moves about in relation to space and time. This suggests that an individual compensates for a loss in space with a gain in time and vice versa. Therefore, the patterns of an individual are manifested through this complementary process. Yet space and time as objective world elements are meaningless to an individual until his/her position in them is expressed by movement.

To Newman, the personal reality comes into existence via patterns of movement. The meanings of space and time are relative to movements of self and of perceived others. In addition, the patterns of movement are expressed within the conscious recognition of body and self. Thus, expressions of self are manifested in movements, and time is "possessed" by an individual through the patterns of movement one develops. Furthermore, since consciousness means awareness of one's life context in space–time dimensions, time measures the level of expanded consciousness. Newman expanded these theoretical ideas by incorporating the assumptions of mutuality of interaction between persons, uniqueness and wholeness of pattern in each client situation, and movement of the life process toward higher consciousness as the evolving pattern of the meaning of the whole (Newman & Jones, 2007, p. 120). Health as expanding consciousness is represented by a pattern that evolves over time and unfolds through interaction with environment.

This conceptualization departs in several ways from the conventional views of health in nursing. To begin with, health is viewed neither in relation to structural integrity nor to functional competency. It is not a property concept, but a process concept. Health is an expression of the level to which an individual's consciousness has expanded and is expanding, influencing the awareness of self, which in turn determines the ways the individual moves within subjective time and space. Time and space are media within which an individual expands self through movement and consciousness. Thus, health is a process in which one finds individualized yet evolving patterns of movement and consciousness, defining "possessed" and "private" space and time and claiming such entities from those that are present in the object world. Indeed, this conceptualization is revolutionary and requires a set of different worldviews. In this view, health is holistic, transcending the notions of illness, disease, or even body and mind. It nearly means life itself; therefore, the conceptualization suffers from a lack of specificity—if health *is* the processes of life, then it must be interchangeable with the concept of life.

According to this conceptualization of health, a state of health cannot be differentiated from a state of life. In addition, this concept equates health with a pattern of consciousness, yet the meaning of consciousness is not explicitly defined in the theory. If consciousness is "knowing," this conceptualization also disregards that aspect of human life which is controlled, regulated, and promoted by the reflexive, autonomic, and unconscious responses. Consciousness equated with the concept of life also raises a philosophical question regarding the intrinsic value of human existence. Certainly, Newman's theory of health opens the way for many other possible revolutionary conceptualizations of health that may be more particularly fitting to theoretical thinking in nursing.

In addition to holistic conceptualizations of health expressed in Rogers's models of unitary humans and Newman's theory of health, there are two more recent ideas that should be noted: (a) existential and phenomenological conceptualizations, and (b) ideological and constructionistic conceptualizations. From the existential and phenomenological perspectives, health is what subjective selves experience that gives specific meaning(s) of wellness.

Gadamer (1996) conceptualizes health as a state of equilibrium between the nature (that is, *animalitas*) and that of being a human person, "a condition of inner accord, of harmony with oneself that cannot be overridden by other, external forms of control, which is hidden and only can be alluded as a feeling of well-being" (p. 112). For Gadamer, health is "a condition of being involved, of being in the world, of being together with one's fellow human beings, of active and rewarding engagement in one's everyday tasks" and is manifested in "a feeling of well-being in which persons are open to new things, ready to embark on new enterprises and, forgetful of ourselves, [we] scarcely notice the demands and strains which are put on us" (1996, pp. 103–113). Gadamer's conceptualization of health rests on the philosophy of human life found in the hermeneutic philosophy, in which all human experiences are individual in context, that is, it is the individual who is experiencing it, although health is experienced unknowingly until a disruption occurs, as health is a hidden harmony. From this perspective, then, a person's health cannot be subjected to a measurement by standards.

These discussions of various models indicate that what is most critical in studying the phenomena of health rests not on the development of a unified concept of health, but on the understanding that different approaches to the conceptualization of health—whether structuralism, functionalism, general systems approach, essentialism, or hermeneutic philosophy—will lead to different sets of theoretical ideas and explanations. Accordingly, health may be understood and explained in relation to such concepts as attitude, value, quality of life, experience, stressful life events, attribution, help-seeking behavior, energy expansion, sensory deprivation, self-image, wellness, etc.

This section has presented a range of diverse conceptual thinking about human nature and health. As indicated earlier, the nursing perspective needs to steer its conceptual development and theoretical analysis into those areas of human affairs and human nature related to health. For nursing to make theoretical sense as a field, it is necessary to develop conceptual and theoretical approaches that can be used for nursing's understanding of human health. At the same time, truly fruitful theoretical advancements may result, not directly from such holistic conceptualizations of humanity and health, but from more focused approaches that are developed to understand more particularistic aspects of humanity and health. This idea is in line with the assertion that nursing may benefit more at the present time by developing middle-range theories of nursing rather than by trying to muddle through grand conceptualizations of humanity and health. What is needed, however, in developing middle-range theories of nursing is a fundamental philosophy about human life and health rather than a well-developed conceptual model.

SELECTED CONCEPTUAL ANALYSIS

In the first section of this chapter, a list of concepts in the domain of client as examples for the nursing perspective was presented. In the present section, however, conceptual analysis of two selected concepts in the domain of client is presented. The main purpose of this section is to show how a first-level analytical approach is used to gain conceptual and empirical understanding of phenomena. Two concepts, restlessness and compliance, are treated as examples for clarifying conceptual ideas about them and their relevance in the framework of nursing. Restlessness is selected as an example of a "problematic" concept, and compliance is selected as an example of a "health care experiential" concept. Each concept is analyzed with respect to (a) definitional clarification and conceptual meanings as reflected in the literature, (b) descriptive features and characterizations as a step toward an empirical analysis, and (c) the concept's relationships with other concepts that are important in nursing. The strategy and rationale for conceptual analysis discussed in detail in chapter 2 is adopted in this section for the analyses of restlessness and compliance. The specific reasons for selecting these two concepts are irrelevant, for actual presentations have no significance to our exercises in theoretical thinking. However, there is a contrast in the level and richness of conceptual development for these two concepts. Restlessness as a concept has received very little scientific attention, whereas compliance has been studied not only by nursing scientists but also by scientists in other behavioral and social sciences in recent decades.

Restlessness

Scenario

Ellen Austin, RN, who is a team leader for this unit of 10 semicritically ill patients, reports about the experiences during the night of two patients: Mrs. Jane Turcotte is a 32-year-old woman who was admitted to the hospital with abdominal and chest injuries resulting from an automobile accident three days ago; Mr. Thomas Taylor is a 68-year-old patient who is diabetic and has chronic obstructive lung disease, and has been on this unit for the past four days. Ms. Austin reports: "Mrs. Turcotte had a very restless night. I do not think she slept even ten minutes. She thrashed about the bed all night long, was agitated and restless. She received the pain medication and the sedative, but these didn't induce her to rest. She took off her TEDS [stockings] several times, almost pulled off her dressing, and attempted to get out of the bed. I stayed with her for a while, which seemed to calm her down a little. Mr. Taylor was out of his bed and walked up and down the corridor more than ten times during the night. He would get into the bed, then get up and sit in the chair, and then walk. This was repeated many times. He took a dose of sleeping medication early in the evening and did not want it repeated. He must be exhausted this morning. I asked him why he was so restless. He couldn't tell me the reason."

Definition

The term *restlessness* is most commonly used in its adjectival form, to describe people's behaviors of agitation. Although the phenomenon of restlessness seems to be a frequent occurrence, it has not been studied extensively as a distinct concept in the literature. Yet the phenomenon of restlessness is found in ordinary life situations and in patients' experiences. We have seen many patients in hospitals, nursing homes, and clinics in a state of restlessness and agitation. We also have experienced restless moments and hours ourselves when we found ourselves wandering about the house without aim, and with a feeling of uneasiness and agitation. Norris (1975) found in her literature review that restless behaviors are found in animals in preparation for migration or hibernation. As described in the above scenario, there are many forms of behaviors that are associated with restlessness.

Agitation is the most commonly used term in combination with restlessness to describe a behavioral state that includes aimless, roving, or wandering movements of the body or extremities. Chevrolet and Jolliet define agitation as "a psychomotor disturbance characterized by a marked increase in both motor and psychological activities, often accompanied by a loss of control of action and a disorganization of thoughts" (2007, p. 214). English and English (1958) define restlessness as "a tendency to aimless and constantly changing movements," and define agitation as "a condition of tense and irrepressible activity, usually rather 'fussy' and anxious." Barnes and Raskind (1980) define agitation as "a broad behavioral term connoting excessive motor activity, often nonpurposeful in nature, and commonly associated with feelings of internal tension, irritability, hostility and belligerency" (p. 112). A person in a state of restlessness tends to move about without purpose, with an unspecified feeling of uneasiness and tension. It is a behavioral state of motor activity accompanied by specific kinds of emotional experiences, and thus is a property concept. Norris (1975) suggests that restlessness may be specified by behavioral indicators: (a) increased, repetitive, aimless skeletomuscular activities; (b) urgency in repeating the activities; and (c) increased muscle tones of body, face, or both. These definitions suggest that restlessness is a state of behavioral movements of muscles, combined with an uneasy feeling state.

Restlessness is a "problematic" concept because it represents a state that requires our questioning of its causes, and because it is an undesirable, troublesome state requiring intervention or support, especially when it lasts for a long duration. Although restlessness of a short duration, the passing restlessness we experience in everyday life, is one in the normal repertoire of human behavioral experiences, when it exists in a person for a prolonged period of time or is exaggerated in its intensity, as apparent in the two patients in the preceding scenario, the phenomenon acquires a "problematic" meaning.

Restlessness, conceptualized interchangeably with "psychomotor agitation,"[7] is considered by many scientists in the context of neuropsychophysiological explanations, as many psychomotor phenomena are treated in the recent literature. Olds (1976) postulates the effects of catecholamines on agitation, especially psychotic agitation, and many recent studies of amines' effects on behaviors have cited restlessness as one of the effects of cimetidine or amphetamines. In addition, nocturnal restlessness of cardiac patients has been explained as the hypoxic response in several recent studies; such explanations might suggest relationships between/ among cerebral hypoxia, catecholamine release, motor activities, and apprehension.

In more recent years, the concept of restlessness has been identified more specifically, as in "terminal restlessness" and "restlessness in dementia." Often used interchangeably with the term *agitated delirium*, these terms combine restlessness with delirium. Delirium is defined in the *Diagnostic and Statistical Manual of Mental Disorders* (*DSM-IV*; American Psychiatric Association, 1994) as an acute change in mental status, or a fluctuation of mood, associated with impaired attention, disorganized thinking, confusion and an altered level of consciousness. Thus, terminal restlessness (agitated delirium) refers to psychomotor agitation in dying patients, frequently associated with impaired consciousness such as confusion and disorientation, emotional instability such as anxiety and irritability, and often involuntary muscle twitching or jerks (Blanchette, 2005; Head & Faul, 2005; Lee, Leppa, & Schepp, 2006). Similarly, "restlessness in dementia" also combines psychomotor agitation and delirium found in elderly persons with dementia.

While it is not too difficult to recognize a person in a state of restlessness, restlessness is difficult to define explicitly, for several reasons. First, it is often used to indicate a state of mind (as in, "I am restless. The spring air must be affecting me!"), even though the person may not exhibit behaviors of restlessness. Second, it is also often used to describe behaviors objectively observed (as in "He is restless today; he acts like a tiger in a cage."). Third, it can be a fleeting or long-lasting experiential phenomenon in which many different kinds of body and motor movements are possible. And fourth, historically it has been described as one aspect of more complex phenomena, such as schizophrenia, depression, anxiety, fear, hyperthyroidism, hypoglycemia, and dysphoria.

Furthermore, it has seldom been treated in scientific fields as a distinct phenomenon. The phenomenon of restlessness, it seems, should be conceptualized with respect to the nature of motor activity and the associated feeling state. Therefore, restlessness may be tentatively defined as a state in which a person exhibits purposeless and irrepressible body movements and activities accompanied by a feeling of tension and uneasiness.

Differentiation of the Concept From Anxiety, Fear, and Delirium

The major aspect that differentiates restlessness from anxiety and fear is the emphasis on motor activities and the specificity of the feeling state.

While all three concepts deal with phenomena that occur in persons in stressful, emotional states, accompanied by neurophysiological and motor behaviors, restlessness as a concept is confined to phenomena in which specific kinds of motor activities are exhibited with a feeling state of uneasiness. In contrast, anxiety refers primarily to the state of an emotion that involves subjectively felt and consciously perceived tension, apprehension, and nervousness. It is usually accompanied by or associated with activation of the autonomic nervous system (Spielberger, 1975). Anxiety may be expressed in many behavioral forms, including restless motor activities. Thus, restlessness as a concept may be considered an element in a more general class of phenomena called "anxiety."

The concept of fear is less similar to the concept of restlessness, but it is possible to imagine the presence of restless behaviors when a person is in a state of mild fear. In general, fear refers to an emotional state in which a person feels the possible, pending imposition of an undesirable, noxious, dangerous, or threatening condition. It is expressed in various behavioral forms through the activation of the autonomic nervous system, ranging from a total frozen state to a frantic flight. The emotional state of fear is focused and usually has a specific object by which fearful emotions are elicited. In these respects, the phenomenon of restlessness differs from fear more definitely than the phenomenon differs from anxiety.

As in the case of terminal restlessness, delirium is a concept that has been combined with restlessness in research and clinical practice. Although a clinical definition of delirium offered by *DSM-IV* makes it clear that it refers to impaired consciousness and arousal disturbances, whereas restlessness refers to psychomotor agitation primarily identified by psychomotor instability, differentiation between these two concepts is blurred because a state of delirium often has motoric presentations, especially in the hyperactive type, and a state of restlessness may accompany impaired cognitive behaviors. Stagno, Gibson, and Breitbart (2004) state that a clear understanding of delirium is lacking often because clinicians and researchers place different emphases on arousal disturbances and motoric presentations. It is the hyperactive delirium that is viewed in relation to restlessness, as in terminal restlessness (or agitated delirium).

Akathisia is a medical diagnosis for a movement disorder characterized by inner restlessness and a compelling need to be in constant motion as well as by actions such as rocking while standing or sitting, lifting the feet as if marching on the spot, and crossing and uncrossing the legs while sitting, often thought of as a side effect of long-term use of antipsychotic medications, lithium, and some other psychiatric drugs. Persons with akathisia typically have restless movements of the arms and legs such as tapping, marching in place, rocking, or crossing and uncrossing the legs, often accompanied by a feeling of anxiety at the thought of sitting down. It is thought to have a neurochemical basis for its emergence, is treated medically, and is differentiated from general restlessness.

Descriptive Features and Characteristics

Nurses in clinical situations have used many descriptions of restlessness, many of which are subjectively derived understandings of restless behaviors. Norris describes restlessness as follows:

> Restlessness seems to be expressed in many ways; by tossing, turning, or twisting in bed, by pacing, tapping with fingers or feet, picking with the fingers, scratching, or other motor activity of a repetitive, seemingly urgent, and not purposeful controlled or directed manner. Facial expressions may be tense, watchful, or fearful. The rate or amount of speech may increase.[8]

Clinical manifestations of restlessness appear to be irregular and are subject to personal interpretations. The diagnostic procedure used in these studies is usually descriptive in nature and is accompanied by a gross measure of judgment with respect to the degree or presence of agitated motor movements.

Blanchette (2005), combining the works by other researchers, specifies the signs and symptoms of terminal restlessness in three dimensions: (a) agitation, fidgeting, tossing and turning, myoclonic jerks/twitching, and moaning or crying out for the physical dimension; (b) hallucinations/paranoia, confusion/disorientation, impaired consciousness for the cognitive dimension; and (c) irritability, anxiety/worry, and sleep–wake disturbance for the affective dimension. Jones and associates (1998) developed an instrument to be used in clinical settings to assess "terminal restlessness," which was based on the characteristics identified by hospice staff. The final version of this instrument contains five items: consciousness impaired, distressed, agitated, anxious, withdrawn. Since these works are on terminal restlessness, which has delirium as one component, these characterizations may not represent restlessness that is devoid of delirium.

Since detailing descriptive features of a concept depends on the explicit definition of the concept adopted or developed, we assume that the characterization or operationalization, given the definition advanced above, requires at least two dimensional considerations: (a) the nature of motor activity, and (b) the feeling state. There are several characteristics inherent in the restless motor activity, including aimlessness of movements, irrepressibility of movements, and fussiness of movements (as in fidgeting, tossing and turning, jerking, and wondering). In addition, an accompanying feeling state of generalized tension, uneasiness, nonspecific distress, irritability, or belligerence is a part of restlessness as exhibited in such behaviors as moaning, irritability, anxiety, sleep disturbances, and labile emotions.

Duration is also an important aspect of restlessness, manifested clinically in patient-care situations. Intensity of restlessness is another aspect of clinical manifestation requiring nursing attention, yet there seems to be no objective way of differentiating degrees of intensity. At best, the measure of restlessness has to be descriptive with respect to motor activities, movements, and feeling states. However, the exact nature of feeling states in association with restlessness is difficult to specify because the experience of restlessness often occurs in situations of distress such as dying, being in critical care units, losing a spouse, and alcohol or tobacco withdrawal.

Relationship to Other Concepts

There is a paucity of research dealing specifically with restlessness in patients, except for studies regarding terminal restlessness. Few studies in the literature deal with the hypoxia hypothesis, which suggests that restless behaviors may be responses to hypoxia. Restlessness also has been considered the response to cerebral anoxia, usually resulting from injury. Norris (1975) alludes to several possible causes of restlessness, such as changes in the rhythmicity of life, anticipation of change, fatigue and boredom, role-deprivation, as well as many pathophysiological conditions.

Conceptualization of restlessness in a global, experiential sense is not found in the literature. Clinical observations and experiences suggest that restlessness is related to such experiences of hospitalized patients as unfamiliarity of surroundings, stress of illness or surgery, symbolic and physical meanings of isolation, and altered perceptions, and has been found in dying patients (especially those with cancer) and in persons who are going through alcohol/tobacco withdrawal as well as in elderly who are experiencing dementia.

There also are some indications that certain drugs are responsible for restlessness, especially in hospitalized elderly patients. A better understanding of restlessness-inducing factors within the person, in the environment, and in experiences can help develop nursing interventions that can be applied to clients who become restless. There may be many experiential and symbolic factors as well as physical ones in hospitalization and illness experiences that tend to arouse restlessness in certain clients. In addition, studies differentiating psychotic/schizophrenic agitation and delirium-associated agitation from simple restlessness should be of interest for a better understanding of neuropsychophysiological propositions, especially those related to catecholamine physiology.

Compliance

The following are but a few examples of noncompliance in health care, as expressed in the literature:

- A bottle full of antihypertensive drug on the night stand having a prescription filling date that is 6 months old.
- Elevated A1C measures of a diabetic client for the past four consecutive visits to the nurse practitioner at a clinic.
- Missed clinic visits by a patient on cardiac medication.
- Two packs of cigarettes smoked daily by a client who has an advanced chronic obstructive lung disease and bronchial asthma.
- A 3,000-calorie diet consumed repeatedly by a client on a 1,000-calorie reducing-diet regime.

Definition

At the conclusion of a Workshop/Symposium on Compliance with Therapeutic Regimens at McMaster University held in May 1974, the group accepted a general definition of compliance as the extent to which the patient's behavior coincides with the clinical prescription (Sackett, 1976). In contrast to this definition of compliance, which is suggestive of neutrality in relation to clinical prescriptions, there have been many definitions of compliance suggested by health care practitioners and scholars that encompass the notion of power influence on the behaviors of conformity. Barofsky (1978) attaches coercion to the phenomenon of compliance, maintaining the negative meaning of the concept. Because of this, compliance raises an ethical issue dealing with client autonomy. The negative connotation of the term has been the focus of many debates among physicians, nurses, behavioral and social scientists, and social workers. Indeed, the connotation of control embedded in the concept has been one of the reasons for the refusal of many researchers and clinicians to use this term.

The primary difference between the definitions proposed by the Sackett group and by Barofsky can be found in the perspectives from which the phenomena are conceptualized. The first approach, in which alignment of client's behaviors with prescriptions is a definition of compliance, views the phenomena as a property concept. Here, the results of compliant or noncompliant behaviors are removed from the definition, and it only refers to the client's behaviors judged against the clinical prescriptions for adherence and conformity. Thus, in the health care field, compliance as a property concept has an accepted meaning that refers to the adherence or matching of a client's behaviors to professional prescriptions. Here, the process by which professional prescriptions are formulated, especially in relation to the degree of collaboration in deciding on the nature of prescriptions, does not enter into the definition.

In contrast, compliance as a process concept refers to the client's behaviors that vary according to the degree with which others influence the behaviors (Barofsky, 1978). This form of definition depicts the process of influence in which power to influence is exercised to produce certain behaviors in the client. Thus, characteristically, the same client behaviors (i.e., by an objective judgment, such as taking medication at certain hours of the day, or making return clinic visits faithfully) may be classified as compliance, adherence, or therapeutic alliance, depending upon whether the behavior is produced by (a) coercion that is thought to produce compliance, (b) conformity that is thought to result in adherence, or (c) negotiation that is considered to bring about therapeutic alliance or concordance. For this definition of the concept, what is central to the phenomenon is not the nature of behaviors exhibited by the client, but the way the behaviors are induced in the client. That is, it is important to differentiate whether the behaviors are produced by coercive pressure, by self-propelled conformity, or by negotiation between the client and the professional in which some type of transaction occurs. It is theoretically important because an understanding of such processes is necessary for predicting future behaviors.

In conceptualizing the phenomenon of compliance, there also has been some debate about what should constitute "clinical prescriptions." Medication orders, return visits, dietary modifications, exercise programs, curtailment of smoking, abstinence of alcohol consumption, and other changes in personal habits have been included as examples of clinical prescriptions in the field. Since the phenomenon of compliance refers to self-administered regimens without the constant surveillance by professional staff that exists in institutionalized care settings, clinical prescriptions generally refer to the kinds of activities and behavior modifications related to daily habits. The object is development of new behavioral patterns or modifications of existing ones. These behaviors are usually embedded at the core of the client's private life.

Sackett (1976) introduces the intended goal (prevention, management, and rehabilitation) as an additional dimension of the clinical prescriptions.

He shows that the studies reviewed suggest different levels of compliance, not only according to the types of regimen but also according to the intended goals of a regimen.

The era of self-determination of the 1970s and 1980s spurred a great deal of debate about the appropriateness of the use of compliance, as the concept is viewed to reflect powerlessness, passivity, and professional control (Chatterjee, 2006; Mullen, 1997; Treharne et al., 2006). Many scholars have offered the concepts of "adherence" and "concordance" in its place (Cohen, 2009; Treharne et al., 2006; WHO, 2003). A shift from the compliance model to the model of concordance has even been officially adopted in the health care system of Great Britain (Marinker, 2003). Although this shift in the use of the term encouraged a shift in perspective regarding power relations between patients and professionals, there has not been a significant shift away from the ideology of compliance in practice (Segal, 2007).

However, although the use of compliance in the literature has waned in recent years, often the terms adherence, compliance, and concordance are still used interchangeably.

It is clear that the phenomenal focus in the concepts of compliance and adherence is the client, whereas the focus in the concept of concordance is the client–professional relationship in which agreement between two parties is emphasized. Therefore, the concept of concordance belongs to the client–nurse domain, as do the concepts of collaboration, negotiation, and therapeutic alliance, while the concepts of compliance and adherence fall within the domain of client. However, the conceptual distinction between compliance and adherence is not clear. Although many scholars prefer the concept of adherence over the concept of compliance, because adherence embraces the notion of self-control and conscious agreement with directives, there are connotations of power and control in both concepts. Whereas Cohen defines adherence as "persistence in the practice and maintenance of desired health behaviors and...the result of active participation and agreement" (2009, p. 27), Bissonnette (2008) in a concept analysis of adherence found no distinct differentiation between the concepts of adherence and compliance. In addition, Kyngäs, Duffy, and Kroll (2000) and Murphy and Canales (2001) found a variety of conceptualizations of compliance in the literature. This diversity in conceptualization of compliance suggests the complexity of the behavioral patterns linked to compliance, and begs for a unified theory of the concept.

Writing from the perspective of social influence on people's behaviors, Cialdini and Goldstein (2004) offer a generic definition of compliance. To them, "compliance refers to a particular kind of response—

acquiescence—to a particular kind of communication—a request" (p. 592). The request may be explicit or implicit, but the person is compelled to respond to the request in a specific way, that is, by a behavior agreeing to the request. In this definition, the focus is on what the person does with a request regardless of how and in what manner such a request comes to be extended. The phenomenal focus is exactly on a person's behaviors regarding requests, demands, or solicitations. In the context of health care, requests are physicians' orders, therapeutic regimens, or health care directives. This definition then focuses specifically on clients' behaviors as the phenomenal contents of the concept.

Figure 5.3 depicts the complications inherent in the conceptualization of compliance. As shown in the flowchart, a set of requests (demands, advices, or recommendations) for desired and/or necessary behaviors exists external to the person of focus, which may remain external or become integrated into the person's cognition, often involving acknowledgement and acceptance. Scholars who object to the term *compliance* usually consider a meaning of control to be inherent in "requests," with resulting conceptualization of the term to encompass the meaning of coercive influence on resulting behaviors. In a generic sense, this way of thinking seems to be biased and will direct theoretical thinking to focus only on the nature of requests or on external forces to explain compliance. This is a limited view, as the process by which compliance/noncompliance occurs needs to be explained from internal perspectives as well. For example, even after external requests (by physicians, nurses, or parents) have become internalized by the person, that person may still engage in noncompliant behaviors, as explained by the action science framework (Argyris, Putnam, & Smith, 1985; Argyris & Schön, 1976). Furthermore, the question of self-control in *how* a person acquiesces to a request, *how* the character of requests influences a person to follow through with a request, and *how* requests are presented to a person (whether or not they are mutually agreed-upon requests) are theoretical questions belonging in the realm of theory rather than in the domain of conceptualization.

Descriptive Features and Characteristics

The essential phenomenal element of compliance is behavior. Behavior refers to how people act or behave in certain ways that are in alignment with requests. Therefore, the key descriptive features of compliance reside in differentiating compliant behaviors from noncompliant behaviors, and in specifying variations in behavioral compliance. When compliance is associated with a request for a single behavior such as a return visit to a

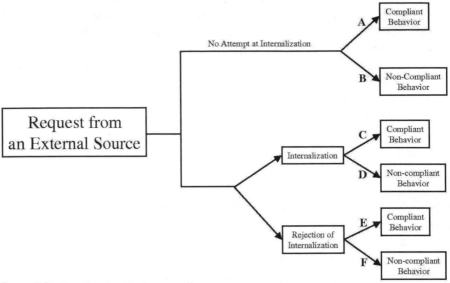

Figure 5.3. Structural paths for compliance as a concept.

health clinic, the differentiation between compliance and noncompliance is not difficult to see. However, when it is associated with a request that contains a set of several behavioral items (such as diabetic self-care directives, which include daily glucose-level monitoring, adhering to a diet, taking medication, and engaging in exercise for continuous behavioral patterns), it is difficult to specify variations in compliance. Because the content of compliance is behavior, there also is a problem with measurement. Although the obvious approach would be observation, often in health care and nursing, behaviors of compliance are not easily observable unless there is a continuous surveillance of the subject for a specified duration. While such technologically oriented tools as the Medication Event Monitoring System (Cramer et al., 1989) have been developed and used with acceptable reliability ratings, there are very few methods of observation that can be used for continuous observation of compliance behaviors. In lieu of observation, there are two methods of detecting behaviors; one is the use of proxy measures and the other is by self-report.

Quantitative expression of compliance using proxy measures has been the major difficulty for researchers in the field. Although there have been many studies using various types of direct or indirect proxy measures of compliance, there is no consensus as to what would explicitly and accurately reflect the degree of compliance. Gordis (1976) surveyed many studies of compliance and found that there is neither a general agreement on a definition that distinguishes compliance from noncompliance, nor is there a measurement system that expresses the true meaning of compliance as an outcome. Direct measures, such as the rate of drug excretion and blood levels of drugs to test the compliance to medication taking, have been found to be more reliable than pill counting or self-reporting. However, it has been suspected that explanations of compliance may be masked by measurement errors in both types of methods.

Many of the indirect measures that use outcomes of regimens (such as blood pressure level, weight-reduction rate, or respiratory capacity) as the criteria for compliance have been found to be influenced by many other physiological and transient variables besides regimen compliance. In many instances, such measurements tend to yield minimal information about compliance.

Another major measurement problem is in the comparability of compliance with one regimen to that of another. For example, there is no conceptual or operational clarity in handling the similarities and differences between compliance to a hypertensive medication and compliance to a low-salt diet. Obviously, the motivational and behavioral constraints that influence compliance to these two regimens are quite different. The complex nature of clinical prescriptions and the requirements these impose on individuals remain the most critical aspects of the phenomenon of compliance, both theoretically and operationally.

Measurement of compliance by relying on self-reporting has received a great deal of criticism for its reliability as well. Many studies found discrepancies between what clients report and their actual behaviors, although there continue to be reports of compliance studies using this form of operationalization, for the lack of a better or more convenient measure.

Relationship to Other Concepts

Compliance literature abounds with research studies that link compliance with different concepts in the domain of client, such as motivation, amount of knowledge, cognitive dissonance, and the presence of serious symptoms. The health-belief model (Becker, 1974) has been used in many studies as the theoretical framework, trying to explain compliance on the basis of clients' internal states and definitions of situations. These explanations are mainly oriented to treating compliance as an essentially self-triggered phenomenon. Thus, compliance is viewed as a behavioral outcome of other personal traits and characteristics, such as (a) how motivated a person is to attain a healthy state, (b) how much a certain state of health is valued by the person, (c) what the extent is to which a person believes his or her conduct will result in a positive outcome, (d) what the extent is to which a person can maintain a cognitively conflicting situation, and (e) how much a person knows about the nature of illness and the effectiveness of treatment. The major theoretical frameworks applied in the study of compliance in nursing include Bandura's self-efficacy model (1997), the theory of reasoned action, the theory of planned action, the transtheoretical model by Prochaska and Vellicer (1997) as well as various theories of motivation, decision making, and emotion in psychology.

In addition, several concepts in the domain of environment with sociological perspectives, such as social support, social pressure, symbolic expectations, and professional dominance, also have been found to have influence on a client's compliance. From the client–nurse domain orientation, characteristics of client–nurse interaction, contracting, and collaborative decision making have also been studied to explain compliance in the client. The degree to which a client receives reinforcement, positive feedback, frequent support, or supportive knowledge from his/her interactions with significant others and professionals, as well as the degree to which a client receives pressure for conformity, have been shown to influence compliance with various types of clinical prescriptions.

This suggests that compliance is related to influences of both internal and external type, as seen from the perspective of the client. The exact nature of the processes by which both internal and external factors mediate compliance has not been studied extensively and needs to be investigated.

SUMMARY

Because this chapter contains a great deal of new terminology and several new ideas in conceptualization, it is perhaps worthwhile to point out the main ideas that have been discussed. The domain of client as the focus of conceptualization is shown to comprise diverse types of concepts and phenomena essential for theoretical thinking in nursing.

Rethinking the models of "human" and of "health" appears to be central to clarifying both the philosophical and the theoretical stances that theoretical thinkers need to assume in nursing. It might be useful to examine many and varied models of humans and health that are currently used as the basis for theoretical developments in other scientific fields so as to attain a greater clarity in the theoretical requirements for nursing models of humans and health. It also would seem fruitful to reexamine nursing models of humans and health that are being used in research and practice, for their theoretical breadth and limitations.

Although there are many different ways of categorizing concepts in the domain of client for studies from the nursing perspective, the suggested typology of essentialistic, problematic, and health care experiential types provides a beginning for examining the conceptual properties in a systematic way. By way of examples, attempts are made to show how to ask important questions in definitional clarification of concept, specifying descriptive features of concept, and in considering relationships of concept to other related phenomena. Restlessness and compliance were discussed to demonstrate the use of these strategies in conceptual analysis.

The main thrust in conceptualization for the domain of client is in developing, ultimately, a nursing theory of humanity or a nursing theory of health that can be the basis for understanding a diverse array of problems presented by the client whom we encounter in nursing, for whom we need to provide services. In addition, the need for development of middle-range theories aimed at understanding boundary-specific phenomena in clients has been implicitly stressed in the discussions of restlessness and compliance. Middle-range theories in nursing that deal with broad, particularistic phenomena in the domain of client will help us accumulate the many layers of theoretical knowledge necessary for the development of grand nursing theories.

NOTES

1. For sociological orientation, see: Skinner, B. F. (1953). *Science and human behavior*. New York: Macmillan; Hull, C. L. (1951). *Essentials of behavior*. New Haven: Yale University Press; Bandura, A. (1969). *Principles of behavior modification*. New York: Holt, Rinehart, and Winston for psychological orientation; and Homans, G. C. (1961). *Social behavior: Its elementary forms*. New York: Harcourt and Brace; and Kunkel, J., & Nagasawa, R. H. (1973). A behavioral model of man: Propositions and implications. *American Sociological Review, 38*, 530–543.
2. See: Cannon, W. B. (1932). *The wisdom of the body*. New York: W.W. Norton and Company; and Selye, H. O. (1956). *The stress of life*. New York: McGraw-Hill.
3. For the similarities and differences between/among the psychoanalytic human models, see the following: Brown, N. O. (1959). *Life against death: The psychoanalytical meaning of history*. Middletown, CT: Wesleyan University Press; Dobzhansky, T. (1967). *The biology of ultimate concern*. New York: The New American Library; Erikson, E. H. (1959). *Identity and the life cycle: Selected papers*. New York: International Universities Press; Erikson, E. H. (1964). *Insight and responsibility: Lectures on the ethical implications of psychoanalytic insight*. New York: W.W. Norton; Fromm, E. (1964). *The heart of man: Its*

genesis for good an evil. New York: Harper and Row; Fromm, E., & Xiran, R. (Eds.). (1968). *The nature of man: A reader.* New York: Macmillan; Hartman, H. (1958). *Ego psychology and the problems of adaptation.* (D. Rapoport, Trans.). New York: International Universities Press; Rieff, P. (1966). *The triumph of the therapeutics: The uses of faith after Freud.* New York: Harper and Row; and Browning, D. S. (1973). *Generative man: Psychoanalytic perspectives.* Philadelphia: The Westminster Press.

4. Simon, H. (1979). *Models of thoughts* (p. 4). New Haven, CT: Yale University Press.

5. Twaddle, A. C. (1974). The concept of health status. *Social Science and Medicine, 8,* 83.

6. Orem, D. E. (1980). *Nursing concepts of practice* (2nd ed., p. 119). New York: McGraw-Hill.

7. *Index Medicus* classifies restlessness as psychomotor agitation, and both terms seem to refer to the same kind of phenomena.

8. Norris, C. M. (1975). Restlessness: A nursing phenomena in search of meaning. *Nursing Outlook, 23,* 104.

Theoretical Analysis of Phenomena in the Client–Nurse Domain

Firstly, there is the unity in things whereby each thing is at one with itself, consists of itself, and coheres with itself. Secondly, there is the unity whereby one creature is united with the others and all parts of the world constitute one world.

—*Della Mirandola*

OVERVIEW

This chapter presents conceptualization of the client–nurse domain and theoretical ideas about phenomena in that domain. As presented in chapter 4, the client–nurse domain is defined as the area of study in nursing related to phenomena arising out of encounters between client and nurse. The client–nurse domain encompasses client–nurse dyad phenomena that exist or are possible when a client is with a nurse or nurses in a health care situation. In specifying this as constituting a specific domain of interest for nursing's theoretical development, I have proposed that "contacts between the client and nurse are occasions in which transfer and/or interchange of information, energy, and affection/humanity occur" (Kim, 1987).

The following section is devoted to discussion of conceptual issues in studying phenomena in the client–nurse domain. Delineation of the phenomenal world for the client–nurse domain is specified with respect to three different ontological foci for the study of human-to-human relations. The rationale and significance for classifying client–nurse relations into three types of phenomena, that is, *contact, communication,* and *interaction,* are discussed as well. This is followed by an examination of selected nursing models in dealing with client–nurse phenomena with respect to their foci of attention and perspectives. The last of these three sections offers conceptual analyses of the phenomena of negotiation and client–nurse alliance as examples of client–nurse domain phenomena.

THE CLIENT–NURSE DOMAIN

Phenomena in the client–nurse domain occur in direct encounters between the client and the nurse. Phenomena that occur between two individuals (sometimes more than two, especially when the client constitutes a group of people as a unit) who have come together into situations because one party is the client and the other the nurse are nursing phenomena. They are nursing phenomena because they require understanding and explanation from the nursing perspective. Here it is necessary to differentiate nursing phenomena in the client–nurse domain from those that are objects of explanation in other scientific fields. For example, a sociologist might consider the patterns of interaction between the client and the nurse as subject matter, properly so, for explanation within a theory of social exchange. The sociologist's focus is necessarily "sociological," and, insofar as it remains to be conceived as sociological, it is a proper subject matter for a sociological explanation. The sociologist is interested in explaining their interaction with respect to how social norms, attitudes, and values influence interactional patterning; how interactions begin, develop, and terminate in such social situations; or how one party's use of social symbols affects others' reactions to them. These are valid and essential questions that sociology tries to answer in its proper relevance structure. The sociological perspective orients such empirical and theoretical examinations so as to gain knowledge about social life with the ultimate purpose of understanding the continuation or disruption of patterns in societies. For sociology, the focus centers on societies and social institutions.

On the other hand, a nursing scientist may take the pattern of interaction between the nurse and the client as subject matter for explanation within a nursing theory or from a nursing perspective that is based on the philosophy of care. The nursing scientist focuses on understanding the phenomena with respect, for example, to: (a) how the patterns of association between the client and the nurse influence the client's reactions to his or her health, problems, and health care situations; (b) what kinds of relations between the client and the nurse and their behaviors help their relations to focus on the client and goals for the client; or (c) what kinds of communicative patterns foster the client's learning of new health care requirements. Nursing focus is apparent in such questions.

The nursing focus on studying client–nurse phenomena is ultimately in how client–nurse phenomena affect clients and their health. The same world, then, is examined on two different planes, that is, from two entirely different perspectives, allowing postulations of scientific problems that are oriented to two different objectives: sociology, in this case, is interested in furthering an understanding of human interaction as social phenomena, whereas nursing is interested in understanding nurse–client interaction as nursing intervention or as a part of nursing actions. For nursing, it is directed toward a knowledge base that can enable prescriptions of the most effective patterns of nursing behaviors in client–nurse exchanges or that provide understanding about the nature of client–nurse dyads as they impact on the client's health-related experiences.

What then are the valid criteria that can be used to point out as appropriate those aspects of reality in the client–nurse domain for study from the nursing perspective? The valid criteria appear to rest with the kinds of questions that are posed in conceptualization. It is in the posture. The main question is this: *Would (or should) a variation of "this occurrence" (that is, any occurrence of a type) that is taking place between the client and the nurse in any way alter or influence the way the client feels, perceives the world relevant to health, or proceeds to make actions regarding his or her health state?* If the answer is yes, then we have successfully conceptualized a nursing phenomenon in the client–nurse domain. In this way, phenomena in the client–nurse domain share two common characteristics:

- They are phenomena "existentially" occurring in situations where a client and a nurse are present in respective roles.
- They are phenomena of which meanings have implications for the client's health and health-related experiences.

Conceptualization of what is happening in such encounters mainly depends on the scope with which specific phenomena are abstracted. An encounter (such as the following) between a nurse and a patient can be used to illustrate how client–nurse phenomena can be abstracted:

Ms. Dumas, the nurse, enters Mr. Smith's room with the IV (intravenous) medication to be put through the IV line, and notices the uneaten dinner, signs of a quiet, depressed mood, and coughing. Mr. Smith's roommate in the bed near the window with curtains drawn around the bed seems to be in a great deal of pain, having had abdominal surgery on the preceding day. He moans and groans aloud at times. Ms. Dumas administers the medication through the IV line and talks to Mr. Smith about his discomfort and coughing.

Each discrete act that occurs between Ms. Dumas and Mr. Smith can be conceived in a different phenomenal term in a particularistic mode of analysis. Thus, exchange of mood, energy transfer, attentiveness, etc., may be considered as particularistic concepts referring to some of the phenomena apparent in this situation. On the other hand, the occurrences in the situation may be conceptualized in a holistic manner, as transaction, as nurse–patient interaction, or as therapeutic relationship. Such differences in conceptualization of the phenomena apparently present in a nursing situation allow several levels of theoretical questioning, yet the locus of occurrence here remains within the context of the client–nurse dyad.

One way of particularizing phenomena in the client–nurse domain is by focusing on specific ontological aspects of humans: *contact phenomena,* with the focus on humans as embodied, "materialized" entities; *communication phenomena,* with the focus on humans as symbol users both of language and of other, nonlinguistic forms; and *interaction phenomena,* with the focus on humans as social agents. Because dyadic relations occur in a holistic manner, engaging all aspects of participants, this differentiation is only an analytical tool to delineate focused features of relations. This means that in all dyadic relations, including those of clients and nurses, we are engaged with each other more or less all at once as embodied selves, using language, gestures, or feeling tones, and being social agents of roles. Some aspects of such dyadic engagements may be conceptualized as *contact, communication,* or *interaction* only for analytic purposes and to develop theoretical understanding.

Contact Phenomena

Contact phenomena as a type in the client–nurse dyad refer to those phenomena involving the participants' embodiment, physicalness, and space-occupying character. The ontological focus in considering dyadic relations as *contact* is in viewing humans as entitative living beings. When we are together with one another, we are close or distant, we touch with hands or with other parts of our bodies, we are present with our beings (that is, with our essences, with energy, prahna, spirit, etc.) and we assume positions relative to each other. In so doing, we exchange energy, make contact with each other, are cognizant of each other's presence, and feel each other's humanness.

A nurse who enters into a patient's room may stand by the foot of the bed to give certain instructions to the patient, turn the patient over to give an injection, massage the patient's feet, or carry out centering and the laying of hands to relieve the patient's pain. In such instances, it is possible to delineate certain phenomena as *contact* between the nurse and the client, as embodied human beings consisting of certain entities that come in contact with each other. It is possible to conceptualize such phenomena as distancing, instrumental touch, energy transfer, and therapeutic touch. This way of conceptualizing certain aspects of the client–nurse dyad is important for nursing, because nursing, unlike much other human services work, entails a great deal of "body work" that involves both patients' and nurses' bodies.

Communication Phenomena

Communication phenomena have received a great deal of attention in nursing, as communication has been considered a critical aspect of nursing practice. Many aspects of nursing practice involve communicating with patients and their families, for example, in gaining information from clients, in providing information to clients, and in exchanging information and sentiments between clients and nurses. Communication phenomena involve the use of language and other symbols.

The ontological focus in considering dyadic relations as *communication* is in viewing humans as acculturated, linguistic, symbol users. Humans as symbol users are grounded in cultures and in socialization, through which shared meanings get established as the basis for understanding and exchanges. Studying communication phenomena is important in nursing, as a large portion of client–nurse relations involve exchange of information and use of symbols. Such concepts as "tailoring," negotiation, therapeutic communication, communicative conflict, and client–nurse communication styles have been identified and studied in the nursing literature for their influence on clients' health, compliance, satisfaction, and learning.

Interaction Phenomena

Interaction phenomena in the client–nurse dyad refer to phenomena that are analyzable by considering clients and nurses as social agents assuming the respective roles in the situation of nursing care. The ontological focus for conceptualizing certain aspects of client–nurse relations as *interaction*

Table 6.1

EXAMPLES OF CONCEPTS IN THE CLIENT–NURSE DOMAIN FOR STUDY IN THE NURSING PERSPECTIVE

CONCEPTS	LEVEL OF CONCEPT DESCRIPTION	
	HOLISTIC	PARTICULARISTIC
Contact concepts	Comforting touch Distancing Interpersonal energy transfer Interpersonal presence Therapeutic touch	Eye contact Instrumental touch Massaging
Communication concepts	Communication styles Communicative conflict Therapeutic communication	Client–nurse negotiation Tailoring
Interaction concepts	Empathetic relationship Mutuality Therapeutic alliance Transaction	Client–nurse collaboration Gift giving Role conflict

is in viewing humans as social agents who are engaged in forms of social life, which vary according to the social situations in which interpersonal engagements occur. Clients and nurses, in assuming their respective roles within health care situations, establish social relations that are unique to such situations.

The interaction phenomena of interest to nursing are "social" in nature and probably qualify (justifiably) as an appropriate subject matter for sociological attention. However, it is important for nursing to delineate and study interaction phenomena in the client–nurse domain with specific attention to their implications for clients, not necessarily from the social patterning perspective often adopted in sociology. Insofar as interactive features of the client–nurse dyad have implications for client outcomes, it is important to develop theoretical knowledge about them from the nursing perspective.

Table 6.1 lists examples of concepts that are appropriate for scientific attention in this client–nurse domain.

CLIENT–NURSE PHENOMENA IN THREE MEANING-ORIENTATIONS

As presented above, client–nurse phenomena exist when two human beings, a client and a nurse, with all of the realities of being humans, are together in the context of nursing care. Such togetherness has three distinct meanings in the nursing context:

1. It is itself a form of nursing therapeutics, by which a specific client outcome is expected, such as relief of pain, alleviation of anxiety, feeling of comfort, or learning of a new self-care technique. This orientation of client–nurse encounters is based on the aspect of nursing that falls under the auspices of the philosophy of therapy.
2. It is a medium through which nurses deliver various nursing actions, therapeutics, and strategies to clients, such as giving of medication, caring for a wound, or providing self-care material. This orientation specifies client–nurse phenomena that are the means by which necessary nursing actions are accomplished.
3. It is a process that occurs within the philosophy of care in which a client and a nurse are connected via the nurse's human service orientation and care focus. Client–nurse phenomena, having the meaning of the philosophy of care, exist to fulfill the nursing mandate of caring.

Though it is possible that an encounter between a client and a nurse have all three of these meanings, a certain aspect of the encounter may be considered to have specific meaning orientation as a nursing therapeutic, a medium, or a philosophy of care. Considering client–nurse phenomena with respect to their meaning orientations is important because of their connections to client outcomes or client-related goals. For instance, client–nurse phenomena with the meaning orientation of nursing therapeutics have direct implications for client outcomes, whereas client–nurse phenomena with the meaning orientation as medium are only contextually and indirectly related to client outcomes. On the other hand, client–nurse phenomena with a meaning orientation in the philosophy of care have implications for client outcomes only in relation to the general care process. Hence, it is essential to differentiate client–nurse phenomena according to their meaning orientations in developing theoretical formulations.

Client–Nurse Phenomena as Nursing Therapeutics

All three types of client–nurse phenomena, that is, *contact, communication,* and *interaction,* may be therapeutic in the sense that nurses' relational behaviors have as their objectives a goal (or goals) of intervention for clients' health-oriented problems. Nurses are in the business of "improving" clients' health, that is, the bulk of what nurses do has to have a therapeutic orientation in the spirit of the philosophy of therapy. Most commonly, nursing therapeutics are physiological, behavioral, or psychological interventions aimed at solving patients' problems. For example, a nursing therapeutic for a patient in dehydration would be an administration of fluid and electrolytes on a hydration schedule based on a physiological theory, whereas a nursing therapeutic for a patient who is noncompliant with diabetic self-care may be the use of patient contracting based on a behavioral theory. However, some of clients' problems require nursing interventions that are based on theories of relations. Hence, nursing therapeutics using specific forms of client–nurse encounters aim to solve clients' problems through relational processes.

Nurses can use relational processes such as touch, communication, or interaction to address specific patient problems. Therapeutic touch has been developed as a modality of nursing intervention used to relieve patient's pain or anxiety. A specific form of communication has also been developed as "therapeutic communication" to deal with patients having difficulties with self-concept, social relations, or the process of adjustment to physical limitations. Role modeling as a form of client–nurse interaction has also been used to teach patients about new style of behaviors. Such processes, for example, therapeutic touch, therapeutic communication, and role modeling, are nursing therapeutics, which use client–nurse relations as the basic forms of interventions. For this meaning orientation, then, specific forms of client–nurse relational process target certain nursing problems of patients and are applied to solve those problems. Hence, this meaning orientation is aligned with the philosophy of therapy in nursing, and points to the need for knowledge development for nursing therapeutics via human-to-human relational theories.

Client–Nurse Phenomena as a Medium for Nursing Actions

Nursing actions, that is, what nurses do in nursing practice, include activities that are carried out either in the presence of patients or away from patients. Although there are many actions which are carried out away from patients, the majority of patient care in which nurses are involved is carried out in actual encounters with patients. In such instances, the encounters themselves do not have specific therapeutic meanings. They are the media through which certain nursing actions are actualized. For instance, when a nurse carries out a complete nursing assessment in a patient, she/he asks the patient certain questions so as to get information about the patient's history, complaints, and habits, listens to the patient's lung sounds or measures the vital signs, and inspects the patient's wound(s) or physical appearance. In this case, the essential aspect of nursing action is a complete nursing assessment. However, this action of assessing the patient involves client–nurse phenomena such as information exchange and physical touch.

Hence, from this context, client–nurse encounters have a meaning orientation as a medium through which nursing actions are instituted and delivered. As a medium, what occurs in the client–nurse encounter has consequences for the way nursing action is accomplished. Communication patterns used in client–nurse encounters may influence the character of information obtained by the nurse in assessment. Or, the way a client and a nurse interacted while the nurse was carrying out colostomy care may influence the way a patient establishes a perception about the nature of colostomy self-care. A subtle difference in a nurse's physical touch of the patient during dressing change, in giving an injection, while doing an endotracheal suctioning, or in adjusting IV chemotherapy infusion can influence the effects of such activity directly or indirectly, immediately or in a delayed fashion.

Client–nurse phenomena from this meaning orientation, then, arise out of client–nurse encounters in which there are primary nursing actions to be performed by nurses and where the encounters function as media for the delivery of such primary nursing actions. The characteristics, processes, and features of client–nurse encounters from this meaning orientation are seen to have impact on the processes and outcomes of primary nursing actions. This view is important for consideration because the effectiveness of nursing actions can be greatly influenced not just by the nature of nursing actions but also by the nature of the medium through which nursing actions are accomplished.

Client–Nurse Phenomena in the Philosophy-of-Care Orientation

Nursing, by its social mandate and professional orientation, has two philosophical orientations, as discussed earlier: the philosophy of therapy and the philosophy of care. As a human practice discipline, nursing work is oriented to helping people in need of service not only by solving their specific health-related, health-experiential problems, but also by providing care to their being as individuals as they go through a process of health care. Hence, the philosophy of care is bifocally central to nursing in conjunction with the philosophy of therapy. The philosophy-of-care focus is actualized in nursing through various forms, such as in nurses' interactions with clients, in upholding the ethical values of human dignity and autonomy in every nursing action, and in defending patients' rights. It is through the nurses' interactions with clients that the philosophy of care is played out in nursing most importantly.

Hence, all client–nurse encounters are thus over-archingly governed by how the philosophy of care is integrated by the nurse. There is embeddedness of the philosophy of care in client–nurse encounters, regardless of whether the encounter is therapy oriented or medium oriented. However, such embeddedness can be analytically separated from the previously discussed two orientations, because the philosophy-of-care orientation points to specific meaning features of client–nurse encounters. Such phenomena as mutuality, empathetic relation, tailoring, therapeutic alliance, collaborativeness, and presence in client–nurse encounters have meanings in relation to the philosophy of care and can be analyzed and understood in this context. Such phenomena in client–nurse encounters shape the governing character of relationship in nursing.

The philosophy-of-care orientation directs us to examine client–nurse encounters relative to the degree with which encounters are client oriented, empathy based, and humane. Hence, the orientation points to the need to develop theories of approaches in client–nurse encounters. Theories of approaches are relevant for understanding nurses' approaches, which differentiate the incorporation of the philosophy of care in client–nurse encounters, and in developing different ways nurses can approach clients in their interactions with them.

Table 6.2 provides examples of phenomena in the client–nurse domain viewed from a matrix formed by three concept-types and three meaning orientations.

NURSING MODELS FOR THE CLIENT–NURSE DOMAIN

Although all nursing theories and conceptual models address client–nurse domain phenomena as relevant aspects to be considered in understanding nursing, there are few models that focus on client–nurse phenomena as the central concepts in their theoretical expositions. Most often, nursing theorists consider and include the presence of the nurse in the delivery of nursing service, often without a specific conceptualization of client–nurse relations as a part of nursing actions. As the conceptual models by Roy and Neuman are specifically oriented to the study of clients and client-domain phenomena, their models do not include specific concepts in the client–nurse domain. For example, to Neuman (1995), the purpose of

Table 6.2

EXAMPLES OF CLIENT–NURSE DOMAIN PHENOMENA ACCORDING TO THE CLASSIFICATION BY TYPES AND MEANING ORIENTATIONS

TYPES OF PHENOMENA	TYPES OF MEANING ORIENTATION		
	THERAPY ORIENTATION	MEDIUM ORIENTATION	PHILOSOPHY-OF-CARE ORIENTATION
Contact phenomena	Massaging Therapeutic touch	Instrumental physical touch	Cradling Distancing
Communication phenomena	Teaching Therapeutic communication	Client–nurse talk Information exchange	Empathetic communication Tailoring
Interaction phenomena	Role modeling	Role conflict	Client–nurse alliance Mutuality Presence

nursing intervention is to reduce stress factors and adverse conditions that either affect or could affect optimal functioning of a client in a given situation. Similarly, Roy's adaptation model also considers nursing intervention as the management of stimuli, and the nurse's role as the deliverer of interventions (Roy & Andrews, 1991). The inherent interactive features involved in carrying out nursing interventions are treated as givens in these models.

Orem, within her self-care model, which is oriented to the study of clients from the perspective of functioning, delineates the nursing system as a separate concept with the understanding that this is a system of actions and interactions designed by nurses for the benefit of clients in nursing practice situations (Orem, 1991). Orem's nursing system thus refers to both the actions of nurses performed to help clients meet their self-care requisites and nurses' interactions with clients in this helping process. Nurses' use of "social and interactive technologies" is seen as essential in producing the outcomes of the "professional-regulatory technologies" applied to clients so as to meet their self-care requisites (Orem, 1991). Thus, Orem's, as well as Roy and Neuman's views of client–nurse interaction derive from the meaning orientation as medium. King (1981, 1990), in her theory of goal attainment, proposes the concept of interpersonal system as the basic system for attaining a state of health for clients, permitting them to function in their roles. Hence she views interpersonal processes between the client and nurse as the media through which nursing goals can be attained.

Among other nursing scholars, Hall (1966) conceptualizes nursing action as care and nurturing, not in an interactive sense but in an "active" sense on the part of the nurse. Orlando's conceptualization of nursing action is an interactional one in which the nurse's action is based on the client's reactions in situations of nursing care. The nursing action is thus viewed as a dynamic relationship (Orlando, 1961). Riehl's interaction model, based on symbolic interactionist orientation, conceptualizes nursing action as that of the nurse taking the role of the other in her relationships with the client (1980). Watson (1979) proposes that nursing action be based on "carative" factors and views the practice of caring as central to nursing. These conceptualizations adhere to the notion that nursing action is not simply doing things for the client or performing actions for the client, but involves the nurse as an interactive agent in a rather total way. On the other hand, theorists like Rogers, Parse, and Newman discuss the inclusive nature of the client–nurse relations in considering client as they view client's experiences or states to have intimate interactions with the environment of which the nurse is an important part. Thus, these authors view client–nurse phenomena from the philosophy-of-care orientation, in which client–nurse relations are viewed to be human-to-human encounters with the involvement of the totality of one's humanity.

Peplau (1962) has a specific interactive orientation in her conceptualization of therapeutic interrelationships in nursing. Wiedenbach (1964) also views nursing action as that directed to the client, for whom actions as a helping process fulfill necessary requirements, which will help restore the client's ability to cope with the demands of a healthy life. Hence, these two authors view client–nurse interaction from the nursing therapeutics orientation. In the following section, mainly, the theoretical ideas of three nursing theorists, Rogers, Peplau, and King, are discussed in detail in relation to client–nurse phenomena.

Rogers's Concept of Unitary Humans

Rogers's conceptualization of nursing action is covertly done within the model of "unitary man." Rogers states that nursing practice is directed toward promoting symphonic interaction between a person and the environment, strengthening the coherence and integrity of the human field, and directing and redirecting patterning of the human and environmental fields for realization of maximum health potential (Rogers, 1970). For Rogers, nursing action is composed of behaviors, operations, and procedures, ranging from the use of instruments to human relationships. They are used with intellectual care in "rhythmic correlates of practice" to help people to achieve positive health or maximum health potential. The basic premises for nursing actions are: (a) the wholeness of a person and his or her integrality with his or her environment; (b) the dynamic, evolutionary, innovative wholeness of individual life pattern; and (c) the energy field for any individual as "an irreducible, pandimensional energy field identified by pattern and integral with the human field" (Rogers, 1992, p. 29).

Health and illness are considered on a continuum, expressed according to the degree with which multiple events as a patterned influence affect the person's life processes at a given space–time. Because each human being is unique and whole, and since a person is conceived to have the capacity to reason and feel, and thus participates knowingly and probabilistically in the process of change, both the client and the nurse are integral participants in the nursing intervention process. The nurse, therefore, is an environmental component for the client, repatterning the energy field of the client's environment simply by being present. According to Rogers's model, nursing action is therefore concerned with the following aspects:

1. *Changing the client's values for probabilistic goal setting that is responsive to the changing nature of the human and environmental fields.* This involves the nurse realizing the client's individual potential and uniqueness for a future maturation relative to health.
2. *Strengthening the person–environment resonancy by rearranging the rhythmic flow of energy waves between a person and his or her environment and by maintaining rhythmic consistency.* This involves the nurse ordering or reordering the nature, amount, and speed of wave dispersion in the human and environmental fields for enhancement of the client's development relative to health.
3. *Attaining the person–environment complementarity in an effort to acquire the best possible patterns of living coordinates for the client in coexistence with environmental changes.* This requires the nurse to help the client come to terms with and realize individual differences and potentialities for directing change that are most beneficial to his or her evolution and the most effective fulfillment of life's capabilities.

These three categories of nursing action in Rogers's model suggest that nursing action is not a discrete activity but a process of holistic, interactive intervention. Thus, the variability of nursing action can be expressed in qualitative terms rather than in nominative terms. Nursing action is conceptualized from the interactive perspective to the extent that the nurse's presence in the environment changes the characteristics of the environmental energy field and has the potential for strong influences on repatterning. The phenomena of mutual, complementary influence between the client and nurse are not distinctively conceptualized as a special case, for Rogers believes not in the human-to-human interaction as an essential phenomenon, but in the human-to-environment interaction, in which other individuals are quality-changing aspects of the environment, as is the nurse.

Because nursing action is not directed at "solving" a health problem, the conceptualization of nursing action is not prescriptive. For that matter, the goal of nursing action is never deterministic. It deals with "correlates" and mutual simultaneity. Hence, the outcomes of nursing action in the client are directed toward the more complex repatterning and organization of the energy field that are expected to occur in a probabilistic and correlative fashion, not in a cause–effect way.

However, there has been a great deal of both theoretical and empirical work on therapeutic touch having the theoretical orientation in Rogers's science of unitary human beings (Biley, 1996; Krieger, 1990; Malinski, 2009; Meehan, 1990; Quinn, 1984, 1989). The theoretical specification for therapeutic touch from Rogers's framework applies the concept of energy fields, field patterning, resonance, and mutuality, and in most cases considers clients and nurses as human energy fields in relation with each other. In many of these works, Rogers's concept of environmental energy field as a holistic, indivisible entity and its relations to human dyadic relationships are not configured into the theoretical specifications. Therapeutic touch as a concept with the meaning orientation of nursing therapeutics has received a great deal of criticism in the literature in its lack of theoretical rigor. This is apparent as many authors who claim to have developed therapeutic touch from Rogers's science of human beings have either interpreted the framework differently or partially applied the framework, creating theoretical confusion.

Peplau's Concept of Interpersonal Relations

Peplau (1952) defines nursing as a therapeutic, interpersonal process that helps the client solve problems and likewise moves the client toward the direction of creative, constructive, productive, personal, and community living. To Peplau, nursing refers to relationships between the client and the nurse in which interactive processes become a maturing force and an educative instrument for both parties. Thus, although the principal aim of nursing is to guide the client toward new learning and a positive change for self-repair and self-renewal, the nurse also experiences growth and maturity through interpersonal involvement. Peplau conceptualizes the interpersonal process in four phases through which the client and the nurse attain therapeutic outcomes. Orientation, identification, exploitation, and resolution are the stages of interpersonal relations, of which nature, length, and effectiveness are determined not only by the nurse's ability to perform the roles of teacher, resource person, counselor, leader, technical expert, or surrogate, but also by the client's abilities and motivations for movement in the relationship. According to Peplau, the major variable characteristics that influence the outcome of the interpersonal process are (a) the sequentiality of the interpersonal relation and (b) the nature of efforts of both actors in their collaborativeness or independence.

Independent variables that prescribe the need for the interpersonal process are psychobiological conditions such as needs, frustration, conflict, or anxiety that are detrimental to an individual's maturing process. Outcomes of nursing action as interpersonal process are oriented to the total person rather than to specific aspects of the individual. The most significant departure in Peplau's ideas of nursing action from those developed by others is in the recognition that experiential growth from the interaction takes place not only in the client but also in the nurse. A resulting postulation is that a nurse will become increasingly proficient and effective in interpersonal relations with clients as the nurse's experiences in nursing action increase. However, this conceptualization does not consider the applicability of interpersonal process as a holistic modality of nursing action, for a variety of problems a client may present, thus it is limited in that way.

King's Model of the Interpersonal System (Theory of Goal Attainment)

King's idea of nursing is based on the conceptualization of the nursing system as comprising dynamic interacting systems. Within the dynamic interacting personal, interpersonal, and social systems, nursing occurs as actions, reactions, and interactions through which information is shared, relationships are created between the nurse and the client, and goals and the means for attaining the goals for the client's health are mutually established (King, 1981, 1990).

According to King, interactional aspects of nursing action accordingly encompass actions of perceiving, thinking, relating, judging, and acting against the behavior of individuals who come to a nursing situation. The client–nurse interaction, the dyad interaction, is one type of interpersonal system in which several processes of the system are used to attain a goal. The processes can be summarized as follows (King, 1981, 1990):

- *Perception*—process used to attain information about each other and the situation
- *Communication*—process for exchange and interpretation of information that each imparts in the interaction
- *Transaction*—process of sharing values, needs, and wants through interaction
- *Role*—process by which the nature of the relationship and modes of communication to be used in the relationship are identified
- *Stressor*—process of becoming energy responses to the other.

These are expressible in variable terms to indicate the quality of nursing. Dependent variables of nurse–client interaction are goal attainment for the client, satisfaction, and enhancement of growth and development. Relationships among the different processes of interaction are hierarchical in that the perceptual process precedes communication, and both perception and communication affect the transaction. At the same time, the processes of role and stressor influence all other aspects of interaction. King's model considers interaction as a descriptive yet normative process, oriented to the client in a holistic way. Interaction is the fundamental mode of nursing action, from which all other subsequent actions and transactions evolve for the attainment of goals.

As shown in these summaries, conceptualizations of client–nurse relation vary in these models in relation to the level of goal specificity (i.e., discrete/global) and with respect to prescriptive versus experiential orientation. These also vary in their meaning orientation: Rogers's unitary human model with the philosophy-of-care orientation, Peplau's model with the nursing therapeutic orientation, and King's theory of goal attainment with the medium orientation. Theoretical explanations of the phenomena of client–nurse relation may take on various analytical forms as well. Client–nurse relation may be a medium through which a discrete activity is performed to correct some deviation in the client. In contrast, it may be the immersion of two individuals, a client and a nurse, in a total experience of interaction. Even at such extremes, the goal is always directed toward the client, notwithstanding any unexpected as well as expected changes in the nurse.

Other Theoretical Developments in Nursing

During the past 2 decades there have been many theoretical proposals at the middle-range level for client–nurse interaction phenomena that are not derived directly from nursing models. Patterson and Zderad (1976, 1988) proposed their theory of humanistic nursing based on existentialism and phenomenology, in which client–nurse interaction conceptualized as intersubjective transaction is viewed as an existential occasion for enhancing clients' well-being through authentic encountering.

In conceptualizing client–nurse interaction generally, Haggerty and Patusky (2003) proposed a theory of human relatedness that encompass four states of relatedness—enmeshment, connectedness, disconnectedness, and parallelism—to explain client–nurse relationships, and Morse, Havens and Wilson (1997) proposed a model of nurse–patient relationship as "the comforting interaction," in which client–nurse relationship is viewed to encompass three interactive processes that involve dynamic interchanges between a nurse with his/her comforting strategies, style of care, and patterns of relating and a client who brings in signals of distress, indices of discomfort, and patterns of relating.

On the other hand, several theoretical ideas have been proposed that apply social interaction theories and frameworks such as Habermas' theory of communicative action (Sumner, 2001), Goffman's social interaction theory (Shattell, 2004), social exchange theory (Byrd, 2006), and the perspective of interpretivism, especially that of Taylor and McIntyre (Scheel, Pedersen, & Rosenkrands, 2008).

As middle-range theories that focus on specific phenomena within the client–nurse domain, Kim's theoretical framework for collaborative decision making (1983) focuses on collaboration between clients and nurses in decision making in nursing practice, Schubert and Lionberger (1995) focus on mutual connectedness as the process through which clients move toward self-healing, and a theory developed through a grounded theory approach by Sahlsten, Larsson, Sjöström, Lindencrona, and Pllos (2007) focuses on mutuality as a key concept in patient participation in nursing care.

Another important area of discussion that has come forward in the literature deals with ethical and moral issues pertaining to the client–nurse relationship, such as discussed by Nortvedt (2001) on closeness and relational responsibilities, the exposition by Peter and Liaschenko (2004) on the paradox of proximity in nurse–patient relationships creating moral distress and ambiguity, and on boundaries in client–nurse relationships by Milton (2008). Naef (2006) also raises a moral question that accompanies nurses "bearing witness" through their interactions with patients.

In the nursing literature, however, there is limited theoretical work that focuses on communication phenomena, whereas in the general area of health communication there has been a rich array of theoretical works that are used to examine communication between health care providers and clients. Babrow and Mattson (2003) review various theoretical issues in the field of health communication, and suggest seven theoretical frameworks specified for communication theory by Craig (1999) as application to address theoretical tensions that are necessary for consideration in the health communication field. These seven theoretical communication frameworks are: (a) the rhetorical tradition that focuses on a practical art of persuasive discourse; (b) the semiotic tradition theorizing communication "as intersubjective mediation by signs and sign systems"; (c) the phenomenological tradition that views communication as dialogue or experience of otherness; (d) the cybernetic tradition of information-processing orientation; (e) the sociopsychological tradition that brings personalities, emotions, sense of self, roles, and beliefs into communication; (f) the sociocultural tradition that views communication as "a symbolic process that produces and reproduces shared sociocultural patterns"; and (g) the critical tradition that questions the possibility of authentic communication in light of material and ideological practices that distort discursive reflections in communication (Babrow & Mattson, 2003, pp. 48–52). There is a great deal of possibility in rethinking these theoretical frameworks for communication to address critical questions in client–nurse communication, such as power and control, misinformation and misunderstanding, effects of communication styles, use and misuse of specialized language, and communicating with patients who have limited capacity.

SELECTED CONCEPTUAL ANALYSES

As in chapter 5, two concepts are examined here as examples of phenomena in the client–nurse domain. The concepts of negotiation and client–nurse alliance are presented. As stated in the earlier chapters, the main purpose of this section is to show how a first-level analytical approach is used to gain conceptual and empirical understanding of phenomena within the client–nurse domain. Each concept is analyzed with respect to (a) definitional clarification and conceptual meanings as reflected in the literature, (b) descriptive features and characteristics as a step toward an empirical analysis, and (c) the concept's relationships with other concepts that are important in nursing. The strategy and rationale for the conceptual analysis were discussed in detail in chapter 2, and that rationale is adopted in this section for the analyses of negotiation and client–nurse alliance.

NEGOTIATION IN NURSING

Negotiation between a nurse and a client as a phenomenon of client–nurse relation has been most frequently discussed with respect to patient compliance. Yet negotiations are found in various nursing situations resulting in client outcomes in informal, incidental ways as well as in a formal, planned fashion. An informal, incidental negotiation may be found in a nurse–client exchange. For example, a nurse prods and cajoles a client, who is in surgical pain, to ambulate while the client implores and pleads against it, and yet after awhile they find a solution together that is agreeable to both, a negotiation. A formal negotiation in nursing may be found in contingency contracting, in which a nurse and a client come to terms regarding the desired or targeted new behavior in the client and the reward in exchange for performance of that behavior, as described by Swain and Steckel (1981).

Negotiation in nursing analyzed in this section only refers to negotiation between nurse and client, rather than client and family, nurse and nurse, or nurse and physician. Although such negotiations occur in nursing, these are not central to the nursing action perspective of the client–nurse domain.

Definitions

According to *Webster's Dictionary,* negotiation is a conferring, discussing, or bargaining to reach an agreement in a generic sense, and it requires two parties, individuals, or groups for the phenomenon to occur. Strauss (1978) accepts the concept of negotiation as one of the possible means of "getting things accomplished" when two or more parties need to deal with each other to get those things done. Negotiation occurs as individuals involved in an interaction attempt to attain certain consequences or outcomes that are realizable only through dealings with another party or parties.

Negotiation may be oriented to many different kinds of consequences, some tangible such as labor contracts, and others intangible such as general understanding of each other's position or rules of behavior. Since negotiations take on different characteristics according to specific structural conditions of interaction—that is, parties (persons), context (time and situation), and subject—negotiations in nursing are special cases of a general type in this respect.

Several characteristics differentiate negotiations in nursing from a general type. First, negotiations in nursing are between two parties having specific social roles, those of nurse and client, and occur in interactions characterized by these role relationships. Second, negotiations in nursing occur in health care situations, in which most clients are more or less "captive," in the sense that they are restricted from walking away freely from the situation. Third, negotiations in nursing are oriented to consequences that are aimed at the client's benefits. Therefore, motivation for negotiation on the part of the nurse is assumed to be inherently "selfless" and other-oriented (i.e., client-oriented).

Negotiation in nursing is a rather new concept. However, since the 1990s there has been an increase in the concept in the context of health care and nursing with concepts such as "negotiated care" and "collaborative practice." Traditionally, clients and professionals are considered to have a one-sided relationship in which the distribution of power and knowledge between the two parties is unequal. Freidson's (1970a) classical analysis of professional dominance in medicine indicates the use of power and expertise in influencing the patient's vulnerability, and the Foucaultian critique of medicine specifies the systemic and structured influence of medical power in both defining health and illness and in determining authoritative ways of behaving in health care (Foucault, 1973). In recent years, however, there has been a growth of popular discussions about the role of the client in influencing the nature of the health care that one receives. With the emerging realization among health care professionals that clients possess resources that can be used to recover and maintain health, and that the client's passivity in health care probably is not conducive to optimal health care outcomes, collaborative models of professional practice have been proposed in various forms. Kleinman's seminal work (1988) expounded on the merit of negotiation in physician–patient relationships as the primary process for empowering patients and families. The current development in mental health care that emphasizes user involvement in care embraces negotiation as its pivotal process.

In nursing, involvement of clients in their care has been a longstanding value and has been emphasized more strongly in recent years, along with the concepts of primary nursing and self-care. The processes by which negotiations occur in nursing and the nature of negotiations in nursing are beginning to be conceptualized formally, and there are efforts and programs that formally incorporate negotiation into nursing practice protocols (Engebretson & Littleton, 2001; Kirk, 2001; McCann et al., 2008;

Polaschek, 2003; Quan et al., 2006; Thorne, 1993). These recent developments are especially prominent in the field of care for chronically ill patients.

Negotiation is a reciprocal, dynamic exchange between the nurse and the client in an effort to arrive at a mutually acceptable solution through a balanced use of expert knowledge, power, human sensitivity, and understanding. As a process, it is interactional and follows a sequence. The sequence of negotiation starts with an initial approach of two parties (a nurse and a client), in which recognition of the need for reconciliation or bargaining occurs. Exchange encounters, in which an option in solutions is not available or permitted, preempt the possibility of their advancing to negotiations.

From the initial state, the process of negotiation becomes diversified in its form and content according to the following six attributes, as described by Zartman (1976) and Strauss (1978):

1. The parties' previous experiences and encounters
2. Patterns and outcomes of previous negotiations between the parties
3. Distribution of actual and perceived power between the parties
4. The values and costs at stake to both parties
5. Expertise in the use of negotiation techniques
6. Personal attributes used for influencing each other.

The final stage of the process culminates in the nature of negotiation outcomes that may be differentiated according to: (a) outcomes' temporal limits, that is, how long the agreement resulting from a specific negotiation is binding to the parties; (b) manifest and latent (tacit) meanings of the agreement; and (c) applicability and transferability of the agreement to other situations or its generalizability.

Buetow (1998) presents four different processes of reaching negotiated agreements: *bridging,* occurring by integration of the interests of involved parties (a patient and a nurse, for example), resulting in an agreement that incorporates strategies that bridge these interests; *trading* one party's interest for the other party's interest so as to reach the mutually agreed-upon goals; *logrolling,* which results in a compromise satisfying only one party, or both parties only partly, with an understanding that monitoring will occur for further deliberation; and *damage limitation,* in which an agreement is for the least damage that will still allow the relationship to be sustained. On the other hand, Engebretson and Littleton (2001) identify specific processes for negotiation in nursing framed within nursing process as: *exchange of expert knowledge* in the assessment stage;

sharing nurse's analysis and interpretation to arrive at nursing diagnoses; *joint decision making* in the planning stage; and *collaborative implementation of mutually derived planned actions* in the implementation stage. In these characterizations of negotiation, the key phenomenal element is the joint work through interaction.

In nursing, then, negotiations occur when the nurse and the client realize difference(s) or a possibility of difference(s) in opinions, approaches, or solutions regarding the client's nursing care. Negotiations may involve joint work regarding goals of nursing care, types of nursing care or interventions in nursing, self-care, and role responsibilities. Negotiations in nursing may be oriented to solving conflicts that are only inherent in one specific situation or that have long-range implications, especially when they are related to lifestyle behaviors or long-term goals. One specific difficulty in conceptualizing negotiation in nursing is in the nature of how it occurs, since any interactive event can contain negotiation as its component and often, unlike in business or politics, there is no declaration that a negotiation will begin.

Descriptive Features and Characteristics

Negotiation as it refers to a process is difficult to characterize because it involves an interactive process. A descriptive characterization, at best, indicates the nature of negotiation as a process. On the other hand, negotiation can be conceptualized as a property concept, which is then characterized by such features as the time it takes to arrive at an agreement or the qualitative change that exists in the final agreement from the original wishes of both parties. In most studies of negotiation, the key features used to specify negotiation are: (a) whether or not negotiation is present in a situation; (b) how long a negotiation session lasts; and (c) what results from a negotiation session. Qualitative operationalization by way of such dichotomies as good/bad, effective/ineffective, or promotive/destructive has not often been considered.

Negotiation as a process involves interactional processes with four phases: (a) *the phase of exploration*, in which both parties are involved in finding out one's own as well as the other's goals, intentions and desires, expertise and knowledge, and assumptions; (b) *the phase of understanding*, in which the involved parties establish understandings about agreements and differences; (c) *the phase of debate*, in which discussions regarding differences and possible solutions to remedy the differences are made; and (d) *the phase of agreement*, in which a final agreement is reached that reflects both parties' satisfaction to follow through with the agreement.

At each phase various interactional processes, such as dialogical patterning, use of language, degree of openness, power sharing, continuity, and commitment are involved, engaging both parties in the process of negotiation.

Differentiation From Other Concepts

Negotiation as a concept has been identified very closely with the concepts of participation and collaboration. Although client participation and client–nurse collaboration are key features of negotiation, these three concepts refer to somewhat different sets of phenomena. Client participation is a client-domain phenomenon that focuses on action involvement of the client in nursing and health care (see, for example, Gallant, Beaulieu, & Carnevale, 2002). On the other hand, collaboration, although a client–nurse domain phenomenon, is usually conceptualized with respect to the client's involvement in decision making (see Kim, 1983). Because some of the phenomenal features of the concepts of negotiation and collaboration are the same, there is a need to clarify these concepts in relation to each other from the nursing perspective.

Relationships With Other Concepts

Zartman (1976) summarizes seven different approaches used in the literature to explain outcomes of negotiation:

- Evolutionary explanation
- Contextual explanation
- Structural explanation
- Strategic explanation
- Personality explanation
- Behavioral explanation
- Process explanation

These seven approaches of explanation identify variables that influence or determine outcomes of negotiation. In nursing, the following considerations may be applicable variables for studying negotiations according to these seven approaches.

Effects of Formality of Negotiation

It appears that formalized negotiation in nursing forces both the nurse and the client to enter into the process, whereas parties involved in informal negotiation may escape from the process without coming to agreements when the process becomes uncomfortable or stressful. Effects of delay or interruption may be significant for the provision of nursing care. Since there are no formal sanctions that either force or prescribe negotiated order in the client–nurse interaction, the form of negotiation in nursing should be considered with respect to client-care outcomes.

Influence of the Context of Nursing Care

Contexts in which the nurse and client come together for negotiation vary according to type of health care organization (ambulatory, acute care, long-term care, or home), type of nursing service system (for example, primary nursing or team nursing), power distribution, organizational philosophy, and so on. Physical and ecological contexts may have influence on certain types of negotiations in clinical settings. The major context of nursing care that has been studied extensively in the literature is the context of chronic illness. A practice developed as "negotiated care" has been used with patients on renal dialysis (Polaschek, 2003) and with diabetic patients on peritoneal dialysis (Quan et al., 2006). Negotiations in the care of chronically ill children for professional and parental role responsibilities (Kirk, 2001) and in community mental health care for user involvement (McAndrew & Samociuk, 2003) are also contextually oriented examinations.

Effect of the Structure of the Relationship

Although tied to the contents in many ways, structures of nurse–client relationships refer to the patterns of communication and influence. Such factors as role orientations of the nurse and the client and their evaluations of the relationship will influence the outcomes of negotiations.

Effect of Strategic Elements

Contingency contracting is a form of negotiation used in nursing in which negotiations focus on the values of "goods" to be forgone and the values of "goods" to be rewarded. Negotiations in nursing involve many different outcomes, ranging from a one-time action of turning in bed to stopping cigarette smoking, or to other major lifestyle changes. In negotiations, tradeoffs are often made among valued objects by the participants in an effort to arrive at an agreement. A personal value structure will influence the way tradeoffs are made in negotiations.

Personality Explanation

Successful negotiations may be attained more often when compatible personalities are negotiating in nurse–client relationships. Other personal characteristics such as affective orientation, independence, and locus of control may also influence negotiations in nursing.

Influence of Behavioral Skills Used in Negotiation

Nurses who have a broad behavioral repertoire, effective in interaction and exchange, may be more successful in nurse–client negotiations.

Process Explanation. Negotiation may be studied as an ongoing process in a phenomenological sense. The symbolic interactionists' approach to explaining what occurs in the nurse–client negotiation will force us to examine negotiation as a special case in social interaction.

CLIENT–NURSE ALLIANCE

One hopes the relationship that develops between the client and the nurse is one that is characterized by mutuality, alliance, and partnership. The nature of client–nurse interaction has an important impact on the way nursing care is provided and the achievement of desired client outcomes (Garvin & Kennedy, 1990; Kim, 1983). Such concepts as collaborativeness, coalition, mutuality, therapeutic alliance, and partnership have been discussed in the literature as desirable characteristics that depict client–nurse relations in which sharing of knowledge, power, understanding, purpose, and feelings exists. However, the concept of client–nurse alliance, or those concepts that seem to refer to the same type of phenomena, has been described as both a state of client–provider interaction and a specific process of client–provider interaction that is oriented toward a client goal.

Definition

Therapeutic alliance as a concept has a long history in psychotherapy and psychiatry as a component of the patient–therapist relationship, and has been used interchangeably with "working alliance." Catty traces the concept's origin to Freud—and to Zetzel, who regarded alliance "as a form of positive transference" in the classical analysis school (2004, p. 256). Elvins and Green (2008), furthermore, identify Carl Rogers as having embraced the concept in his work in humanistic psychotherapy. In psychoanalysis and psychiatry these two terms—therapeutic alliance and transference—embrace psychological bonding that occurs during therapeutic relationships. However, there has also been a great deal of controversy in this discipline over the differences between therapeutic alliance and transference, over the question of overlap between these two concepts in psychoanalytic relationships, and over whether or not transference is a desirable component of patient–therapist relationship (Catty, 2004). For example, Meissner (1992, 2006) notes conceptual distinctions between therapeutic alliance and transference, and between alliance and the real relation.

In nursing, however, therapeutic alliance has taken up a somewhat different meaning as applied to general client–nurse relationships, with an emphasis on collaboration and partnership building. Hummelvoll (1996) describes a nurse–client alliance model for helping clients in a psychiatric setting to access and gain insights into their subjective experiences. Somewhat differently, Wills (1996) suggests nurse–client alliance as forming a partnership to move toward mutually agreed goals of care. The phenomena of a client and a health care professional being in concert with each other have been conceptualized in many different ways in the literature. For example, Madden (1990) reviews the use of the term "therapeutic alliance" in relation to patient compliance, and indicates that often this concept refers to the interactive process between the client and the professional that is oriented to producing behaviors in the client that align with the therapeutic goals. Through the application of the hybrid model for concept development proposed by Schwartz-Barcott and Kim (2000), Madden arrived at the definition of the concept of therapeutic alliance as:

> [A] process that emerges within a provider-client interaction in which both the client and the provider are (1) actively working toward the goal of developing client health behaviors chosen for consistency with the client's current health status and life style, (2) focusing on mutual negotiation to determine activities to be carried out toward that goal, and (3) using a supportive and equitable therapeutic relationship to facilitate that goal.[1] (Madden, 1990, p. 85)

Hougaard (1994) distinguishes two conceptual components of therapeutic alliance: (a) personal alliance based in the interpersonal relationship between a client and a health care professional and (b) the task-related alliance that is oriented to the contractual aspects of treatment planning and goal orientation. On the other hand, Zigmond (1987) suggests that mutuality between the client and the professional is achieved through the development of empathy that is possible through a dialectic fusion and merger of framework of experiences and a construction of common language oriented to empowerment, dignity, and self-responsibility.

Jordan (1986) also emphasizes mutual empathy and mutual intersubjectivity as the key aspects of developing mutuality between two individuals. Henson identifies mutuality as "a connection with or understanding of another that facilitates a dynamic process of joint exchange between people" (1997, p. 80). Briant and Freshwater (1998) emphasize equality and boundary maintenance as the key features of mutuality. Mutuality is viewed as a form of relationship between nurses and clients, in which they can be actively involved to work together for the attainment of mutually identified goals. Sullivan (1998) views the phenomenon as coalition, which develops a spirit of cooperation and partnership building. Interpersonal coalition is viewed as a power-sharing partnership characterized by collaborative empowerment, mutual respect, trust, and mutual goals. Ponsi (2000) illustrates the collaborative relationship as the key feature of therapeutic alliance, which needs to be regulated through various interactive processes. Jonsdottir, Litchfield, and Pharris (2003 and 2004) have advanced the concept of client–nurse partnership to have the same meaning as nurse–client alliance, stating that the partnership is the relational core of nursing practice developed through dialogue, mutuality, and patient-centered concerns.

The literature is rich with descriptions of the concepts of mutuality, collaboration, participation, coalition, and therapeutic alliance as referring to the aspects of client and provider relationships that pertain to sharing of feelings and orientation (mutuality), joining efforts to achieve goals (collaboration and participation), establishing a common power base (coalition) which is often posed as an affronting force to an opposing party, and building a mutual understanding of therapeutic goals (therapeutic alliance). However, these concepts, especially the concepts of mutuality, coalition, and therapeutic alliance, are viewed here as subaspects of the concept of client–nurse alliance, which is considered to refer to a broad conceptualization of client–nurse relationship, encompassing the conjoining of two partners in a bond of understanding, knowledge, power, and goals.

The concept of client–nurse alliance is viewed here as a property concept depicting a state of relationship that is oriented to having a conjoint front. According to *Webster's Dictionary, alliance* is a state of being united in interest, in which two parties establish relationships for mutual objectives. Empathy, mutuality, and coalition in client–nurse relations are the basis for *alliance* and encompass not only an understanding of and commitment to the client's needs and goals but also the building of a concerted power base and sharing of knowledge. However, the concept of *alliance* in a health care context must be considered as a state in which the major orientation of the alliance is for the client's benefit. Hence, the alliance results from interactive processes that are oriented to helping clients to attain health care goals.

Descriptive Features and Characteristics

As there is no specific work in the literature that specifies the concept of client–nurse alliance as defined above, the concept's descriptive features and characteristics must be considered by consolidating the conceptualizations of mutuality, coalition, and therapeutic alliance. The key empirical aspects of client–nurse alliance then include the following:

- A feeling of mutual understanding
- A mutual appreciation of possibilities and limitations that exist in the situation of nursing care
- A culmination into mutual acknowledgement of the client's health and health care goals
- A sharing of power and knowledge for the client's health and health care goals
- An achievement of a joint "voice" for the client's health and health care goals.

This is an empowered state both for the client and the nurse in relation to adversities that may arise in health care situations, making it possible for the movement toward the attainment of goals for the client.

However, many measurement instruments for therapeutic alliance have been developed within the field of psychoanalysis and psychiatry. Elvins and Green (2008) reviewed 64 different measures of therapeutic alliance beginning with one developed in 1962. They state that this proliferation of measures represents the genealogical development trajectory of the concept of therapeutic alliance, as measures seem to have embraced different sets of conceptual constructs that have emerged over time (Elvins & Green, 2008, p. 1169). Hatcher and Barends (1996) in their critical review of three therapeutic alliance measures (The HAQ, The WAI, and the CALPAS) found six factors common to these scales—confident collaboration, goals and tasks, bond, idealized relationship, dedicated patient, and help received—as judged by a sample of patients regarding therapeutic alliance. But it was the subscale of confident collaboration that emerged as an integrated view of the core of alliance, suggesting collaboration as the critical feature of alliance. There is a need to specify the key features and characteristics of nurse–client alliance, identifying similarities to and differences from the concept of therapeutic alliance as found in the field of psychoanalysis and psychiatry.

Relationships With Other Concepts

Although client–nurse alliance has not been studied specifically in relation to other concepts, the concepts of mutuality, coalition, and therapeutic alliance have been identified as having effects on attainment of a goal that is satisfactory to involved parties (Henson, 1997), patient satisfaction (Hall, Roter, & Katz, 1988), compliance with therapeutic regimes (Barofsky, 1978; Deering, 1987, among others), medication adherence in psychiatry (Julius, Novitsky, & Dubin, 2009), outcomes of various psychological interventions such as cognitive–behavioral therapy (Shirk, Gudmundsen, Kaplinski, & McMakin, 2008), diabetes education outcomes (Anderson & Funnell, 2008; Reach, 2003), positive client outcomes (Frieswyk et al., 1986), and mental health case management (Howgego et al., 2003). In a review of 79 studies, Martin, Garske, and Davis (2000) found a positive, moderate, and consistent relationship between patient outcomes and therapeutic alliance.

In addition, alliance concepts are in turn influenced both by interactional processes and the nature of commitment that exists among participants of relationships. The establishment, quality, continuation, and characteristics of a therapeutic alliance have been found to be influenced by interpersonal problems (Puschner, Bauer, Horowitz, & Kordy, 2005), by therapist—but not patient—variability (Baldwin, Wampold, & Imel, 2007), by cultural differences (Vasquez, 2007), and by interpersonal distress as well as hostility/submissiveness in patients (Constantino & Smith-Hansen, 2008). These findings, although preliminary, suggest the variability in alliance as the process, which then can affect patient outcomes.

Theoretically, then, the concept of client–nurse alliance must be examined in relation to (a) how such a state as the client–nurse alliance may develop, and (b) what impact the client–nurse alliance has on client. Explanation of client–nurse alliance can be posed by considering the participants' characteristics, such as the willingness to share, openness, empathy, power dynamics, and comfort in self-disclosure (Jordan, 1986). In addition, it can also be posed by focusing on the nature of interactional processes as factors that result in client–nurse alliance. Such processes as empathic interaction (Jordan, 1986); dialectical fusioning in which shared meanings and common language get established (Zigmond, 1987); equalizing of power differentials (Henson, 1997); and the interaction of mutual support, negotiation, and active participation (Madden, 1990) seem to be critical to alliance.

Possible consequences and impacts of client–nurse alliance need to be thought of from the perspective of clients. Since implicitly the state of alliance is desired for the client's health goals and health care outcomes, the theoretical significance of client–nurse alliance resides in the concept's relationship to client outcomes. Client–nurse alliance may influence at the primary level the kinds of decisions made on behalf of patients—not only by nurses but also by other health care professionals—by affecting negotiation and collaboration. Such effects may in turn have an impact on the ultimate client outcomes of care. In addition, client–nurse alliance may create a sense of empowerment in the client. The concept of client–nurse alliance refers to an important aspect of client–nurse phenomena, and should be fully developed theoretically.

SUMMARY

The ideas presented in this chapter focus on phenomena that occur in situations in which a client and a nurse are together. It is difficult to conceptualize phenomena in the client–nurse domain, distinctively distinguishing them from those belonging to the client (the client domain) and those belonging to the nurse (the practice domain). Phenomena in the client–nurse domain must be considered analytically distinct from the phenomena in the client and the practice domains, by viewing them as belonging to both the client and the nurse in the context of relation. Although what is felt, experienced, and acted belongs empirically to the actors of interaction, these phenomena are also relational because their existence is not possible without the coexistence of the actors in the context of interchange.

I have proposed an analytical schema to differentiate phenomena of the client–nurse domain as contact, communication, and interaction types. Although this schema is useful to partition out different aspects of client–nurse relations analytically, there may be strong opposition to such particularization from holistic scholars. This schema is proposed as a way to clearly delineate different aspects of client–nurse relations and to think theoretically from a pluralistic perspective. This schema points to the possibility of focusing on specific ontological aspects of human relations in developing theoretical ideas about client–nurse phenomena.

In addition, three meaning-orientations of client–nurse phenomena have been identified: (a) the medium orientation, (b) the therapy orientation, and (c) the care orientation. Viewing client–nurse phenomena from these three orientations allows conceptual and theoretical examinations of them from different perspectives of impact.

The major thrust in conceptualization for the client–nurse domain is to view client–nurse relations as human-to-human engagements with a specific emphasis on the features of client and nurse as participants and with the consideration of the nursing context as the locus of occurrence. This thrust makes the knowledge development from a nursing perspective for the client–nurse domain unique and essential.

NOTE

1. Madden, B. P. (1990). The hybrid model for concept development: Its values for the study of therapeutic alliance. *Advances in Nursing Science, 12,* 85.

7

Theoretical Analysis of Phenomena in the Domain of Practice

[M]aking and acting are different...; so that the reasoned state of capacity to act is different from the reasoned state of capacity to make....The origin of action—its efficient, not its final cause—is choice, and that of choice is desire and reasoning with a view to an end....and such an origin of action is a man.

—*Aristotle*

OVERVIEW

This chapter presents theoretical ideas about phenomena of nursing work (that is, practice), particularly "located" in the person of the nurse as she/ he is engaged in delivering nursing care. I propose a view of nursing work to encompass what nurses do and experience in clinical situations in relation to clients and in addressing clients' health-related experiences and problems that are subject to nursing attention. Nursing work refers to nurses' practice, which includes the cognitive, behavioral, social, and ethical aspects of professional actions and activities performed and/or experienced by nurses in relation to patient care. This view is a somewhat limited view of nursing work, disregarding those aspects of what nurses do as organizational role-players, such as making out unit assignments, working with unit budget, working on a committee, and engaging in clinical research. Discussions regarding the conceptualization of nursing practice focus on the need to develop systematic and theoretical ideas about the nature of phenomena in the nurse as she/he is practicing nursing. A framework to analytically delineate two aspects of nursing practice is presented as a way to examine the complex nature of practice. A separate section is devoted to discussion of issues related to the concept of nursing diagnosis. Recent developments in the area of nursing diagnosis make it necessary to give an exposition on theoretical considerations regarding the concept and its referents, as well as on the role of the concept in theory development in nursing.

The last section offers conceptual analyses of the phenomena of clinical expertise and aesthetics of nursing practice as examples of phenomena in the practice domain.

MEANINGS OF NURSING PRACTICE

This domain embraces what and how nurses carry out and perform those actions called "nursing." Our interest lies in understanding and explaining nursing practice and in improving the way we practice nursing.

As discussed in chapters 5 and 6, many phenomena within the client and client–nurse interaction are of critical importance to nursing; yet, to make nursing practice scientific, theoretical development for the domain of practice is essential. With knowledge of this domain, we can come to a full understanding of how nurses make a difference for clients and their health. Obviously, theoretical concerns for this domain are determined by the definition of nursing adopted in this study. If we consider nursing as a "particular way" of managing human health affairs, it is precisely this "particular way" that requires definition and by which relevant phenomena are identified for scientific explanation. Through scientific explanations of what goes on in the world of "nursing practice," we are able to system-atize our ways of acting and to design and carry out specific actions to fit nursing requirements.

The ultimate objective of the science of nursing is to understand and explain scientific problems specific to the domains of client and client–nurse. However, since the contents of nursing work affects clients, there also is a need to develop knowledge about nursing practice through theoretical and empirical work. More specifically, those theoretical postu-lates and empirical questions that have ultimate significance for the con-tents of nursing work can be considered to be within the nursing frame of reference, and require scientific answers from the nursing angle of vision. The starting point, then, for a scientific study of nursing is in thinking of nursing activities as "purposive."

In ordinary nursing terminology, nursing practice refers to many different things and is often used interchangeably with "nursing skills," "clinical practice," or simply "nursing." Most often it is used, in a comparative sense, on a par with nursing theory and nursing research. Nursing as a discipline is viewed as having three structural components in this usage: theory, practice, and research. In addition, by definition, nursing practice may refer to the phenomena of the nursing profession, the phenomena that occur with the individual nurse in everyday practice in general, or the phenomena of specific action(s) performed by a nurse in a given specific situation. Nursing practice can also be specified according to the type of nursing action, such as in nursing practice of communication or nursing practice of preoperative teaching. It also may be categorized according to client characteristics, such as nursing practice for children, nursing practice for healthy adults, etc. Departing somewhat from such common-sense uses of the term, the conceptualization of nursing practice specified as nursing work here refers to phenomena related to what nurses as agents of nursing work do and experience.

In a generic sense, practice is considered as actions, both mental and behavioral, that are carried out or performed by individuals in a specific situation of health care. The term is used differently from that common usage of "practice," as in "You will improve with practice," in which it is synonymous with "drill." A theoretical conceptualization of "practice" as used in nursing practice or professional practice is closely linked with another common usage, as in "Your idea is a good one, but it won't work in practice."

In proposing situation-producing theory as the proper form of nursing theory, Dickoff and James (1968) implicitly equate practice with activities that "produce a situation." To them, practice is the vehicle by which a desired situation in nursing is produced, and it is theoretically influenced by goal content, prescription, and a survey list. Theoretically, a survey list infers situational variables relative to prescribed nursing activity. In turn, they also conceive that practice, the activity performed in reality, is the base for descriptive theories (factor-isolating theories) as well. In a similar analysis, Wilson (1977) proposed that the grounded theory approach advanced by Glaser and Strauss (1967) may be adopted to develop theories that are applicable to explaining and predicting processes of nursing practice. Beckstrand (1978a, 1978b) also defined practice as a class of phenomena that includes all actions that bring about changes in an entity for a realization of a greater good. Phenomenologists have considered practice as experiences in clinical situations and as engagement in lifeworld, having subjective meanings and contextual significance (Benner, 1984, 2009). Phenomenologists often use the term "comportment" to refer to practice, within the general category of human engagement in situations. In more recent decades, many other frameworks have been applied to conceptualize and theorize about nursing practice, drawing from Aristolean philosophy, the work of hermeneutic philosophers in social sciences such as Taylor and Bernstein, the critical philosophy of Habermas, and postmodernism.

The concept of "practice" has been proposed by several authors in a general perspective (Benne, Chin, & Bennis, 1976; Bourdieu, 1977, 1990; Freidson, 1970b). The concept of practice that refers to the cognitive aspects of professional actions, along with the behavioral and social aspects, appears to be a significant departure from earlier ideas about professional practice in which professionals are presumed to behave according to what they know. Variability in professional actions related to the professional's use of knowledge and cognitive processes that are used for translating "what one knows" to "what one does" is at the core of questioning about the concept of practice. Argyris and Schön (1976) define professional practice as a sequence of actions undertaken by a person to serve others who are considered clients. In this sense, the term "practice" consists of the following characteristics:

- Practice as a phenomenon is a broader term than action but encompasses action; its conceptualization is based on a set of assumptions.
- Practice presupposes the presence of a mental image of what will be or need to be enacted. It assumes that a mental picture, a cognitive understanding, or knowledge is antecedent to action.
- Practice is situation-specific.
- Practice is social in that it belongs to actions associated with being a social agent.
- Practice is ethically and morally entrenched as an aspect of a human agent's life in the Aristotelian sense that it refers to life forms as free agents in an ethical sense.

And it is precisely this notion that is vital to scientific study of nursing actions within the practice domain. This focus of theoretical questioning is interested not only in "what" the nurse does with or for the client but more importantly in *"how the nurse arrives at given action choices"* and *"how such action choices turn into human activities."*

Nursing practice in general is accepted as a set of activities performed by a nurse (an agent) toward the good of the client in specific situations. The concept involves: (a) knowledge of how to arrive at "good" outcomes of nursing, (b) knowledge of what is "good" for the client, and (c) performance of prescribed nursing actions in reality. The goal of action is always in the client established by the nurse as the originator of "provisions" for the client. Of course, this does not deny that a nurse can come to establish a goal for a client through various processes—on one's own initiative, through collaboration with the client, by following a directive established by others (such as other nurses, supervisors, or physicians), or by using pre-established templates. The actions in nursing practice are special types of human enactments performed in the context of the service requirements of a client. Practice exists in a given nursing situation as a discrete case apart from all other cases and is primarily oriented to the values that define what is normatively good for the client.

Donaldson and Crowley (1978) indicate that nursing scholars generally are in agreement on what nursing should be concerned with, and Riehl and Roy (1980) found commonalties among five nursing models examined by them with respect to the characteristics of interventions prescribed as nursing. For example, they found that nursing interventions prescribed by these nursing models allow for the client's expression of feelings, are aimed at maintaining whatever independent behaviors are possible for the client, and provide new ways for increasing the client's independence (Riehl & Roy, 1980). Furthermore, there is a movement toward developing a common conceptual scheme for nursing, beginning with the work of the North American Nursing Diagnosis Association on nursing diagnosis and also with scholarly work to systematize nursing interventions (Bulechek & McCloskey, 1992) and nursing outcomes (Moorehead et al., 1997). Nevertheless, fuzziness still exists in conceptualizations, especially with respect to defining the boundary within which actions are classified as nursing. This fuzziness can be attributed to the fact that most of what nurses do is not significantly different from what ordinary people do in their everyday lives. What are different are not the acts themselves, but when, how, and why they are carried out. In nursing, the same acts take on special meanings in their enactment.

A nurse sits with a dying patient as a wife sits with her dying husband. The "act" of attending the last hours of a dying person may appear the same for these two individuals. However, the meanings of that act to the "attendees" as well as to the client would be different, and the actual contents of the act of attending may be very different in behavioral, affective, informational, and technical senses. Theoretical efforts in nursing, then, need to focus on how such ordinary actions take on professional, nursing meanings and in what ways they become different from ordinary human actions. In a non-deliberate effort to make nursing actions "unordinary," that is "technical," the current nursing world has become preoccupied with bringing into the core of nursing those actions that require competent use of technological instruments. Though this preoccupation results from the current use of technology in health care, technology has to be considered as a tool for nursing, not the content of nursing itself. The core of nursing actions within nursing work resides in the human-to-human actions performed by a professional nurse for goals that are oriented to the client's health-related affairs.

For theoretical thinking in this chapter, then, I propose a definition of nursing practice as acts of a person under the conscious aegis of "nursing." Although this definition appears to be circular, the labeling of the act as "nursing" is necessary for both subjective and objective endorsement of the actions within nursing practice in a social sense. Because nursing is a social role, the content of the role, that is, the performance of it, has to be designated formally as belonging to that role. Since acts enacted in a given role may be different in many ways, it is difficult to describe the acts without enumerating every kind. It is more of a conceptualization issue than a definitional one to be concerned with what kinds of acts are of a nursing type.

By this way of thinking, then, a nursing act takes on a specific meaning with respect to its locus of occurrence, that is, in the nurse agent. Hence, nursing acts include those performed in the presence of a client or by the nurse in solitude, away from clients but on behalf of them, such as consulting with physicians, conferring with family members, making decisions about what needs to be done for clients, or negotiating with referring agencies on behalf of clients. These certainly are behaviors or acts that need to be considered appropriate nursing actions.

A FRAMEWORK FOR THE PRACTICE DOMAIN

Nursing practice is configured by three sets of structures: the philosophies, the dimensions, and the processes, as shown in Figure 7.1. The *structure of philosophy* provides the fundamental guidelines for how nursing practice is to be carried out, and consists of three philosophical orientations: the philosophies of therapy, of care, and of professional work. The *structure of dimension* refers to the characteristics that make up the nature of nursing practice and is constituted by the scientific, aesthetic, and ethical dimensions. The *structure of process* refers to how nursing practice is carried out, specifying human processes that produce actual contents of nursing practice, and is composed of two processes: deliberation and enactment.

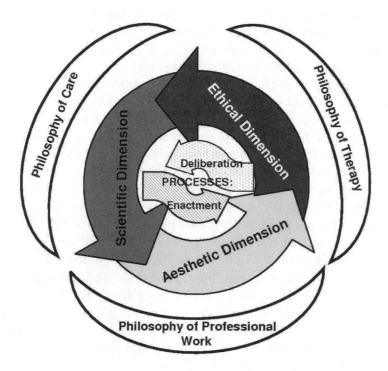

Figure 7.1. Philosophies, dimensions, and processes of nursing practice.

PHILOSOPHIES OF NURSING PRACTICE

Philosophical orientations for practice are the systems of over-arching value constructs that provide fundamental guidelines for how nurses are to "be" in their practice. Nursing practice has three philosophical orientations in its relationship to nursing clients and to its work. Nursing clients represents two aspects of attention for nurses: clients' specific clinical problems and clients as human persons. Nurses must address "problems" the client experiences in the health care situation with nursing therapeutics and at the same time deal with the client as a human person. Hence, nursing practice must coordinate two philosophies of practice related to its attendance to clients: the *philosophy of therapy*, focusing on clients' problems, and the *philosophy of care*, focusing on clients as human persons in their totality. In addition, a philosophy of nursing practice is related to how nurses work as agents of health care provision to individuals and groups and is referred to here as the philosophy of professional work. The third philosophy of practice, the *philosophy of professional work*, guides the way nurses practice in responding to clients and clinical situations of patient care as professional, social agents.

The philosophy of therapy provides the guidelines for the aspect of practice that are goal-oriented and strategic and are aimed at solving or attending to clients' specific problem(s). Nursing is mandated professionally and socially to address, intervene, and treat clients' health-related problems in the realm of nursing responsibilities. Clients' problems such as fatigue, pain, dyspnea, cognitive deficit, immobility, or noncompliance are viewed as targets (that is, the objects of nursing attention) requiring certain sets of therapeutic actions, interventions, or strategies. This occurs as an aspect of nursing practice from the philosophy-of-therapy orientation with the major aim of remedy and treatment. The philosophy of therapy orients nurses in practice to the values of therapy embedded in effectiveness, efficiency, timeliness, and appropriateness. The therapeutic aspect of nursing practice has to be guided by this philosophy. The philosophy of therapy therefore guides nurses to select and implement nursing actions that are effective, efficient, timely, and appropriate in given nursing situations. The values of effectiveness, efficiency, timeliness, and appropriateness constitute the philosophy of therapy.

On the other hand, the philosophy of care orients nursing practice involving the whole of clients' experiences as human persons. The focus of attention for nursing practice with this orientation is not clinical problem(s) but is humans in specific situations. Engster (2005) defines caring as doing "directly to help others to meet their basic needs, develop or sustain their basic capabilities, and alleviate or avoid pain or suffering in an attentive, responsive, and respectful manner" (p. 55). This means that nursing practice involves caring for clients as human beings, upholding the values of individuality and wholeness with attentiveness, responsiveness, and respectfulness as the foundational guidelines. Nursing practice with this orientation involves approaches to clients as human persons situated in the service settings of nursing. The major aim with this orientation is in providing "care" to clients as human persons, with specific and unique histories, personhood, and experiences.

In addition to these two philosophies of practice that are directly related to providing nursing care to specific clients, nursing work is also framed by the third philosophy: the philosophy of professional work. Because nurses function as players of a social and professional role, their practice is guided by the philosophy of professional work, which is oriented to meeting the standards of professional conduct in nursing. The philosophy of professional work for nursing practice provides the guidelines for prioritizing for one client as well as for a group of clients, coordinating one's work with other members of health care systems, seeking out the best available solutions and approaches, and following the established ethical standards for practice. Although the focus of professional work of nursing is the client, the philosophy of professional work addresses how nurses deal with situational contingencies, the representation of clients' problems, and the requirements for effectiveness and efficiency in practice. This means that the major orientation of the philosophy of professional work is a "clinical situation" that involves clients. It addresses such issues as expertise, management, and coordination. Nursing practice is framed by three philosophies: of therapy with the focus on clinical problems, of care with the focus on the person, and of professional work with the focus on clinical situation. Nursing practice, then, must coordinate these philosophies in providing individual patient care.

THE DIMENSIONS OF NURSING PRACTICE

Nursing practice as human action encompasses three dimensions that must coexist and be integrated into a specific type of human service to fulfill its goals for clients and service. Nursing practice guided by the philosophies of therapy, care, and professional work is configured by three dimensional characteristics specifying the integrated nature of human praxis. This configuration of three-dimensional characteristics of nursing practice revises the syntax of nursing proposed by Donaldson and Crowley (1978). Donaldson and Crowley (1978) suggested that the syntax of nursing is composed of two sets of value systems, that of science and that of professional ethics. The aesthetic dimension is added to these two dimensions, with the assumption that nursing practice as a human, moral practice must contain the characteristics representing how self-presentation is configured as a part of the practice. This idea of three dimensions of nursing practice is different from the classification of the patterns of knowing in nursing identified by Carper (1978) into four types, because the orientation here is on the characteristics of nursing practice, not on the types of knowing necessary for practice.

Nursing practice is represented by a scientific character because of its instrumental orientation and its basis in scientific disciplinary knowledge. "Scientific character" refers to making practical decisions guided by science and scientific knowledge. In the tenets of evidence-based practice, the science to be applied in health care decisions in a general sense refers to what may be termed "sound science" or knowledge based on research. Although there are debates regarding what sorts of principles of rationality and of evidence are appropriate in the use of scientific knowledge in applied and practice sciences as well as in nursing (Hansson, 2007; Kim, 2006), it is generally accepted that practice in human services disciplines utilizes scientific knowledge in designing and enacting with a view toward specific ends, goals, or *teleos*. However, scientific character of nursing practice as in other practice disciplines is not solely dependent upon direct transfer of scientific knowledge into practice, but on the assessment of science for its heuristic and explanatory power as well as by applying practical rationality regarding desired outcomes and situational requirements.

The ethical dimension of nursing practice refers to the character of practice representing what the nurse *ought* to do so as to uphold the principles of morally good and right practice. The requirement is for the nurse to hold and integrate ethical standards and moral beliefs regarding professional conduct and nursing care in her/his everyday practice. The ethical character of nursing practice reveals choices nurses make regarding nursing care so as to achieve the goodness and rightness for clients, which in some instances modify or circumvent decisions made based on scientific knowledge. The ethics of practice is revealed in the everyday conduct of nursing practice in which the nurse in her/his "doings" in practice both relates to and affects the client (Gadow, 1996).

The aesthetic dimension of nursing practice refers to the mode of self-presentation revealed in the nurse's practice. Nurses are engaged in presenting themselves in clinical situations through various actions revealing a degree of harmony with situations that include clients. The aesthetic character of nursing practice is in the way the nurse manages herself/himself in relation to the requirements of a clinical situation to achieve harmony with the client. Harmony is revealed in the use of creativity in relation to individuation, values, and desires.

Nursing practice, thus, is composed of these three characteristics, which are integrated to represent effectiveness/efficiency, goodness/justice, and harmony/desirability. Nursing practice consisting of these characteristics, especially as it occurs in a specific patient care situation, needs to be examined to determine its quality regarding each characteristic and its integration.

THE PROCESSES OF NURSING PRACTICE[1]

As discussed in the preceding section, nursing practice conceptualized as such points to a rather complex picture. It involves both mental and behavioral aspects of actions, which are interlinked with the agent of practice, the client and the client's situation, the context of practice, and the nursing perspectives.

Nursing practice encompasses actions that are performed by nurses either alone without the physical presence of a client or with the physical presence of a client involving or not involving the client actively in the actions. Yet the goals of such actions are always oriented to the client. These actions refer to intellectual or cognitive as well as behavioral actions involved in providing nursing care to clients. The clearest example of such actions is what we call "nursing process." The concept of the nursing process refers to a set of intellectual and behavioral actions performed by a nurse in systematizing actual nursing-care actions. The purpose of the nursing process and relevant features of the nursing process are inherently tied to the client's problems; nevertheless, the actions of the nursing process belong to the nurse agent. As an agent, the nurse performs the following activities within the process:

- Gathers information.
- Makes judgments about the nature of information available.
- Arrives at problem statements based on many information networks.
- Examines available and possible kinds of strategies for the solution of problems.
- Selects certain types as appropriate and effective interventions.
- Carries out those interventions or approaches, adopting scientifically selected operational procedures.
- Evaluates outcomes of the intervention.
- Modifies the existing information based on the client as well as the future *modus operandi* regarding the solution of the client's problems.

The nursing process is the most global way of conceptualizing nursing practice, for it includes nearly all aspects of nursing's intellectual and behavioral activities. However, this view of nursing practice within the frame of nursing process is linear and does not take into account the complex and comprehensive features inherent in actions of nursing practice. The framework presented below is a way to elaborate on the complexity of nursing practice. This framework is an elaboration of the work presented earlier (Kim, 1994).

The complex nature of nursing practice indicates that the practitioner is involved in a set of actions—mental activities and enactment activities in a specific situation of practice encompassing aspects that pertain to: (a) the client, (b) the context, (c) the agent-self, and (d) the nursing frames.

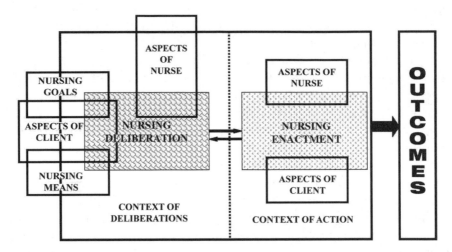

Figure 7.2. Analytic representation of the conceptualization of nursing practice.

Nursing practice is a complex series of actions that can be partitioned into two processes: deliberation and enactment, as shown in Figure 7.2, as the basic processes that can be *analytically* partitioned for a full understanding of how nursing practice is actualized in clinical situations.

Nursing practice is deliberative in that it is designed and intended to address the goals for patients. It requires nurses to know how to mobilize their own resources, both instrumental and cultural (such as knowledge, skills, techniques, attitudes, and values), as well as resources in patients and in the environment, deliberatively and intentionally. In practice, nurses need to be aware of and take into consideration the consequences of their actions in patients through their deliberations. Deliberation is making choices, as Aristotle says that we deliberate about things which are in our power and which could be done in one way or another to achieve a given end. Aristotle articulates the characteristics of excellence in deliberation as that which is aimed at an end, involving an inquiry into "a particular kind of thing," as "a kind of correctness," and involving reasoning; he summarizes this by stating that "excellence in deliberation in a particular sense is that which succeeds relatively to a particular end...[*and*] will be correctness with regard to what conduces to the end of which practical wisdom [*phronesis*] is the true apprehension" (Aristotle, 1980). In this sense, deliberation is what occurs in a situation of practice aimed at a goal or an end that is viewed to be "good" in nursing, the "goodness" being located in the outcomes in patients.

The process of deliberation involves the practitioner engaging in mental activities to develop a program of action, manifestly or latently (that is, consciously or unconsciously), as analytically separated from the enactment of action. It focuses on the structuring of information the practitioner gains of the situation, the practitioner's judgement about the meaning of information, and the arriving at decisions as to what the nurse should do or needs to do to meet the demands of the situation. This may involve a situation with a specific, single problem to be addressed, or one that is entrenched with coexisting, multiple problems and issues requiring decisions not only for problem-solutions, but also for coordination of judgements and choices. Deliberations are viewed to be analytically connected to a network of five structural units: (a) aspects of client, (b) aspects of nurse-agent, (c) nursing goals, (d) nursing means, and (e) context of nurse-agent.

Nursing practice is *doing* and *acting* that eventually counts in practice. Practice occurs as nurses are engaged in actions such as assessing patients, observing, carrying out treatments, caring, teaching, or counseling. And such *doings* require doing them correctly and skillfully, doing them at right moments, doing them in concert with other things happening at the same time, doing them with foresight, and doing them valuing patients' identities, worth, wants, and humanness. Nursing practice as doing is *praxis* in the sense that it is originally articulated by Aristotle, who differentiates *praxis* as doing and acting guided by a moral disposition to act truly and rightly with a commitment to human well-being from *poiesis* as making of something or producing (*Nicomachean Ethics*, Book VI, Chapter IV; see also Lobkowicz, 1967, pp. 9–15). *Praxis* to Freire (1970/1992) means "reflection and action upon the world in order to transform it" and refers to "the dialectic relation between the subjective and the objective in which men engage and confront reality by critical intervention for transformation of it" (pp. 36–37). Along the same lines, Holmes and Warelow (2000) proposed nursing "as a form of praxis" in which it is "seen as a standard of excellence, an ideal ethical goal for which to strive; it is also what Marxists would describe as an attempt to make an irrational world more rational, or a way of making useable sense of one's practice world" (p. 175). Nursing practice as "doing" in this sense transcends mere acting or performing and is elevated to the realm of morally committed human actions of nurses.

The process of enactment of "doing" is analytically separated from the process of deliberation, and involves acting and behaving in a specific practice situation involving the practitioner, the client as a recipient of service as well as a responding human "other," and the contextual frames within which the actions take place. In this process, nursing action is analytically connected to three structural units: (a) the client, (b) the nurse-agent, and (c) context of nursing action. Enactment is bound by time, space, and physical locality in relation to the acting agent, that is, the practitioner. Although conceptualized to be analytically separated from the process of deliberation, it does not mean that the process of enactment does not have mental elements, as human actions cannot be considered devoid of mental contents. Separating this process from the deliberation process allows us to examine nursing practice for what is actually done and accomplished concretely in clinical situations. Although I conceptualize these two as analytically separate processes, the occurrence of these processes is neither linear nor are they independent of each other, and the two processes are connected intricately and interactively in actual practice situations. This means that a nurse may be engaged in a sequence of activities in a given clinical situation, in which the activities are all deliberative, deliberative and enactive, or a series of enactments.

The Process of Deliberation

Deliberation in nursing practice refers to phenomena in the nurse-agent as she or he is mentally and intellectually addressing the clinical situation in anticipation of actual delivery of nursing services. Aristotle discusses the meaning of deliberation in relation to practical wisdom (prudence or *phronesis*) as:

> Practical wisdom on the other hand is concerned with things human and things about which it is possible to deliberate; for we say this is above all the work of the man of practical wisdom, to deliberate well, but no one deliberates about things that cannot be otherwise, nor about things which have not an end, and that a good that can be brought about by action. The man who is without qualification good at deliberating is the man who is capable of aiming in accordance with calculation at the best for man of things attainable by action.[2]

Hence, deliberation is connected to action and is oriented to a result. The nurse in the process of deliberation (a) considers the meaning and nature of information, (b) processes a given set of information vis-à-vis existing relevant structures, (c) surveys and draws on both the public and personal knowledge arenas, (d) contemplates future courses of action and establishes intentions, and (e) makes judgements and choices about conceptual and action decisions. The nurse in this process of practice may be involved in such mental activities knowingly or unknowingly, but regardless, she/he is engaged in deliberations by involving the following five sets of structures:

1. **The structure related to aspects of the client** is the focal framework upon which the significance of nursing for that client is established situationally, that is, for a given situation or an event, and holistically for that client's nursing care. This structure encompasses those elements that are related to the nature of specific problems confronting the client, that provide the client with meanings and perceptions about the problems and situations, and that are related to personal resources present and available in the client. As shown in Figure 7.3, these elements can be differentiated as general or specific, identified in relation to health problems and health-related experiences, personal history, motivation and commitment, attitudes, knowledge, and capacity. This structure thus defines the elements that the nurse must bring into a varying focus in deliberating about a program of nursing actions. It is the major frame that provides information to the nurse during this phase. Since what the nurse knows about or becomes exposed to with respect to aspects of the client rather than what "actually" exists within this structure is of significance for deliberation, the critical issue being what information regarding the client the nurse brings into the process of deliberation. The concept of knowing the patient has been discussed in the literature to address processes by which nurses gain comprehensive understanding about the patient, which is brought into deliberation (Jenny & Logan, 1992; Liaschenko, 1997; Radwin, 1996; Tanner, Benner, Chesla, & Gordon, 1993; Whittemore, 2000). The concept of "knowing the patient" refers to developing an in-depth understanding of the patient as an individual located in a specific health care situation with a unique background and specific modes of living. This means that the process of deliberation is a continuing process that is used to build up the content of "knowing the patient."

2. **The structure of nurse-agent** refers to the aspects of variability in the nurse, which are possible for activation in the process of deliberation. As shown in Figure 7.3, it is organized into two aspects of the practitioners (i.e., the general and specific situation-bound) with respect to six categories:

   ■ The frame of reference the nurse is adopting in providing personal meanings regarding nursing practice in the form of standards, commitments, locus of interest, philosophy, and worldviews.
   ■ Motivation and feeling states.
   ■ Value commitments from the ethical and moral perspective that guide the nurse's practice.

Structure of Client		Structure of Nurse	
General Aspects	Specific Aspects	General Aspects	Specific Aspects
Problems & Their Meanings		Personal Frames of Reference	
Motivation/Commitment		Motivation/Commitment	
Values and Value Standards		Values and Value Standards	
Knowledge and Experience		Knowledge and Experience	
Capacity/Abilities		Capacity/Competency	
History and Contextual Grounding		History and Contextual Grounding	

Figure 7.3. Structures for deliberation: Aspects of client and nurse.

- Personal knowledge existent in the nurse both as organized and as unorganized entities.
- Experiential history both as a nurse and as a human being.
- Personal capacity for practice as resources such as energy, skills, and modes of thinking.

The structure of nurse-agent is critical in the process of deliberation since professional practice requires the agent's primary focus on others (i.e., clients) and other-directed actions (i.e., actions for the benefit of clients). The practitioner has to negotiate with herself/ himself regarding the paradox that ensues with the coexistence of this other-directedness in orientation and the fundamentally self-centered nature of human actions. It means that the practitioner, in having the goals of practice embedded in the client, engages in the phase of deliberation both with and without the conscious recognition of the extent to which the nurse's own aspects are involved. The elements identified within this structure are what the nurse brings into the nursing practice setting, and are basically attained, accumulated, and transformed through professional socialization and experience. Their mobilization in and impact on the processes of this phase are selective and variable in different clinical situations.

One critical concept in the aspects of the nurse that has received a great deal of attention in the literature is the concept of *phronesis* (or practical wisdom) as specified by Aristotle, referring to practical wisdom, which is viewed to be a necessary quality for deliberative praxis to attain goodness (that is, human flourishing) in human life. Connor (2004) suggests that phronesis is the key concept that undergirds various praxiological discussions in nursing. Svenaeus (2003) on the other hand proposes hermeneutical phronesis, which is based on interpretation, as the way to know the best thing to do for a particular patient in a particular situation and time. Benner (2000) emphasizes phronesis as the essential feature of nursing practice with which the nurse as an embodied and socially embedded moral agent produces good practice. Flaming (2001) in a similar way proposes phronesis, which involves the combined use of intuitive reason from the knowledge of the particular and the knowledge of universals, as the basis for deliberation to arrive at an ethically correct nursing action in a particular nursing situation. Phronesis is viewed vis-à-vis scientific, research-based thinking that is generally oriented to knowledge of universals and generalities, with the conception domain phronesis focuses on the knowledge of particulars and situationally embedded understandings with a concern for producing socially and morally good actions (i.e., praxis).

As phronesis is viewed to be a quality associated with intuition and morality, it is sometimes viewed as a more critical quality than the possession of scientific knowledge. However, the current culture of evidence-based practice claims the critical importance of both the possession of scientific knowledge and the ability to use the knowledge that exists in the public domain. Certainly professional practice must be based on the knowledge of the discipline, and the expectation is for the nurse to possess a rich decisional base that can be used in deliberation.

3. **The structure of nursing goals**, as shown in Figure 7.4, encompasses the goals inherent in a clinical situation, both latent and manifest, and is differentiated on two dimensions: scope and orientation. Goals in clinical situations may be general from the nursing perspective, such as promotion of health or attainment of client autonomy, and specific to the situation and problem at hand, such as maintenance of airway patency or attainment of competence in diabetic self-care. In addition, goals may exist differently from the perspectives of the client, the nurse, and others such as family members and other health care professionals. For any given clinical

Structure of Nursing Goals		Structure of Nursing Means	
General Goals	Specific Goals (Situation or Problem Specific)	General Means and Approaches	Specific Means or Strategies
ORIENTATION		*AVAILABILITY*	
Goals defined by Client		Repertoire at Large	
Goals defined by Nurse		Personal Repertoire	
Goals defined by Others		Conjectured Means & Approaches	

Figure 7.4. Structures for deliberation: Aspects of nursing goals and nursing means.

situation in which nursing actions must take place, there exists a set of goals identifiable as a varying combination of the generalized and specific goals for the client, the nurse, and others. There may be alignment or misalignment among these goals, as the client, the nurse, and others (such as family members) could be oriented to primarily different aspects of the client's well-being, different priorities, or different motivational structures. How the nurse becomes cognizant of and puts emphasis on different sets of goals in deliberation is one of the problematic aspects of the process of deliberation.

4. **The structure of nursing means**, in a similar manner to the structure of nursing goals (as shown in Figure 7.4), is differentiated into two aspects: the scope of application and availability. Nursing means include strategies of nursing applicable in clinical situations to bring about some ends that are relevant to nursing practice. Nursing means, from the view of the scope of application, can be general in that the target for the application is the client as a human person, or specific to the situation or problem. Nursing means can be available in the public arena, mostly as validated forms of strategies; or privately to individual nurses, attained mostly through personal experience; or as conjectures existing only as tentative ideas. The nurse-agent thus also brings varying combinations of means emerging from this structure into the process of deliberation. The process therefore must involve juxtaposing the elements within this structure with the elements of the structure of nursing goals with a view

toward establishing a program of action that makes the practice coherent, meaningful, strategically effective, and sensible.

5. **The structure of the context of nurse-agent** is the background upon which the nurse's deliberation is processed and refers to elements in the physical, social, and symbolic spheres of the practice environment. Deliberation takes place in the context of a practice situation that contains not only the environmental entities but also the meanings of such entities. Noise, conflicting demands present in the situation, value structure or culture of the situation, an institutionalized form of practice (what Bourdieu [1977, 1990] calls institutional *habitus*), level of institutional integration of roles, a lack of staff, and being assigned to several complex clients—these are examples of the elements within this structure that impinge on the deliberation process.

Deliberations involving these five structures are not only oriented to making choices for actions to be pursued, but in doing so the present situation of deliberation is contiguously linked to the future in association with the chosen actions. Normatively, it is expected that a practitioner be engaged in the deliberation phase with a commitment to achieving fidelity of strategy, competent delivery, timeliness and relevancy of program, and efficacy of outcomes. This view points to the idea that the process of deliberation necessarily needs to be rational and prescriptive; however, the phenomena as they exist in actual practice may be more haphazardly or intuitively organized than programmatic or intentional.

Clinical decision making, clinical judgement and diagnosing, information processing, surveilling, priority setting, and nursing care planning are examples of phenomena in this phase.

The Process of Enactment

The process of enactment refers to the phase at which the nurse performs activities in nursing. The phenomena of enactment in nursing are conceptualized as human action being carried out and performed behaviorally by a nurse-agent in the context of nursing care. If one believes that the reality of enactment has a direct and complete causal relation with intention, and intentions are sufficient explanation of enactment, then it would not be necessary to consider this phase separately from the phase of deliberation. However, I believe this view is not tenable from the theoretical considerations but also because the conceptualization of human action within the disciplines of human service practice requires us to consider human action in a much more complex way. Enactment in human service practice is not only realized by the nurse-agent, but also invariably involves another human being (the client) that is also an engaged, enacting agent. In addition, certain aspects of nursing practice require deliberation as separate activities of the nurse. Furthermore, the connections between deliberation and enactment are not uniform and linear, and can take various forms according to differences in the nature of practice setting. For example, a critical care situation often requires on-the-spot, immediate action responses, whereas in a home-care setting enactment of nursing actions may be separated from deliberation by a prolonged time lag. Or a nurse may do a deliberation whereas the enactment needs to be done by a third person through delegation of actions.

Facts of enactment are nonetheless time-bound, possibly have multiple meanings, and are fleeting, as depicted by Bourdieu (1990) in describing game playing as an example of practice:

> A player who is involved and caught up in the game adjusts not to what he sees but to what he foresees, sees in advance in the directly perceived present....He decides in terms of objective probabilities, that is, in response to an overall, instantaneous assessment of the whole set of his opponents and the whole set of his teammates, seen not as they are but in their impending positions. And he does so "on the spot," "in the twinkling of an eye," "in the heat of the moment," that is, in conditions which exclude distance, perspective, detachment and reflection. He is launched into the impending future, present in the imminent moment, and abdicating the possibility of suspending at every moment the ecstasies that project him into the probable, he identifies himself with the imminent future of the world, postulating the continuity of time.[3]

Enactment is connected to deliberation but is accommodated by on-the-spot adjustments that connect what exists at the present of enactment to the immediate future. We feel the urgency of human enactment, as it is bound to the present and future at the same time but becomes a thing of the past instantaneously. We also feel the immediacy of human action in the human agent's engagement, as well as the finality of action once it is enacted. Action science proposed by Argyris, Putnam, and Smith (1985), and the notion of reflective practice advanced by Schön (1983) examine the reasons for practitioners' failure to achieve intended consequences in their practice and possible disparity that exists between what practitioners believe they are doing and what they actually do.

Enactment is conditioned by three structures: (a) aspects of nurse-agent, (b) the client, and (c) the context of nursing action. As an enactor in this process, the nurse brings into the situation of enactment the agent-self with all of its capabilities and limitations, desires and hesitancies, sensibility and hardiness, habits and quirks, history and background, and beliefs and knowledge. Such aspects of the nurse accommodate how actions become actualized, by making them good or bad, skillful or cumbersome, with passion or without, coordinated or disjointed, organized or disorganized, efficient or inefficient, ethical or unethical, and artful or mundane.

The client—often as a coengager in enactment of nursing actions—brings into the situation all aspects that makes her or him a specific individual, also engaged in her or his life of the specific situation that is ongoing for him/her. Through the client's responses, behaviors, and presence, enactment is also accommodated as nursing actions are being performed in clinical situations.

The contextual aspects of the situation of enactment are the physical, social, and symbolic aspects of the environment that is bound to the enactment in a spatiotemporal sense, both immediately and remotely but significantly. The context of enactment both confines and allows forms of nursing actions that are possible. Bourdieu's work (1990) on organizational *habitus* points to the effects of the context as an enduring and sustaining influence on human practice. Furthermore, nurses, regardless of their deliberation, need to adapt actual performances of nursing actions to situational contingencies that exist at an immediate environment. For example, a nurse may "end up" delegating a specific action to a health-care assistant even though her intention was to do it herself. A nurse may need to stop teaching a patient about diabetic self-care in midstream, as she is being paged for immediate attention to another client.

Technical competence, nursing aesthetics, delegation behavior, nursing documentation and nursing description, ritualized practice, caring, ethical practice, nurse talk, and tailoring nursing actions are examples of phenomena in the practice domain with a focus on the enactment phase.

PHENOMENA IN THE PRACTICE DOMAIN— HOLISTIC OR PARTICULARISTIC CONCEPTUALIZATIONS

This differentiation advanced in the preceding section allows us to view nursing practice analytically with an orientation to two different processes, partitioning out phenomena that are particularly mentalistic from those that are action oriented. This, for analytic purposes, serves us to look toward developing theories, which are oriented to characteristically different types of human processes. However, many of human experiences and

Table 7.1

EXAMPLES OF CONCEPTS IN THE PRACTICE DOMAIN		
ANALYTIC FOCI	LEVEL OF CONCEPT DESCRIPTION	
	HOLISTIC	PARTICULARISTIC
Focus on deliberation phase	Clinical decision making Information processing Nursing care planning	Clinical inferencing Nursing diagnosis Prioritization Surveilling
Focus on enactment phase	Caring Ethical practice Nursing aesthetics Skillful comportment	Delegation Nursing assessment Nursing description Nursing documentation Ritualization Tailoring Technical competence
Holistic focus	Clinical competence Clinical expertise Innovation adoption Knowledge utilization Nursing process Role overload	

human practice phenomena are so totally, intricately, and pan-dimensionally interwoven with both mental and action aspects that it is impossible to partition out even analytically with a phase orientation. Such are phenomena that require more holistic conceptualizations. For example, the concept of innovation adoption refers to both mental and action-oriented phenomena of knowledge utilization. Similarly, the concept of clinical expertise as advanced by Benner (1984, 2009) has a holistic orientation. In addition, many of the professional role-related phenomena in the nurse relevant to clinical nursing practice are not amenable to the phase conceptualization. These include such phenomena as role overload. Table 7.1 shows examples of phenomena in the practice domain.

These are beginning conceptualizations of many aspects of phenomena in the practice domain. It appears that it is useful to adopt two distinct approaches to conceptualizing phenomena in the practice domain, as there are in other domains. The first approach is a holistic one by which the total process is perceived as nursing practice or nursing process. The second approach is a particularistic mode by which many phenomena are distinctly perceived as separate concepts, especially in relation to two different processes of practice.

Conceptualization of phenomena in the practice domain either in the holistic or the particularistic approach points up two distinct characteristics of the phenomena: quality of nursing action and methodological difference in nursing action. Hence, for example, the phenomena of the nursing process can be considered for scientific explanation with respect to the qualitative nature (e.g., good/bad; effective/ineffective; or efficient/inefficient) and to the techniques or adoption (i.e., sequential application; frequency of use; time of use; independent/team approach). Nursing decision making can also be thought of in these two ways: (a) good/bad, appropriate/inappropriate, or adequate/inadequate, which are qualitative aspects of decision making, regardless of actual techniques adopted in the process; and (b) adoption of specific techniques of decision making, such as optimization, "satisficing," or balance techniques.

MODES OF INVESTIGATION FOR THE PRACTICE DOMAIN

Nursing scientists have to be in a somewhat different position from that of pure scientists, for whom detachment and debunking are, of necessity, essential attitudes toward their subject matter, especially in studying phenomena in the practice domain. While maintaining scientific objectivity and detachment, nursing scientists have to work in balance with the attitude of advocacy for "good practice." Indeed, the science of nursing is in finding ways to discard trivial and frivolous acts from the ordinary repertoires of what nurses perform in "doing nursing," and to replace these acts with approaches, interventions, and therapies that have significant purpose and rationality.

To do this, it is necessary, first, to know (or find) ways of separating those nursing acts that are trivial or frivolous from those that are meaningful, in that they are "nursing" acts. Implied in this statement is an acceptance of the reality that all of what nurses do in ordinary nursing situations is not necessarily "nursing," and that nurses are neither goal-oriented in all their acts nor able to make all their acts have nursing meanings. It is probably neither necessary nor possible to program (i.e., prescribe) every action of a nurse, that is, every act performed in a nursing situation. Nonetheless, the essential objective for the science of nursing is to strive for a system of knowledge that will increase the proportion of rational and explained acts in the total repertoire of what the nurse does in nursing.

One primary way of arriving at this understanding is through deciphering the meanings of acts performed by nurses. This points us to an inductive method of study in which the description of the nursing world allows us to attach meanings to nursing acts and discover patterns of occurrence. For example, if we find that different nurses entering a termi-nally ill patient's room assume certain body postures and utter certain words to the patient, we would be in a position to question their meanings as well as effects on the patient. The inductive approach for the discovery of patterns and meanings of nursing acts is important for the science of nursing in its current developmental stage as a scientific field. This is not to say that the deductive approach is not useful for development in the science of nursing. Both approaches need to be applied appropriately in nursing.

Scholars with interpretivist orientations have raised a debate during the last three decades regarding how to view and study nursing as human practice. Nursing practice has been viewed as human engagements in situations and studied as lived experiences, such as by Benner for skillful comportment in nursing practice from the Heideggerian existential phe-nomenology (Benner, 1984, 1991, 2009; Benner & Wrubel, 1989), and by Bishop and Scudder (1990) from Gadamerian hermeneutic philosophy focusing on the meaning embedded in practice. These perspectives of nursing practice provide descriptive and interpretive understandings re-garding nursing practice as it occurs.

Various modes of inquiry applicable to the study of nursing practice point to the nature of theories that may be developed for phenomena in the practice domain. For the practice domain, two types of theories (i.e., descriptive and normative theories) are needed to have a comprehensive understanding of the nature of nursing practice and also to guide nurses to design their practice to be "good" and effective. Descriptive nursing theories are those discovered and advanced through inductive, field meth-ods or through interpretive methods by studying what is in practice, and provides the foundation for understanding the characteristics, processes, and meaning embedded in nursing practice. Ellefsen and colleagues (Ellef-sen, 2004; Ellefsen & Kim, 2004, 2005; Ellefsen, Kim, & Han, 2007; Kim, Ellefsen, Han, & Alves, 2008) have developed a descriptive theory of nursing practice from a cross-national fieldwork study of nursing practice in acute care hospitals. From this study they identified three components of practice as nursing gaze, clinical construction, and clinical engagement, which are interrelated and interlooped processes that reveal how nurses practice patient care. Another example of descriptive theory of nursing practice is one by Benner regarding nursing expertise (Benner, 1984, 1991, 2009; Benner & Wrubel, 1989).

On the other hand, normative theories of nursing practice are those developed with the goal of producing good practice. Often normative theories are developed by deductive methods or applying prescriptive modes of theory development. Normative nursing practice theories are aimed at how nurses ought to practice so as to produce certain types of outcomes or end points. Although it is not a theory in a rigorous sense, the model of nursing process that has become the epitomized model for patient care is a normative theory of nursing practice.

Watson's theory of human caring (1979, 1985a, 1999) is an example of normative theory, as the theory dictates what and how nurses "ought" to be healing and caring. So is the theory of nursing art proposed by Chinn (2001) that gives ways for nurses to engage in nursing art in nursing practice. There are several prescriptive theories of knowledge utilization in practice, among which is the theory of research utilization in practice developed by Stetler (2001). In addition, various theoretical models for clinical decision making are normative in nature, aimed at producing the best or the "correct" clinical decisions in practice.

MODELS FOR THE PRACTICE DOMAIN

Conceptualization of phenomena in the practice domain is rarely done by nursing theorists in a systematic way. Most conceptual models of nursing treat phenomena in the practice domain as natural occurrences, neither requiring specific conceptualization nor theoretical explanations from a specific nursing perspective. Otherwise, it is considered as encompassed within the idea of nursing process that the profession has come to accept as a universally correct *modus operandi* for providing nursing care. During the last three decades, nursing process has become well incorporated into the nursing knowledge system and is considered the systematic way of giving care. The American Nurses Association's Standards for Practice are based on this form of problem solving and action in nursing. Nursing process as an accepted "theory" or "principle" for provision of nursing care is treated by most nursing theorists in their writings as such. Application of the nursing model in the nursing process is discussed in great detail in many writings.

The attitude that nursing action follows naturally from nursing assessment is particularly prominent in models in which nursing action is viewed in a prescriptive manner. For example, according to the Roy Adaptation Model, the nurse knows what to do if the behavior of the client has been clearly specified, linking it to its predominant stimuli in the nurse's assessment, since the "intervention is based specifically on the nursing assessment" (Roy & Roberts, 1981, p. 47). Further on, they state that:

> Based on this model [the Roy Adaptation Model], some nursing interventions will be traditional techniques such as comfort measures or health teaching. However, our theoretical work may allow us to discover entirely new activities that are the unique responsibility of the nurse when she is viewed as the promoter of patient adaptation.[4]

What they do not consider "problematic" in these statements is "how a nurse will discover a new activity" or "how a nurse makes a choice of a new activity over an old one" or even "why a nurse might want to seek new activities." In this model, the nurse is required to make "judgments" about ineffective processes influencing the client's adaptation level so as to come up with a diagnostic label for an ineffective behavior. It is exactly this phenomenon of nursing judgment that is problematic when a nurse scientist shifts the focus from the client to the nurse. The phenomenon of nursing judgment is an example of constructs that belong to the practice domain, requiring scientific explanations. Nursing assessment also refers to a set of phenomena in the nurse, pertaining to specific processes and features.

Similarly, Neuman (1995) considers the use of the assessment/intervention tool designed according to the Neuman Health Care System model to offer a prescriptive base for nursing action. Like Roy, Neuman views the selection of nursing action as deterministic of the adoption and careful use of an assessment tool.

Rogers is somewhat more specific and states that professional nursing practice is creative and imaginative and is considered to be rooted in "abstract knowledge, intellectual judgement, and human compassion" (Rogers, 1970, p. 122). She believes that nursing action is not determined by set formulas and that the nurse's ability to select appropriate tools of practice is an intellectual skill. Rogers identifies three variables as those influencing the safe practice of nursing (i.e., how the nurse selects appropriate actions and how selected actions are put together): (a) the nature and amount of scientific knowledge; (b) the imaginative, intellectual judgment; and (c) human compassion.

> Intellectual skill in selecting those tools and procedures best suited to a given situation and artistry in utilization of mechanical and personal resources are important dimensions of nursing practice. However, it must be thoroughly understood that tools and procedures are adjuncts to practice and are safe and meaningful only to the extent that *knowledgeable nursing judgements underwrite their selection and the ways in which they may be used.*[5]

She continues:

> Nursing practice must be flexible and creative, individualized and socially oriented, compassionate and skillful. Professional practitioners in nursing

must be continuously *translating theoretical knowledge into human service* and participating in the coordination of their knowledge and skills with those of professional personnel in other health disciplines.[6]

Although these are pointed out as essential elements for good nursing practice and refer to both the deliberation and enactment processes of nursing practice, Rogers does not follow through with this idea in her model, nor does she translate the meaning of this idea within her model of unitary human beings. Conceptualization in which an explanation of variable conditions of such phenomena as "translating knowledge" or "using the tools of practice" apparent in the practice domain is not offered in the model of unitary man. Theoretically, Rogers' statements are rhetorical and fall short of scientific explanation. Although she identifies phenomena requiring scientific explanation, she neither offers exact definitions of elements critical for variations in the nurse's actions nor describes the way these elements are related to each other and related to the contents of nursing action. However, various scholars who have been developing Rogers' science further in recent decades have proposed nursing practice as transformatory process between nurse and client—a participatory process based on the principles of homeodynamics, and mutuality involving intentionality (Malinski, 2006).

King's (1981) notion of nursing practice is incorporated into the concept of give-and-take, the interaction that is the basis for nursing decision making in the model. Thus, the variables influencing nursing practice are what the nurse brings into the client–nurse interaction situation. These are nurse's perceptions; skills in communication; values for transaction, role concepts, and stress. These same elements as variables in the client are also brought into the interaction. Nursing practice varies not because of what the nurse processes in isolation from the client, but only as a result of the nature of the interactional evolution that takes place with what the nurse and the client bring into the situation and how they work together. This suggests that King considers nursing practice only from the interactional orientation. Nursing action as a process does not exist in the nurse; the nurse is a variable for nursing action for what the nurse is and how she or he participates in interaction.

In a more specific fashion, Orem (1991) proposes the concept of nursing agency, denoting the nurse's specialized abilities. Nursing agency includes (a) specialized education, (b) specialized knowledge of the nursing situation, (c) mastery of technology of nursing practice, and (d) motivation for practice. The characteristics of nursing practice are expressed in the art of nursing and nursing prudence. The art of nursing means creating systems of nursing assistance and care, and depends upon the quality of the nurse for creative investigations and analyses and syntheses of information within the nursing situation. On the other hand, nursing prudence means rightly doing selected acts in a given situation based on one's knowledge of the situation. It depends on that quality of a nurse that is related to the ability to seek and take counsel in new or difficult nursing situations, to make correct judgment for action under changing conditions, to decide to act in a particular way, and to take action. The art of nursing and nursing prudence are influenced by experience primarily, but interactively also by such variables as a nurse's talent, personality, developed and preferred modes of thinking, stages of personal and moral development, ability to conceptualize complex situations of action and to analyze and synthesize information, and life experiences (Orem, 1991).

Thus, according to Orem's conceptualization of nursing practice, an activated nursing agency produces nursing operations and actions that vary according to the art of nursing and nursing prudence. The basic postulation is that nursing agency, in combination with other personal characteristics of the nurse, influences the nature and mastery of those nursing actions performed. This model, however, neither deals with how the nurse selects and performs nursing actions in certain ways nor addresses contextual features of nursing practice. Orem conceptualizes the phenomena in the practice domain in a holistic manner.

Somewhat differently from the above theoretical models, Watson (1979), beginning with her initial proposal of the theory of human caring, posits nursing practice in a caring perspective, focusing on human-to-human responsiveness rooted in upholding human values. Through the evolutionary progress of her theory, Watson (1979, 1985a, 1999, 2007) proposes a perspective of "clinical carative processes" for nursing practice. Her concept of clinical carative processes is the basis of the transpersonal caring theory. Watson (2007) furthermore suggests that clinical *caritas* (labeled in her earlier theoretical works as carative factors and identified as the basic units of her theory of human caring) is the core for clinical carative processes that are central to nursing practice in the revised model of transpersonal caring. To Watson (2007), the core of nursing is constituted by such clinical caritas that potentiates "therapeutic healing processes," and is not in what she calls the "trim" of nursing and not in what it "does" in given health care occasions. Watson views clients not as problems, but as human persons. In this model, nursing is a practice of healing through love (caritas) and of caring through human-to-human engagements, rather than responding to specific clinical problems. Thus, in this model the focus is not on what nurses "do" in practice, but in how nurses are present with clients.

The above section surveyed the approaches used by selected theoretical works in conceptualizing nursing practice and treating phenomena in the practice domain within the proposed theoretical models. As shown, these theoretical frameworks (except one by Watson) treat phenomena in the practice domain tangentially rather than as their primary foci for description and explanation. In the nursing literature during the past 2 decades, there have been several approaches to the study of nursing practice, not from nursing's grand theoretical models but from philosophical orientations of viewing practice as human actions. Two key developments among these approaches are the hermeneutic perspective based on Heideggerian philosophy and the reflective practice framework.

Heideggerian hermeneutic phenomenology, with its ontological orientation for an understanding of the meaning of Being through interpretation, was adopted by Benner in the study of nursing practice probably as the first deviation from the logico-positivistic orientation of the 1970s and 1980s in studying nursing and nursing practice (Benner, 1984, 1991; Benner & Wrubel, 1989). These authors present a descriptive understanding of nursing expertise as skillful comportment. Although this work was influential in opening a view of interpretation as a new way of understanding nursing practice, there have been strong criticisms of Benner's work for its misrepresentation of Heidegger (Cash, 1995; Connor, 2004; Draucker, 1999; Horrocks, 2000; Mackey, 2005). However, this approach to the study of nursing practice shifts the focus from acts or activities of nursing practice to the totality of being in practice and from acts themselves to the meanings of being in actions. This perspective embraces nursing practice as one sort of Being in lifeworld, thus to be understood from the general understanding of Being and interpreted as such (Mackey, 2005). From the tradition of philosophical hermeneutics, Allen (1995, 2007) suggested that it is critical to study nursing practice without escaping from nursing's historical background.

The reflective framework for nursing practice has developed with a focus on phronesis and adopting the tenets advanced in Schön's work (1983, 1991) on reflective practice. Nursing practice is analyzed from the position that the relationship between theory and practice in actions is not linear and direct but is intertwined, and often circumvented by personal knowing and situational contingencies. Phronesis and personal knowing are seen to play a critical role in shaping nursing practice (Allmark, 1995; Flaming, 2001) and at the same time reflection is viewed to be a necessary part of developing practice (Holmes, 1992; Kim, 1999; Penny & Warelow, 1999; Rolfe, 1993, 1997a, 2005). An element from the critical philosophy, especially from the Frierian reflection, is incorporated into this framework for self-emancipation from distorted views of self and world and from misuse of power in practice. The framework goes beyond descriptions of practice, getting into the desirability of reflexivity in practice.

In addition to these theoretical models and approaches, there are many other theoretical orientations that are applied to study phenomena in the practice domain. These include various action frameworks, including behavioral, cognitive, and ethical theories. In addition, Gidden's social structuration theory (Hardcastle, Usher, & Holmes, 2006; Purkis, 1994), Bourdieu's theory of practice specifying *habitus* (Hall, 2004; Lauzon Clabo, 2008; Rhynas, 2005), as well as the emancipatory perspectives of Habermas and postmodernism have been applied to study nursing practice.

ISSUES IN THE CONCEPT OF NURSING DIAGNOSIS

The discussions offered in the preceding sections of this chapter bring us to conceptual issues regarding the concept of nursing diagnosis. The reasons for dealing with this concept in a separate section are twofold. In a definitional sense, nursing diagnosis is a label that is attached to a phenomenon (or a cluster of phenomena) present in a client, indicating that the phenomenon requires a nursing solution. Moreover, phenomena referred to in nursing diagnoses are present in the client domain. However, since it is the concept developed to refer to "naming" of client phenomena by nurses, the "labeling" aspect is in the practice domain. Thus, the naming of client phenomena has to depend in the first place on the way "client" is conceptualized and, second, on the definition of a nursing solution vis-à-vis a medical solution, or pharmacological solution, or social service solution, and so on. In addition, a nursing diagnosis as a phenomenon is a "created" phenomenon, that is, it is a concept constructed to fulfill specific needs of the profession. A nurse has to perform a labeling act in examining the reality that is present in the client and by selecting relevant facts. Nursing diagnosis is a way of translating "natural phenomena" so that they have a specific, professional "nursing" meaning. It is a systematic conceptualization of phenomena in the client system from a nursing perspective, not only for descriptive understanding but necessarily also for prescriptive purposes. Nursing diagnosis is necessary only because one is interested in also making decisions about a specific nursing solution (i.e., nursing intervention, nursing approach, or nursing therapy).

In accepting the nursing process as the major scientific approach for delivering nursing service during the past 5 decades, the nursing profession has also basically accepted the concept of nursing diagnosis as a process through which a nurse arrives at a judgment regarding the client's problems requiring nursing solutions. However, there still is an interchange in the use of the terms nursing diagnosis, nursing problems, and nursing needs.

Whether or not a nurse comes up with an exact name for the client's problem in nursing terms, the diagnosing act for the nurse has been included firmly and formally in the nursing process. In general, nursing theorists, nursing researchers, and nursing practitioners agree that a nurse, in delivering a systematic nursing service to the client, should go through the step of identifying the client's problems and arriving at a list (i.e., nursing problem statement, list of nursing needs, or nursing diagnosis) that is then scrutinized for nursing solutions. Nursing diagnosing also has been politically integrated into the system of nursing practice so as to claim legitimation for service provision by nurses in the current economic culture of health care, especially for the purpose of reimbursement.

The first organized movement to develop a standardized language system of nursing diagnoses occurred in the early 1970s with the establishment of the North American Nursing Diagnosis Association (NANDA). During the past 4 decades there has been a rigorous development of nursing diagnosis categories through the systematic procedures developed by NANDA-I, culminating into the most current set of NANDA-I Approved Nursing Diagnosis 2009–2011, numbering 201 diagnoses in 13 domains and 47 subclasses (Herdman, 2009). The development and codification of nursing diagnoses through NANDA-I as an evolving process was followed by the development of the classification systems for nursing interventions (NIC; the first edition of the compilation published in 1992 and the 4th edition in 2004 by McCloskey-Dochterman & Bulechek of the University of Iowa) and for nursing outcomes (NOC; the first edition of compilation published in 1997 and the 4th edition in 2007 by Moorehead, Johnson, Maas, and Swanson).

These three sets of classification systems for nursing have become the core of nursing's minimum data set used for documentation purposes, and has also become the base for the development of the International Classification for Nursing Practice Project at the worldwide level (Clark, 1998; Coenen, 2003). In addition to these national and international classification systems developed for nursing practice, there are also many other systems developed by individual nurse researchers based on specific theoretical frameworks. Although such developments have been instrumental in developing and standardizing terminologies used for nursing practice, especially in relation to patient care, there still remain some issues pertaining to the basic concept of nursing diagnosis, especially in relation to knowledge development. The major issues are related to (a) varying views regarding "clinical" referents of nursing diagnosis, and (b) a nursing diagnosis classification system.

NANDA-I defines a nursing diagnosis as "a clinical judgment about individual, family or community response to actual or potential health problems/life processes which provides the basis for definitive therapy toward achievement of outcomes for which a nurse is accountable" (Herdman, 2009, p. 367). This definition aligns with the lexical meaning of diagnosis, that is, discrimination. What is inferred in this definition is that the act of clinical judgment results in a specific statement, which is in turn labeled as a nursing diagnosis. Therefore, the term comprises two meanings—discrimination and labeling. The second meaning is applied in specifying three types of nursing diagnoses in the most current NANDA-I system—actual, risk, and syndrome. Each "actual" diagnosis consists of a name, a definition, and defining characteristics, whereas each "risk" diagnosis consists of a name, a definition, and risk factors. A "syndrome" diagnosis is represented by a group of diagnoses, and consists of a name and a definition. Although a clinical judgment can result in a narrative account rather than a label, labeling has become a necessary part of the act (i.e., clinical judgment) in nursing practice during the past four decades for professional and political reasons and needs, and is the basis for the development of the classification system.

Referents of Nursing Diagnosis

It has been generally accepted that nursing diagnosis refers to health problems or health states that are treated by means of nursing intervention from the early stage of the nursing diagnosis movement (Gebbie & Lavin, 1975). Health problems that are the referents of nursing diagnosis have been conceptualized from nursing perspectives in a variety of ways. As an attempt to differentiate nursing diagnosis from medical diagnosis, Aspinall, Jambruno, and Phoenix (1977) view health problems in nursing diagnosis as impaired body functions, whereas others (for example, Roy, 1975) view health problems as a response to illness or to pathological conditions. Jones (1979), on the other hand, states that a nursing diagnosis is the statement of a person's responses to a situation or illness that is actually or potentially unhealthful and that a nursing intervention can help to change the direction of health, a concept adopted from Mundinger and Jauron (1975). This diversity in the early conceptualizations of nursing diagnosis still persists, although the position taken by NANDA has dominated the definition regarding nursing diagnosis, which now focuses on "responses to actual or potential health problems/life processes."

The definition proposed by the theorists at the Third National Conference is more global and made in the spirit of holism that undergirded various grand nursing theories proposed during the 1970s and 1980s: "Nursing diagnosis is a concise phrase or term summarizing a cluster of empirical indicators representing patterns of unitary man" (Kim & Moritz, 1982, p. 219). Although this definition has been developed by a group of nursing theorists and suggests general agreement in viewing problems of human health, the actual application of this definition in "creating" conceptual labels (or terminology) for nursing diagnostic states is at variance with the concept of wholeness and holism. In addition, nursing's grand theories already have included their own definitions of health problems within the theories: adaptation (Roy), self-care deficit (Orem), patterns of unitary man (Rogers), responses to stressors (Neuman), and behavior (Johnson). As indicated by Gordon and Sweeney (1979), there is a lack of consensus on the referents of nursing diagnosis.

There is general acceptance of the idea that nursing diagnosis does not (or should not) refer to pathological deviations or disease states, which belong to medical diagnoses. However, nursing diagnosis may refer to health problems and health states, focusing on many different aspects of human experience. Stevens lists the following five examples (1979, p. 95):

1. Experiential states
2. Physiologic deviations from the norm
3. Problematic behaviors
4. Altered relationships
5. Reactions of others

Stevens' observation was based on the list established by the National Conference Group's work in the early 1970s. Three decades later, having gone through several revisions, however, the most current list (Herdman, 2009) still consists of nursing diagnoses in several different conceptual categories that are not too different from those abstracted by Stevens in 1979. In a different way from Stevens, the list can be categorized into several conceptual types according to phenomenal constituents referred to in the diagnoses:

1. Physiological states (deviations from norm, such as decreased cardiac output, impaired liver function, and urinary retention)
2. Psychological states (problematic states, such as anxiety, fear, and low self-esteem)
3. Experiential states (problematic experiences such as confusion, pain, and social isolation)
4. Existential states (problematic states, such as delayed development, disturbed energy field, moral distress, and powerlessness)
5. Behavioral patterns (problematic behaviors, such as ineffective breastfeeding, deficient diversional activity, and self-care deficits)

6. Psychological and cognitive processes (such as coping and grieving)
7. Social processes (such as dysfunctional family processes and unilateral neglect)
8. Functioning (such as impaired mobility, parenting, ineffective role performance).

This delineation suggests that nursing diagnosis categories refer to different sorts of human phenomena, ranging from purely physiologic (decreased cardiac output) to holistically existential (disturbed energy field). The persisting problem with the presence of multiple types lies, I believe, in the definitional confusion regarding the meaning of health problems and the apparent lack of conceptual differentiation between health problems and "responses to health problems." If we take the concept of "responses to health problems" literally, then such diagnostic categories as constipation, diarrhea, dysfunctional family processes, ineffective infant feeding pattern, and insomnia, to name a few from the list, would not qualify as nursing diagnoses since they are *not* responses to health problems but are themselves actual health problems.

Thus, there are two issues with delineation and proposals of nursing diagnosis categories (among those that have already been institutionalized through NANDA-I and those that may be proposed in the future): (a) the definition of nursing diagnosis is conceptually too unclear to offer a fundamental base from which to delineate various types of nursing diagnoses; and (b) there is *no* unitary, foundational perspective from which to view clients' nursing problems so as to tease out relevant phenomenal and experiential elements for the delineation of diagnoses. This means that the focus of nursing's problematization of human condition is multifaceted and is directed to various aspects of human states and experiences. There seems to be a need to delineate an ontological focus regarding what nursing aims to address in humans as clients. The overarching focus is health; however, what sorts of deviations from health nursing aims to take care has not been well articulated in the development and delineation of nursing diagnosis, especially from the NANDA-I framework. There is a need for an identification of common threads that unify these classes of diagnostic concepts, especially because the classification is an ongoing effort and the list is not complete. As nurses in practice apply nursing diagnosis as labeling act and labels, it is critical that they have a perspective to view client situations for identification of nursing diagnoses and also to engage in conceptualizations for those phenomena, which do not yet have labels.

Another issue related to the referents and the diagnostic categories has to do with the notions of normality, positive experiences, and resources. For example, Avant (1979) developed a set of criteria for nursing diagnosis of maternal attachment early on. In proposing this as a nursing diagnosis, Avant submitted a vast array of nonproblematic phenomena as possible referents for nursing diagnosis. Indeed, this is philosophically correct, since nursing is concerned with enhancement of health and healthful behavior. However, making diagnoses about nonproblematic phenomena raises a question of suitability: Should nursing diagnosis indicate the results of differentiation and abstraction of problems that require nursing interventions only, especially if the term "intervention" is to be used when addressing problems? Or should nursing diagnosis indicate concise statements descriptive of human conditions from the nursing perspective? The question also is how rigorously we should follow the criteria for rejection: "Any rejection [of a category from the list of nursing diagnoses established by NANDA-I] should be based on clinical evidence that the diagnosis provides no basis for nursing intervention" (Gebbie & Lavin, 1975, p. 57).

This position continued through the early part of the 1990s by approving nursing diagnosis categories only for problematic phenomena, denoted by such phrases as "alterations in," "impairment of," "abnormal," "dysfunctional," "inadequate," "lack of," and "disturbance in," referring to deviant and problematic states in structural (i.e., alteration, lack, disturbance, and inadequacy) and functional (impairment, abnormality, and dysfunction) aspects of human phenomena. NANDA-I still requires a connection between nursing diagnosis and intervention in its definition.

However, NANDA-I has addressed this issue of developing nursing diagnosis categories for non-problematic phenomena partly by creating a type of diagnosis called "risk" diagnosis for potentially problematic sets of phenomena and another so-called "wellness" type, with labels that include the phrase "readiness for enhanced," referring to positively inclined sets of phenomena. The most current list contains many such diagnosis categories (Herdman, 2009). These two types of nursing diagnosis categories referring to nonproblematic phenomena are constructed in the spirit of the need for nursing intervention. Therefore, as long as the definition of a nursing diagnosis consists of the idea that it has to be the base for selecting nursing interventions, human conditions that are resources for health and resources for recovery are neglected. This raises a related question regarding the role of nursing diagnosis in the process of nursing assessment. There may be a need to consider various components of nursing assessment that go beyond nursing diagnosis.

Nursing Diagnosis Classification System

The impetus for development of a classification system of nursing diagnosis stems from the positions that "without such a system, nurses will continue to experience difficulty in educating beginning practitioners, designing and performing research, and communicating nursing care within the nursing profession or across the health system" (Gebbie & Lavin, 1975, p. 1) and that "the development of a diagnostic classification system for nursing is an essential next step in the development of the science of nursing" (Roy, 1975, p. 90). These positions are congruent with the ideals and hopes of the profession, and seem to suggest a diagnostic classification system as a way of defining the content of nursing's subject matter. This attempt is also thought of as a step in theory development in nursing (Henderson, 1978; Kritek, 1978; Roy, 1975). Kritek (1978) believes a nursing diagnosis classification system is a factor-isolating theory, on which the next level of theory development is based.

The North American Nursing Diagnosis Association, as the official body formed to advance the systematization of nursing diagnoses and the development of a nursing diagnosis classification system, has adopted the inductive approach of what they termed a taxonomic classification of nursing diagnosis initially (Gebbie & Lavin, 1975). By adopting the inductive method, NANDA bypassed the question of "theoretical orientation" for the classification system, notwithstanding their later adoption of the conceptual framework of "unitary man." Their position was to arrive at an agreement on the problem label, etiology, and signs and symptoms (i.e., defining characteristics for diagnostic categories by using language that is not theory-based). By being atheoretical in its approach, the classification system may be accepted, tested, and used by nurses with different theoretical orientations.

This initial approach was revised with the acceptance in 1986 of Taxonomy I as the classification system for nursing diagnoses. Taxonomy I includes nine human response patterns (choosing, communicating, exchanging, feeling, knowing, moving, perceiving, relating, and valuing) developed and proposed through consensus among nursing theorists (Fitzpatrick, 1991). The term *human response* was adopted by the group in line with the definition of nursing diagnosis and in accord with the ANA's social policy statement that defines nursing as the diagnosis and treatment of human responses to actual or potential health problems. A re-examination of Taxonomy I took place in the latter part of the 1990s in response to the general rejection by clinicians of the human response patterns for being too abstract and because of the difficulty classifying diagnoses that may belong to more than one pattern (Gordon, 1998). This re-examination ultimately culminated in Taxonomy II, which is in use at present and includes 13 domains (health promotion, nutrition, elimination/exchange, activity/reset, perception/cognition, self-perception, role relationship, sexuality, coping/stress tolerance, life principles, safety/protection, comfort, and growth/development) comprising 47 subclasses (Herdman, 2009).

The term *taxonomy* in NANDA-I refers to a classification system that is not based on a specific theory or logic. The meanings of the categories in Taxonomy II range from human needs (nutrition) to human process (coping/stress tolerance) to human characteristics (life principles). A need for a philosophical, theoretical, or logical framework for Taxonomy II is apparent for further refinement of this classification system, as the arbitrariness that permeates the nursing diagnoses efforts is rooted in this system of classification.

The advent of three classification systems for nursing practice during the last two decades—NANDA-I, NIC, and NOC—also calls for clarification of foundational perspectives for such systems, as the current position in the application of nursing diagnoses is to link diagnoses to interventions and to outcomes. The use of NANDA-I nursing diagnoses, NIC, and NOC in nursing practice should not remain at the level of documentation, but should influence actual practice behaviors of nurses. Rutherford (2008) stresses and reiterates the evidence for the benefits of using standardized nursing language for "communication among nurses and other health care providers, increased visibility of nursing interventions, improved patient care, enhanced data collection to evaluate nursing care outcomes, greater adherence to standards of care, and facilitated assessment of nursing competency." However, it is not evident how the structures of the classification systems in nursing affect nurses' practice. In adopting the proposal that diagnosis categories be developed based on theories (Gordon, 1990), NANDA-I requires a nursing diagnosis to be delineated with a definition, operationalization of the term (defining characteristics), and a causal or explanatory statement as to why such a phenomenon occurs (supported by theoretical and empirical evidence). This means that each diagnosis is based on a theory, however tentative that theory may be. This means that the total system of nursing diagnoses contained in Taxonomy II represents multiple theories, requiring a framework for the articulation of multiple theories. This raises questions such as: To what extent would alternative classification systems of diagnostic terms that are based on specific nursing theories be acceptable and be used interchangeably with other systems? Could a unified nursing diagnosis classification system incorporate alternate "explanations of etiology" that are based on other theoretical assumptions and postulations?

There are also voices criticizing the label development work of nursing diagnosis itself, for example, as possible grounds for erroneous reification of phenomena or as a means of professional stereotyping and labeling of clients (Mitchell, 1991). These are questions nursing scientists and practitioners should deal with and debate if we are not to be stifled by "a need to have a system" and if we are to allow multiple approaches to theoretical development in nursing.

SELECTED CONCEPTUAL ANALYSES

As in chapters 5 and 6, two concepts are examined in the present chapter as examples of phenomena in the practice domain. The concepts of *clinical expertise* and of *nursing aesthetics* are analyzed as examples of such phenomena. As stated in the earlier chapters, the main purpose of this section is to show how a first-level analytical approach is used to gain conceptual and empirical understanding of phenomena within the practice domain. Each concept is analyzed with respect to (a) definitional clarification and conceptual meanings as reflected in the literature, (b) essential descriptive features and characteristics as a step toward an empirical analysis, and (c) the concept's relationships with other concepts that are important in nursing. The strategy and rationale for the conceptual analysis were discussed in detail in chapter 2, and that rationale is adopted in this section for the analyses of clinical competence and nursing aesthetics.

THE CONCEPT OF CLINICAL EXPERTISE

Definition

Since the publication of Benner's work, *From Novice to Expert: Excellence and Power in Clinical Nursing Practice,* in 1984, and its revision in 2001, the term *clinical expertise* has been used quite extensively in the nursing literature. It often refers to a state that results from an extensive clinical experience that culminates in a special state of "know-how" in clinical situations. *Clinical expertise* is often used interchangeably with *clinical competence.* Because nurses begin to practice as professional practitioners in clinical situations upon graduation from educational programs, their practice is considered to foster increasing expertise and competence through experiences and acquisition of advanced knowledge. As any professionals, nurses learn and accumulate new knowledge through experience. Through each clinical case and each incidence of clinical experience, nurses are able to validate and/or refine existing knowledge and have the opportunity to create new knowledge. In addition, through experience nurses become comfortable and skillful in executing clinical techniques, and develop shortcuts in thinking and deliberating about clinical problems. Expertise and competence have been depicted as intuition, skillfulness, and adaptability to new clinical situations.

Benner (1984, 2001), specifically drawing from Dreyfus and Dreyfus (1986), espouses the notion of expertise from the perspective of "skillful comportment" in clinical situations. Benner uses the concept of clinical expertise within the context of a conceptualization of levels of practice, adopted from Dreyfus' model of skill acquisition, which includes beginners, advanced beginners, competence, proficient practice, and expert practice. Within this model, expert practice is shaped through experiences and is notable for the use of a mode of pattern recognition based on exemplars and intuitive knowledge developed from holistic grasping of situations and understanding. Benner's conceptualization of clinical expertise views nursing practice with a focus on initial grasping of clinical situation as the foundation for a stream of both deliberation and enactment that become actualized as an integrated, nonseparable whole.[7]

In reviewing the nursing literature, Jasper (1994) notes that the expert nurse is understood to be a person who has acquired and exhibits advanced levels of knowledge and skills which have usually resulted from experience, and who has developed intuition that allows her/him to respond to clinical problems with holistic, non-compartmentalized "know-how." In the view of many scholars, intuition is a key to expertise; is differentiated from analytical, structured knowledge; and is even identified as "tacit knowledge" (Polanyi, 1964).

From the cognitive perspective, "expertise" refers to the development of knowledge structures underlying a professional's practice. Schmidt, Norman, and Boshuizen (1990) suggest that expert physicians develop sequentially different sets of knowledge structures, which are used as the basis for their practice. Different knowledge structures are developed sequentially, beginning with the elaborated causal networks, building up to a compilation of abridged causal networks, a network of illness scripts, and a network of instance scripts.

In most of these conceptualizations, professional expertise focuses on the thinking aspect of practice, with a view that the way a clinical situation is initially grasped and recognized leads to different sets of nursing activities. Defining clinical expertise solely as intuitive knowing was raised as problematic for its lack of "truth value" and validity claims (Cash, 1995).

Furthermore, the concept of clinical expertise derived from experience also points to the problem of routinization, as shown by Argyris and Schön (1976) and Argyris, Putnam, and Smith (1985).

Hence, although the concept of clinical expertise is used frequently in the literature to designate a specific form of practice, a definition of the exact nature of clinical expertise remains elusive. One area of agreement seems to be the difference in the nature of problem solving between experts and novices.

Descriptive Features and Characteristics

Identifying the exact features of clinical expertise has not been done well in the literature, indicating the difficulty embedded in its definition. The qualitative features identified for clinical expertise, such as intuitive knowing and holistic pattern recognition, are themselves difficult phenomena to pin down. In addition, there is a controversy as to the emphasis placed on skillfulness in technical execution of nursing activities, possession of advanced knowledge, ability to produce correct outcomes, and recognition by peers as the features of clinical expertise. Adams and associates (1997) identified intuition, skills and competencies, and role functions as the major characteristics of expert practice, whereas Christensen and Hewitt-Taylor (2006), incorporating the tenets of evidence-based practice, identify expertise as composed of knowledge, experience, and the assimilation of these, which contributes to intuition and the ability to use this to make appropriate and prompt clinical decisions.

Benner (1984, 2000, 2009) has used the recognition by peers and supervisors as one criterion for recognizing clinical expertise. Bonner (2003) also suggests that expertise requires recognition by others of the expert's status in addition to the possession of knowledge and experience. In addition, Benner, Tanner, and Chesla (1992) identified three other aspects of expert practice in addition to pattern recognition: (a) the sense of urgency and the grasp of what lay ahead; (b) the ability to manage multiple, complex demands of a situation with skillful maneuvering; and (c) a realistic sense of responsibility. Edwards (1998) found that a group of accident and emergency nurses perceived the notion of expert practice to be characterized by empirical knowledge, supportive team building, assertive clinical leadership, and patient-focused involvement. Bonner (2003), in a study of nephrology nurses, also found being trusted, being a role model, and teaching others as additional dimensions of expert nurses beyond the possession of knowledge and skills. On the other hand, Jasper (1994) identifies possession of a specialized body of knowledge or skill, extensive experience in that field of practice, highly developed levels of pattern recognition, and acknowledgement by others as the major defining attributes of expertise. From another perspective, Schvaneveldt and colleagues (1985) suggest that expertise can be specified by the use of cognitive processes that identify the important, critical information and associations, yielding a simpler network.

Intuition has been identified as the core element of expertise in nursing practice in the initial work by Benner. To Benner (1984, 2000) and Benner and Wrubel (1989), intuition refers to the ability to grasp the meaning of situations and act without the use of conscious reasoning. Similarly, Rew (1990) refers to intuition as knowing that allows practitioners to make decisions without engaging in conscious analytical processes of decision making and deliberation, most often applied in nursing assessment and implementing care. Intuition, which is differentiated from knowledge, is thought to be gained through experience, and has the characteristics of grasping and perceiving situations wholistically rather than analytically (King & Appleton, 1997; Schraeder & Fisher, 1986). Gobet and Chassy (2008) characterize intuition by rapid perception, grasp of the situation as a whole, lack of awareness of the mechanisms leading to an action, and participation of emotions. They suggest that this definition is embraced in Benner's work, and is also applicable to the Template Theory they propose for expert intuition. However, Cash (1995) questions whether intuition is a distinctive characteristic of expertise, as intuitive skills may be the result of experience regardless of whether that experience results in expertise. And Rolfe (1997b) suggests that intuition may be explicated as the use of fuzzy logic and application of the logic of abduction in practice by expert nurses.

Skills and competencies as another component of expertise point to the nature of nursing practice in which various types of skills are required, including cognitive, psychomotor, technological, managerial, coordination, and relational skills. The skills and competencies of expert nurses are often identified in relation to Benner's seven domains of nursing practice. Skills and competence are viewed to be domain-specific, and there are other qualities that are more general and applicable to expertise in general. Adams and associates (1997) identify several different roles and functions that have become identified in relation to the practice of expert practitioners, including leadership roles. The caring function emphasized by Benner and Wrubel (1989) and the role of advocacy have also been implicated in expertise. Somewhat differently, Hardy, Titchen, Manley, and McCormack (2006) identified five attributes of expertise as skilled know-how, holistic practice knowledge, saliency, knowing the patient/client, and moral agency. They added, "being risk takers" and "being catalysts for change" as two characteristics of expert nurses, which may be personal attributes rather than attributes and abilities that can be developed through experience.

Clinical expertise vis-à-vis attitudes toward clients and toward the profession of nursing have not been addressed extensively, although nursing experts are described often not just as skillful, intuitive practitioners but also as compassionate, caring, and trustful professionals. The work by Johnston and Smith (2006) on palliative nursing identifies different sets of attributes for nursing expertise on the part of patients and nurses, suggesting that patients' views of nursing expertise focus mainly on their needs for care, safety, and comfort as well as an assurance of control, whereas nurses tend to emphasize superior knowledge and decision-making skills. The work by Benner and other scholars in the same epistemological tradition has dominated the conceptualization of clinical expertise to emphasize the "decision-making" aspect of practice. It seems the views of clinical expertise from the perspective of problem solving alone are limiting and do not take into account the general features of nursing practice that encompass the scientific, ethical, and aesthetic aspects. It is critical to consider the conceptualization of clinical expertise, including specification of its phenomenal features from the general perspective of nursing practice that encompasses all dimensions pertinent to determining "good," "skilled," and "exemplary" practice, especially if we believe that clinical expertise is something that epitomizes the highest level of nursing practice.

Relationships With Other Concepts

Most of the studies dealing with clinical expertise in nursing have been descriptive and specify the length of clinical experience as the major determining factor. Benner's model of clinical practice, which distinguishes levels of practice, is based on the length of experience, identifying expert practice as a professional having at least 5 years of experience (Benner, 1984, 2009; Benner, Tanner, & Chesla, 1992). This consideration of the length of experience as the major determining factor for clinical expertise poses a controversy in light of the literature on action science and reflective practice. The action science proponents (Argyris, Putnam, & Smith, 1985; Argyris & Schön, 1976; Schön, 1983, 1991) suggest that there is a tendency in professional practitioners to adopt what they call the Model I theory of practice (a practice that tends to be self-sealing and nonprogressive). This model suggests that the length of experience alone may not lead to clinical expertise.

Another concept that has been discussed in relation to clinical expertise is experience as the basis for learning. Benner, Tanner, and Chesla (1992) suggest that expertise is developed through a progressive construction of clinical worlds. Experiential learning as the basis for developing such clinical worlds is closely tied to emotional responses to actual situations. From this hermeneutic phenomenological perspective, different emotional responses to experience are seen to guide the types of learning and construction of clinical worlds. On the contrary, Eraut (1994) suggests that professionals' case-specific learning may not contribute to the development of advanced professional knowledge unless each case is regarded as a special case and deliberation about its significance is consolidated into any general theory of practice. This means that experience must be reflected and thought through if its contents are to be consolidated into a personal knowledge system.

Hardy and colleagues (2006) carried out extensive research examining enabling factors for nursing expertise identified through a review of the literature. The enabling factors for expertise identified include reflectivity, organization of practice, autonomy and authority, good interpersonal relationships, and recognition from others.

More important, the relevance of clinical expertise must be considered in relation to client outcomes. Although it is understood in general that the notion of clinical expertise must make some claim to the effectiveness of nursing care and health outcomes in clients, there is a very little work that specifically addresses the relationship between expert practice and client outcomes. There are only cursory findings from narrative accounts regarding the positive impacts of expert nursing practice (for example, Johnson & Hauser, 2001; Ritter, 2003). It is imperative that we examine to what extent and in what ways clinical expertise influences client outcomes and the process of nursing care.

THE CONCEPT OF AESTHETIC NURSING PRACTICE

The art or aesthetics of nursing has been claimed by many nursing scholars to be a necessary and rightful aspect and counterpart to the science of nursing. However, nursing has been preoccupied during the past four decades with the development of scientific knowledge in an effort to "come of age" as a legitimate scientific discipline. We are beginning to hear voices raised, calling our attention to the aspects of nursing that transcend prescriptions, therapies, and interventions. Among these voices are the ones that consider the aesthetic nature of nursing practice to be its essential component. Carper (1978) raised this point by citing "esthetic pattern of knowing" as one of the four essential patterns of knowing in nursing. Another voice is that of Katims (1993), who proposes nursing caregiving as an aesthetic experience that needs to be founded upon the "felt" qualities of care and excellence. Holmes (1992) offers a view of nursing as a "form of aesthetic praxis," refering to nursing action as performance expressive of a nurse's values and beliefs, embracing a reflection upon theory and practice. Aesthetic nursing practice thus refers to the doing, performing, and engaging that are involved in nursing work.

Definition

Art and aesthetics are very difficult concepts to define. The uses of these terms also vary. In the nursing literature these two terms are often indiscriminately used to refer to the same thing, and at the same time are used to convey different ideas. For example, De Raeve (1998) differentiates the terms "art" and "aesthetics" from a philosophical perspective, and suggests that the art of nursing cannot be represented by the language of aesthetics. Although the term "aesthetics" is philosophically oriented and used to specify the quality of human appreciation, it is used interchangeably with the term "art" in nursing to refer to the aspects of practice that transcend the control or immersion by scientific knowledge. In this exposition, the concepts of art and aesthetics are used as synonyms referring to the same phenomena, as it is extremely difficult to tease out three camps, namely, an "art" camp, an "aesthetic" camp, and an art/aesthetic camp. However, one of our tasks is to clarify the differences between these two concepts and offer specific conceptualizations of them.

Johnson (1994) delineates from the literature five separate senses used to describe nursing art as:

- The nurse's ability to grasp meaning in patient encounters
- The nurse's ability to establish a meaningful connection with the patient
- The nurse's ability to skillfully perform nursing activities
- The nurse's ability to rationally determine an appropriate course of nursing action
- The nurse's ability to morally conduct his or her nursing practice[8]

On the other hand, I have differentiated the conceptualizations of aesthetic nursing practice that appear in the literature from three different perspectives (Kim, 1993c). These perspectives are based on a different conceptualization of aesthetics and human action. The conceptualization of aesthetic nursing practice with an emphasis on creativity focusing on the "form" of practice as a product is based on the Kantian notion of aesthetics as oriented to an "experiencing aesthetic" or an "art" (Crawford, 1974). From this perspective, the "art" of nursing is in the contents of nursing practice as they communicate aesthetic ideas to perceivers, especially to clients.

From the Kantian perspective, nursing practice may be considered as the object of aesthetic experiences, as it satisfies judgements of taste regarding the beauty and felt pleasures, both by nurses as the creators and by clients as the observers. Here, creativity is an essential component arousing aesthetic experiences. Chinn, Maeve, and Bostick (1997) define the art of nursing as a spontaneous, in-the-moment act that requires deliberate rehearsal. Chinn and Kramer define nursing art with a focus on the art form as "the nurse's synchronous arrangement of narrative and movement into a form that transforms experiences into a realm that would not otherwise be possible. The arrangement is spontaneous, in-the-moment, and intuitive" (Chinn, 2001, p. 291). Chinn and Kramer (2007) further suggest that both the patient and the nurse can experience possibilities and transformations through artful nursing.

The second perspective comes from the view of the totality of nursing practice as aesthetic experience (Katims, 1993). The lived experience of nursing is considered art to the extent that nurses are able to "keep experience through aesthetic practice in which self-reflection and creativity are emphasized in the presentation of self by the actor from falling toward meaningless ritual or yawning chaos" (Alexander, 1987, p. 204). This view aligns with the idea of creativity as "the fusion in an experience of the pressure upon the self of necessary conditions and the spontaneity and novelty of individuality" (Dewey, 1934, p. 286). LeVasseur (1999) insists that the art of nursing is only compatible with Dewey's emphasis on art as experience that involves both the nurse and the client.

On the other hand, Wainwright (2000), from the Deweyan perspective, suggests aesthetic nursing is commensurate with aesthetic quality in experiences. Aesthetic nursing practice, hence, results from coordinated creativity and is involved with the totalizing process that unifies the knowledge, thoughts, feelings, meanings, connections, and performances embedded in nursing experience. Austgard (2006), citing the Norwegian nursing theorist Martinsen, suggests that aesthetic experience is central to nursing practice, which refers to how nurses encounter and respond with patients. From this sense, aesthetic experience is not in the judgements of actions as products but in the experience itself. Carper's (1978) notion of empathy as an essential aspect of an aesthetic pattern of knowing also belongs to this conceptualization. The nurse as an actor can make the experience aesthetically meaningful through interpersonal engagements that uphold care, empathy, and an integrated coordination of points of views of participants in the experience.

The third perspective emerges from critical philosophy and the emancipatory theory of aesthetics. Aesthetics is considered in alignment with the notion of human practice that emphasizes self-reflection and human freedom. Holmes (1992), from this perspective, proposes "art as a form of value-expression" and suggests aesthetic nursing praxis as "a performance in which the values and ideals of nursing practice are embodied" (p. 946). Nurses' actions as art are the vehicles through which nurses are able to express personal meanings and values in actions and secure personal identity and mutual understanding. Aesthetic nursing practice as presentation of self is represented by the emphasis on self-reflection and creativity through the rejection of meaninglessness and alienation.

A definition of aesthetic nursing practice may be possible that encompasses this diversity in the conceptualizations of aesthetic nursing practice. The following definition is offered as a generic form:

> Aesthetic nursing practice refers to the aspects of nursing practice that are involved in "careful" individuation of actions and harmony with the acting of another person (i.e. the client), the world in which the actions take place, and the acting self (i.e., the nurse). This harmony is produced through creative presentation of the self in consideration of what is desired, meaningful, and beautiful in practice.[9]

Descriptive Features and Characteristics

Although the literature abounds with expositions on aesthetic nursing practice from descriptive points of view, there is a paucity of discussion regarding the exact features of aesthetic nursing practice. Carper (1978) suggests that empathy, "the capacity for participating in or vicariously experiencing another's feelings," is an important mode for aesthetic pattern(s) of knowing that "enable the creation of a design for nursing care that eliminate or would minimize the fragmentation of means and ends." She also suggests that aesthetic nursing must be accompanied by the design of nursing care with a sense of form that is controlled by "the perception of the balance, rhythm, proportion and unity of what is done in relation to the dynamic integration and articulation of the whole" (Carper, 1978, p. 18).

Aesthetic nursing practice, on the other hand, has been considered in relation to creativity, emphasizing the description of creative process in nursing. This is in line with the work by Rothenberg (1992), in which the form and structure of creative process are thought to be critical features along with the contents of the process.

For Holmes (1992), aesthetic praxis is evident when the practitioner as a reflective practitioner shapes her/his practice by becoming aware of the interplay between self and performance, applying creativity and genuine value expressions. It is performance in which the practitioner aims to realize the optimal potentialities of one's being through the engagement in practice that is good in itself.

Johnson's survey of the literature (1994) illustrates the diverse, multiple, and complex nature of what constitutes aesthetic nursing practice. The elements of aesthetic nursing practice include intuition, insight, authenticity, skillfulness, rational ability, and moral commitments, depending on the conceptualization of nursing art. In a concept synthesis study of the meaning of an art of nursing based on the literature Finfgeld-Connett (2008a) identified five attributes: (a) expert use and adaptation of empirical and metaphysical knowledge and values; (b) relationship-centeredness involving sensitive adaptation of care to meet the needs of individual patients; (c) use of creativity in a discretionary manner in the face of uncertainty; (d) insights into circumstantial elements; and (e) values-based risk taking. The art of nursing promotes beneficent practice and results in enhanced mental and physical well-being among participants, and results in professional satisfaction and personal growth among nurses. These findings not only point out the multiple perspectives with which aesthetic nursing practice is conceptualized, but also the diversity in designating the essential features that specify aesthetic nursing practice.

Relationships With Other Concepts

The major questions pointing to further understanding and explanation regarding the phenomena of aesthetic nursing practice are: When is nursing practice aesthetic? How can we know that aesthetic nursing practice exists? What brings about aesthetic nursing practice? (and) What is the impact of aesthetic nursing practice on clients and nurses, and on the culture of nursing practice? Although these are important questions requiring systematic investigation, there is a fundamental question regarding the epistemology of aesthetics. Aesthetics or art refers to personal experiences, which are situationally and often fleetingly experienced. They are accessible only through subjective reflections. Hence, the methodology for studying aesthetic nursing practice needs to be identified carefully to address such major questions, especially those inquiring into the descriptive nature of aesthetic nursing practice.

A nurse's personal qualities and experiences (such as creativity, intuition, and knowledge) as well as a nurse's mode of practice (oriented to reflection and emancipation), moral commitment (to caring and authenticity), and relational abilities have been discussed as possible factors associated with aesthetic nursing practice. Caring and empathy are considered either as the intrinsic features of aesthetic nursing practice or as those aspects of practice that lead to the experience of aesthetic nursing practice (Appleton, 1993). However, understanding the nature of aesthetic nursing practice in its relationships with specific phenomena in the nurse, experiences of the clients, and the context in which nursing practice takes place is at a beginning stage.

Chinn (2001) in her theory of nursing art specifies four ways by which nursing art evolves: refining synchronous narrative skills, refining synchronous movement skills, rehearsal and connoisseurship, and reflective practice in nursing with a critic or connoisseur. This is a normative theory of nursing art, specifying how nurses can achieve the art form that is transformative and integrative of all aspects of nursing practice.

SUMMARY

The main idea for this chapter has been to bring about closure to a circle used for conceptualizing nursing phenomena. Knowledge about nursing practice is one of the central aspects of nursing knowledge. My contention throughout the chapter has been to offer a systematic framework for conceptualizing nursing practice phenomena. Once different phenomena are classified into like categories, it becomes clear to theoretical thinkers that discovering and developing theories for nursing phenomena can be pursued in a systematic fashion.

Nursing's theoretical development up until now has paid more attention to developing models to understand phenomena in the domain of client. As shown in this chapter, conceptualizations of phenomena in the practice domain are descriptive at best. Theoretical linkages explaining the nature of phenomena in the practice domain in relation to both intrinsic and extrinsic forces, and development of normative theories for practice must be developed. We also are still struggling with boundary-defining tasks. Subject matter for nursing study and definitions of nursing phenomena can only result from rigorous conceptual and theoretical specifications of the domains of nursing knowledge.

NOTES

1. This section is an expansion and elaboration of Kim, H. S. (1994). Practice theories in nursing and a science of nursing practice. *Scholarly Inquiry for Nursing Practice: An International Journal, 8,* 145–158.
2. Barnes, J. (Ed). (1984). *The complete works of Aristotle: The revised Oxford translation* (Vol. 2, pp. 802). Princeton, NJ: Princeton University Press.
3. Bourdieu, P. (1990). *The logic of practice* (pp. 81–82). Stanford, CA: Stanford University Press.
4. Roy, C., & Roberts, S. L. (1981). *Theory construction in nursing: An adaptation model* (pp. 47–48). Englewood Cliffs, NJ: Prentice-Hall.
5. Rogers, M. E. (1970). *An introduction to the theoretical basis of nursing* (p. 126). Philadelphia: F.A. Davis. [Italics are mine.]
6. Rogers, M. E. (1970). *An introduction to the theoretical basis of nursing* (p. 128). Philadelphia: F.A. Davis. [Italics are mine.]
7. Debates regarding Benner's conceptualization of expertise are found in English (1993), Darbyshire (1994), Cash (1995), Paley (1996b), and Benner (1996a).
8. Johnson, J. L. (1994). A dialectical examination of nursing art. *Advances in Nursing Science, 17,* 3.
9. Kim, H. S. (1993c). Response to "Nursing as aesthetic experience and the notion of practice." *Scholarly Inquiry for Nursing Practice: An International Journal, 7,* 281.

8 Theoretical Analysis of Phenomena in the Domain of Environment

[T]he man of flesh, bone, and illusions will always experience unexpected difficulties as he tries to adapt to the real world, which is often hostile to him.

—René Dubos

OVERVIEW

In the preceding chapters, the theoretical nature of phenomena in humans, in the client–nurse encounters, and in nursing practice is examined from the nursing perspective. The purpose of the present chapter is to shift the focus to the nursing "environment" and examine the relevance of environment and environmental factors to the consideration of human health and nursing practice. The fundamental question for the purpose of this chapter is: In what ways and to what extent is it useful to analyze environment from the nursing perspective? This chapter deals with this question in four steps. In the first section, delineation of the general characteristics of the domain of environment is carried out, paying attention to spatial, temporal, and qualitative meanings of environmental elements. Expositions also deal with essential aspects of environment with reference to client and nursing practice. In addition, the holistic approach to conceptualization of human environment, especially that advocated by Rogers (1970, 1980, 1992), is examined for its theoretical and methodological adequacies.

In the second section, each qualitative component of environment—physical, social, and symbolic—is analyzed theoretically. Distinct bodies of knowledge and specific theoretical perspectives exist for each component, making separate expositions helpful. Health care environment as a concept that is important for nursing is discussed. In the third section, four perspectives are presented by which environment can be, and is, applied theoretically to address issues pertinent to nursing.

In the fourth and final section, three concepts (sensory deprivation, social support, and sick-role expectation) are analyzed as illustrations of conceptual analysis applied to the domain of environment. These analyses show different ways of conceptualizing selected aspects of environment and how such conceptualizations are linked to different phenomena in nursing. Relationships between these selected concepts from the domain of environment and several important phenomena in the domain of client are examined in this section as well. The aim is to show the extent to which explanations of human phenomena may be attributed to environmental factors from a nursing perspective.

THE DOMAIN OF ENVIRONMENT

Human living is carried on in a changing context that we call environment. Our feet rest on the ground that is a part of the planet Earth because we are unable to float about in the air; we breathe the air, of varying degrees of cleanliness; we sometimes are able to claim many acres of land as ours, but we are sometimes forced to occupy only several cubic feet of space for our body; we can see a setting sun and feel pleasantly affected by its beauty, or depressed by the burden of a lost day; we pray to God for salvation, but we at other times participate in a dance to chase away demons; and we wake up in the morning next to a loving person, as we run away from our parents, friends, or enemies at other times in desperation. And such factors cause us to be malnourished or fat, to have goiter or scurvy, to be healthy or sick, to be lonely or content, and to feel secure or anxious. Environment is an essential part of human existence.

Environment is defined as the entity that exists external to a person or to humanity, conceived either as a whole or as that which contains many distinct elements. This definition does not include what Claude Bernard called *milieu interieur* as a part of environment. A person's functioning and development are partly constrained and determined by the nature of the environment in which the person finds or positions him or herself. Many human health conditions have been found to be associated with environmental factors. For example, regional differences have been found in studies of the prevalence of dental caries (Ludwig, 1968). Effects of ecology on nutritional stress (Newman, 1968), black lung disease among miners, and neurosis in industrial societies highlight the effects of environment on people's health. Feibelman delineates the relationship between human nature and the environment in a spirit similar to Dobzhansky's (1967) and Dubos's (1965) espousal of the environmental control of human conditions:

> Where he [man] begins is determined by the equipment he brings with him to his birth, and it is considerable. He inherits the past of his ancestors, and thus acquires all sorts of capabilities and limitations; but he acquires during infancy the responses to artifactual [tool and language] and social stimuli. He is in contact with tools from the cradle, and adults make signs to him in it [language].[1]

Yet, it does not suffice to say only that the environment affects human conditions and experiences such as health, illness, happiness, or growth. It is necessary to go one step further and consider that human nature also entails conscious and purposeful use of environmental conditions for the benefit of its existence. Control of environment has been one of the many persisting human preoccupations, especially for Western humanity. Modern civilization and technology, specifically, exemplify the advances people have made in controlling their environment. People have created changes in their environment over time—and likewise have been affected by those changes.

Demonstrations against the proliferation of nuclear weapons and demonstrations in various sites in the United States against the construction of nuclear power plants, as well as the "Green" movement's response to "climate change," identify particular concerns about the influence, actual and potential, of an "artifactual" environment on human life. At the same time, factors in a person's more immediate environment, such as crowding or pollution, can be said to have an influence on the person's state of health, growth, and feelings. In a real sense, human existence cannot be considered distinct from the context of environment.

For our analysis, environment is considered in relation to three characteristics, which describe environment as a complex entity: (a) spatial, (b) temporal, and (c) qualitative. These three characteristics provide different frameworks for conceptualizing environment.

Environment in a *spatial* sense can be conceptualized in concentric circles around the person in the center, indicating relative proximity of environmental elements to the person. Spatial aspects of the environment also circumscribe the size of its boundary. Thus, if we consider the universe as the total environment of a person, some of its elements are parts of the immediate milieu, located within the inner ring. Elements in the immediate environment (such as one's home) have a rather direct impact upon a person's life. On the other hand, many elements are remote, existing in the outer circles. These elements influence the person only in marginal or other indirect ways. Yet all these elements in the environment in their totality represent a spatial context within which one lives.

The *temporally* defined environment encompasses aspects of environment with respect to (a) duration and (b) manner of presence. Hence we may have environments of which elements exist (a) continuously, intermittently, or fleetingly; and (b) regularly or randomly. The first characteristic of the presence of elements in the environment is related to duration and is suggestive of either permanence or temporariness. The second characteristic (regularly or randomly) is related to the manner of presence, that is, whether elements exist in the environment in a patterned, systematic way, or in a haphazard, irregular manner. Whether or not an environmental element is present in one's surroundings rather permanently will determine to a certain degree the extent of its influence on a person, although certainly the element's quality will affect the degree of its influence.

The third way of conceptualizing environment focuses on the *qualitative* aspect of the environmental elements, thought of as physical, social, and symbolic qualities. Accordingly, environment can be classified into three subenvironments—physical environment, social environment, and symbolic environment—by dividing the environmental elements according to their characteristics in these three respects. This differentiation is similar to the conceptualization offered by Murdock (1980) in which he distinguishes physical, social, and ideational environment. Parsons' notion (1951) of the "object world" of an individual, thought to be composed of physical, social, and cultural objects, is also akin to this categorization. Parsons defines the object world as a situation of social interaction in which physical objects are means and conditions of one's actions, social objects provide specific orientations of interaction, and cultural objects provide symbolic elements for definition of interaction (Parsons, 1951). For our conceptualization, the object world (i.e., environment) is considered not only in regard to situations of social interaction but also in regard to situations of human living of all sorts.

Physical environment consists of the energy-generating, matter-based aspects of milieux that are in various forms of biotic and abiotic elements. Social environment, on the other hand, refers to individuals and groups

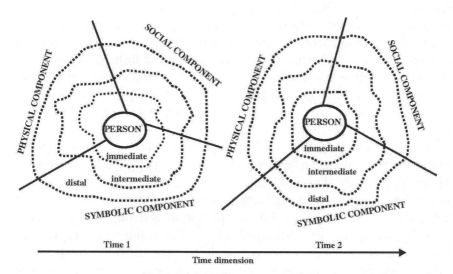

Figure 8.1. Aspects of client's environment: Time, space, and components (physical, social, and symbolic).

with whom a person interacts and communicates. Family members, friends, colleagues, neighbors, and other people who may be remotely situated constitute one's social environment. In contrast to these two categories of environment (physical and social), which are more concretely based in the empirical world and are in concrete forms, the symbolic environment consists of: (a) ideational elements such as ideas, values, beliefs, history and knowledge; (b) normative elements such as rules, laws, expectations, and constraints; and (c) institutional elements such as roles, organizations, institutions, society, and culture. These are elements that have no physical or concrete forms and exist only in people's minds. The symbolic environment is the specific artifact of human history, in that contents of the symbolic environment are the products of life stories of successions of ancestors and contemporaries.

Figure 8.1 shows the relationships among the three aspects describing and defining the environment, and suggests variability in its compositions in three dimensions. Contracting and expanding natures of the three components, physical, social, and symbolic, depicted in Time 1 and Time 2 sequences, are characterized by spatiality and by temporal effects that change the manners with which the qualitative constituents of the environment are present in it.

The concept of environment proposed here implies that environment can be perceived either as a whole, encompassing the totality in the three dimensions, or as separate spheres or milieux viewed according to size (spatiality), continuity (temporality), or constituents (qualitative components). Specifically, this three-dimensional differentiation points to possible qualitative variability in an environment. For example, an environment can be indicated as a specific physical territory containing physical elements that stay or disappear randomly, as a vast symbolic and social field such as a scientific community, or as a home within which there are people, history, rules, and activities.

There are two specific ways by which environment exists for specific persons. Environment can be viewed to exist "for" people generally without existing specifically "for" individuals. This means that although the reference point of environment is a human person, it is not for specific persons that the environment exists, but for people in general, such as society, the universe, culture, ecosystem, ocean, etc. Environment conceptualized in this general way is the objective world to individuals, which is shared and coexperienced in various ways. Gaining knowledge about the environment in this general way does not necessarily involve specific persons. For example, the level of social integration or the types of shared beliefs differentiate one culture from others as general environment, and such differentiation of culture may be applied in the study of individuals' health-related behaviors. In this application, different culture types shared by many persons are conceptualized as general environmental concepts. On the other hand, environment does exist for individuals by having specific persons as the reference points. It is *my* environment, which is different from Mary Smith's environment. An individual's or a group's environment comes to be that in relation to specific persons or groups. Therefore, when we talk about family as an environment, it is an individual-specific environment, which can be highly integrated, fragmented, or dysfunctional as types. The effects of family types can be studied in relation to an individual's health-related behaviors. The difference between how this concept is applied differently from the general concept is methodological. Family types are identified for specific individuals by knowing what exists in the persons' family environment, whereas culture types are identified through aggregates and specific types get attached to individuals by their backgrounds and affiliation.

At the philosophy-of-science level, there are two ways of conceptualizing environment in relation to objectivity and human perception. Objective reality, especially physical reality, has been the subject matter of physics for decades, leading to the question of objective existence of physical reality addressed in the theory of relativity and quantum theory (Mermin, 1992). Although this question applies to all phenomena, it presents a critical issue in the conceptualization of environment, as the existential features of an individual-oriented environment have to be referred back to specific individuals. Hence, objectivists will determine an individual's environment by obtaining information about what exists in the person's environment objectively, regardless of whether the person him/herself acknowledges the existence of them.

On the other hand, environment may be conceptualized to be subjectively constructed, meaning that it is constituted by what is perceived to exist by the person at the reference point. This is an interpretive and subjectivist perspective of an environment. Inherent in this way of conceptualizing human environment is the idea that elements of the environment are perceived by the person through the senses and consciousness and are evaluated according to the affective and cognitive structures developed within the person. Therefore, sensory perception is the basis of knowing what exists, whereas cognitive and affective evaluation allows the person to attach meanings to whatever is perceived to exist. Thus, we like the setting sun, interpret a touch as caressing, etc. However, both of these ways of conceptualizing have problems. On one hand, elements in the environment that are neither perceived consciously nor evaluated to have a specific meaning may nevertheless exert influences on one's life, but on the other hand, what one perceives and the way one perceives the environment may determine both the way it affects the person and how the person approaches it. These two ways, therefore, have both theoretical and methodological implications.

What, then, are useful ways of examining environment and phenomena of environment in the nursing perspective? The nursing perspective requires conceptualization of environment in two specific ways: (a) environment having the client as an individual at the core of the concentric field; and (b) environment as nursing care environment in which the environment takes on specific symbolic meaning, that of a health care environment, to both the client and the nurse.

For the first concern, environment of client is the external reality that is identifiable according to the three dimensions proposed in the preceding section. Analytically, the environment of the client needs to be considered with specific references to his or her health. This orientation is basically related to examining Dubos's proposition that "the states of health or disease are the expressions of the success or failure experienced by the organism in its efforts to respond adaptively to environmental changes."[2] Theoretical interests, then, are in extracting those aspects of the client's environment (or human environment in general) that are more closely tied to human conditions of health. Dubos (1965) views the environment as physical, biological, and social forces and qualities, and defines health as a person functioning in a given physical and social environment. Inherent in his notion is the idea that environment not only provides the circumstances and forces for a person's adaptation that is expressed as health, but is also a context in which health as "functioning" is defined for the individual. The environment is seen as a whole in which a person acts, reacts, and interacts within the confines of genotypic and phenotypic givens and of the potentialities of self-determination, and through which one occupies changing states of health.

Rogers (1970, 1980, 1992) conceptualizes the environment in a holistic way, although her approach is more totally unitary than that postulated by Dubos. Dubos (1965) maintains the separateness of different components of the environment analytically helpful in examining specific effects of different environmental forces on the human condition. Rogers (1970) views environment as one open system that should be considered in its totality as an energy field. Rogers's conceptualization of environment may be best understood within the current worldview of physics, the theory of relativity. Einstein's general theory of relativity suggests that the universe as a construct of space, in a relativistic sense, is curved, and that the flow of time in that universe is "relative" to the timekeeper's state of motion (1961). Since this assumption holds for the general case, that is, with a holistic worldview, and is tied to the notion of "dematerialization" (or transformation) of matter into energy (i.e., matter as concentrated patterns of energy), environment in this view is a spatial, temporal entity consisting of energy patterns.

Accordingly, Rogers proposes that the universe is an energy field within which the human field and its environmental field coexist only in a relativistic sense. Environment is conceptualized as "a four dimensional, negentropic energy field identified by pattern and organization, and encompassing all that are outside any given human field" (Rogers, 1980, p. 332). It is also considered to be unique to each human person. To Rogers, environment is that possessing a spatial and temporal boundary, and expressed as a patterned and organized field of energy. It is seen as a totality, an entity that is only expressible as a whole. Therefore, to Rogers, environment is a variable only with respect to energy patterns and organization.

Operationalization of this conceptualization has been found wanting, because the energizing and wave-patterning of an environmental field as the manifestations of the totality are empirically difficult to grasp for understanding as well as for measuring. However, Rogers's global posture of conceptualizing environment may be a fruitful way of looking at the world, especially if we are interested in considering human health in a holistic manner. According to Rogers's model, nurses and nursing actions as elements of the external world of a client are imperceptible, totally interfused aspects of the environment. The environment as a totality is represented as an energy field, having certain kinds of patterns and organization. What is rather confusing in Rogers's conceptualization of environment is her conceptualization that both human and environmental systems are expressed as energy fields. Possible differences in the characteristics of energy fields have not been clearly conceptualized. For instance, the human energy field is said to be more complex because of human consciousness and creativity, yet the exact nature of that complexity and its difference from the environmental energy field, which is composed of both animate (including humans) and inanimate elements, is not specified in the model. Specifying similarities and differences between the human field and the environmental field will yield a greater explanatory credence.

Other nursing theorists view environment in a rather casual manner. King (1981), for example, conceptualizes environment as the world that is perceived by a person, composed of people and things that are sources of stress (stressors) for the person. This view is useful insofar as it is adopted in the interactional contexts with which King is mainly concerned. In a similar fashion, theorists such as Neuman (1998), Roy (Roy & Andrews, 1991), and others having a theoretical orientation in systems models of stress/adaptation also view environment as that from which stresses and stimulations are generated to the individual and with which the individual tries to attain balance. The exact nature of environment and the mechanisms by which stresses originate in the environment are neither defined nor explored in these models. For such conceptualizations, nurses and nursing actions are capable of generating stresses and stimulations to the client as parts of the environment.

Such observations make apparent the difficulty in viewing and analyzing environment in a holistic sense. For this reason, a particularistic approach, taking physical, social, and symbolic environments as separate phenomena, is adopted as an analytic posture in the following sections. Although no environment may be conceptualized as having only one of these components apart from the others, completely, it appears useful to take different characteristics of environment as the point of departure for theoretical considerations in an analytical sense.

THE MAJOR COMPONENTS OF ENVIRONMENT

Physical Environment

Concepts of physical environment are most appropriately found within the domain of a field called human ecology. The main concept in the field of human ecology is ecosystem, which is defined as a system of interactions between the various human groups themselves and with the physical and chemical components of the environment. The basic process of an ecosystem is usually considered as a form of energetics, having energy transfer between and among elements of the environment as the basis for changes that evolve. Inherent in this idea of environment is that elements in the environment are capable of generating and exchanging energy and that energy transfer is the elementary form of interaction between elements.

Physical environment has been categorized in various ways. Air, water, and places as used by Hippocrates are persistently used to describe the universalistic world of living. The concept of "place" can be all encompassing with regard to the constituents that are connected with a spatially and/or geographically defined area. Therefore, a "place" may mean an urban location of congestion with polluted air, limited open space and vegetation, and crowded with heterogeneous sorts of people, or as an immediate situation of one's presence.

In general, physical environment is thought to be composed of biotic and abiotic elements. Biotic elements come in various forms, ranging from viruses to human beings. Symbiosis as a process has been identified as producing peaceful, mutually advantageous coexistence and growth among many species. A human being as a physical entity in the physical environment takes conceptually a quite different meaning from that of a social being in the social environment. As a physical entity, a person produces and uses heat; occupies space; generates, regenerates, and degenerates its chemical constituents; and has a contiguous surface. Territoriality and crowding are the most commonly studied phenomena in which human beings are taken as physical objects in the environment. Of course, the process by which a person handles the problems of territorial competition and crowding are far more sophisticated than those of other biotic organisms.

Abiotic elements may be distinguished as natural or as artifacts. Although our external world is composed of many and various types of natural physical elements, such as air, water, mountains, rivers, stars, sounds, and so on, civilization has created and deposited many more abiotic artifactual elements in the environment of modern humanity. We are surrounded by artifacts, starting with clothing as the most proximal one and extending to satellites orbiting the earth. In addition, we are continuously trying to change the nature and forms of the natural physical elements in an attempt to control our surroundings, such as building canals and dams, creating gardens and parks, using various lighting fixtures, and playing music.

Currently, in the field of genetic engineering research, biotic artifacts such as variant DNA-spliced *Escherichia coli* forms are being created, arousing suspicions and concerns about contaminating the biosphere with previously unknown living organisms whose potential effects on humans and the universe are not predictable. Genetic engineering poses problems, not only those related to changing the fundamental genetic makeup of organisms, but also associated with the consequences of such manipulations on human existence. Yet, a fascination with control and understanding persists. In a way, the diversity in the available forms of artifacts in modern societies suggests the high level of control of its physical environment humanity has attained, and also suggests more of the same in the future. Maskit (2007) presents an interesting argument regarding the treatment of postindustrial sites that have been abandoned after their uses, such as mines, quarries, factories, and rail yards. These are the remnants of human doings, which have outlived their usefulness, presenting "depressing holes in the spatial fabrics of a place" and disturbing people's experience of time and space. He suggests conversion of such sites through environmental aesthetics, by which the scenes of such postindustrial sites can come to have different meanings to people who experience them. The concept, environmental aesthetics, thus leads to shifting the quality and character of natural as well as artifactual environments for human's aesthetic experiences.

Physical environment affects people's health in a variety of ways. Nutritional disturbances produced by an undersupply of foodstuffs in different regions of the world are the most obvious. Environmental diseases, such as lead poisoning, asbestosis, or high altitude headache, as well as infectious diseases, are also well-recognized byproducts of the harmful elements in the physical world. In addition, many physical elements of an environment are also responsible for patterning specific life styles, activities, and habits of people, indirectly influencing individuals' statures, physiques, longevity, and health. Furthermore, artifacts produce stimulations such as noise, heat, radiation, and crowding as well as convenience, efficiency, and effectiveness in living conditions. These, in turn, influence an individual's health in both positive and negative ways. We are currently struggling with how to address the changes in air quality and climate that are threatening human health, lives, and conditions as well as the viability of the earth's long-term existence.

Dubos (1965) has made the most impressive arguments regarding a person's relationships to the environment and his or her capacity to adapt to various environmental elements:

> At a higher level of integration, the organism responds adaptively to many kinds of stimuli by behavior patterns designed to abolish or neutralize the stressor stimuli, or to withdraw from it. Organisms with a highly developed nervous system have several alternative mechanisms of behavioral responses

and, furthermore, they possess the ability to ignore some of the stimuli that impinge upon them. The higher the organism is in the evolutionary scale, the more numerous and varied are the types of responses at its disposal and the greater its ability for selecting limited aspects of the environment to which it responds. The most evolved types of responses are the processes of social adaptation, through which the individual organism and the group modify either their environment or their habits, or both, in order to achieve a way of life better suited to their needs and tastes.[3]

In addition, Dubos postulates that a person's ability to adapt to the environment is influenced by the kinds of symbolic meaning the person attaches to elements in the environment and by the manner with which he or she responds emotionally, that is symbolically, to other human beings. A person's capacity for adaptation is seen as boundless, yet this potentiality can become stifled if a state of adaptedness to environmental conditions is attained and maintained for a prolonged period. A person's adaptive potentiality is stimulated by challenges of unforeseeable threats and changes in the environment, although sudden and profound changes in the environment always pose adaptive difficulties, however transitory they may be. In this perspective, Dubos (1965) indicates that health as a state free of pain and disease is a mirage, but when viewed as a state in which environmental challenges are met adaptively for human functioning, it conveys a dynamic meaning.

These ideas suggest that physical environment may be conceptualized in a variety of ways:

1. Milieu for functioning
2. Source of stress and stimulation
3. Source for adaptive challenge
4. Symbiotic-interdependent system
5. Spatial construct
6. Object of human control

In this way, environmental influences on health are thus perceived differently according to the perspectives taken to view the environment. Furthermore, the nursing care environment, as a temporary physical environment for a client, may also be considered in different ways, such as: (a) a milieu for the client's functioning that possesses many restrictive objects; (b) that containing objects and people providing stimulation to the client (e.g., beeping sound of the cardiac monitor); (c) that providing unexpected as well as expected difficulties to the client, such as an uncomfortable bed; (d) a system of interdependence in which material, energy, and information are exchanged between the elements in the environment and the client; (e) a confinement where there is a limited freedom of movement; or (f) that containing objects for control by the client. Thus, the environmental forces in a nursing care environment are additions to a person's ordinary environment, posing temporary threats to and amenities for a client's life and health.

Social Environment

The physical and mental health of an individual depend to a great extent on social factors: the socialization process to which he was submitted by his parents; his present work situation, family life and group affiliation; and the modes of medical treatment he can economically afford and which are culturally prescribed. There is a dynamic relationship between the physical condition of a person and the social structure of which he is a part. Health as a normal condition of the body does not mean the absence of disturbances but rather an effective bodily reaction toward them, which continuously reestablishes the precarious equilibrium between different physiological functions.[4]

The basic propositions by which we consider social environment an important factor for human health are that a successful and satisfying social life is partly responsible for health, and that the quality of social life is determined by characteristics of social environment and a person's handling of social environmental forces.

Physical and mental health of an individual is known to be closely tied to one's attitudes toward life and living, one's style of coping, and the amount of understanding, love, and companionship one receives. In postulating the notion that effective social adjustment is positively related to health and longevity, Wolf (1981) states that "one prototype of the healthy, long-lived, fulfilled person may be the fine symphony conductor, an individual who is persistently responsive to physical, intellectual, and aesthetic challenges and, also, who is more or less continuously the recipient of approbation from his audiences" (p. 11).

More specifically, an individual's health is affected by the quality of social forces: opportunities for and quality of social interaction and affiliation; affective quality in dominant social situations, such as family, work, or neighborhood settings; and stresses generated in social life. A person learns how to cope with stresses and develops patterns of behaviors in dealing with life tasks and crises through the socialization process that takes place mainly in family and primary social groups (Kaplan, Cassel, & Gore, 1977). In addition, a person also learns to behave according to social expectations, expectations of self and others that may be universal to all situations or particular to a given context. In this view, people having the same "diagnostic" condition may be healthy or sick according to the way they respond within the prescribed, expected, and desired rules of their social contexts of actions and interactions.

Conceptualization of social environment is rooted in the tradition of sociology. As stated earlier, Parsons considers social objects, that is, individuals and collectivities of individuals, as making up significant aspects of the object world in which an individual is engaged in actions and interactions. One crucial distinction between social environment and physical environment is the ability of social objects to act according to will. A person acts upon and reacts in a situation not only to "stimuli" given to him or her, but also, more importantly, according to symbolic interpretations of the stimuli, which are made both unconsciously and consciously. Thus, social environment represents multiplicity of human characteristics composed of organism-personality complexes.

In a social environment, a person brings with him or her different genetic and developmental characteristics, personality, social capabilities, and personal history. But because a person moves within society, that is, within carefully defined systems of power, prestige, and expectations, the social environment of any given individual at any given time takes on somewhat predictable characteristics. In addition, the structures of society in which we live provide reasons for the coming together of certain individuals in a social situation. Hence, many children and adults are in the immediate home setting of a child in an orphanage, and this setting comprises the ordinary social environment for that child. In contrast, one sibling and one or more parents probably make up the immediate social environment of a child of an ordinary American family.

The fabrics of social environment are reflected not only by individual characteristics but also by the meanings that are attached to them. To Parsons (1951), individuals in interactions are oriented to such actions in three respects: cathectic, cognitive, and evaluative orientations. This conceptualization can be extended for our exposition to classify conceptual meanings of social objects in an environment, to wit, each individual in a social environment projects to another person certain meanings through his or her presence, actions, or interactions with respect to affection (cathexis), information (cognition), and appraisal (evaluation). In turn, such meanings are translated by the second person as forces having certain values to him or her according to the social rules under which most social acts take place. In this way, social objects and the significance of them to the person become personalized within the boundary of social rules.

Thus, recognizing social objects, a person literally embraces those individuals into his or her environment and accepts affective, informational, and evaluative meanings from them. For example, a girl in a crowd takes in meanings and orientations of a special form when she sees or knows the presence of a close friend among them, which also would be entirely different from the meanings and orientations she takes in when she believes that she is totally among strangers.

Analytically, the social environment can thus be conceptualized in two ways: (a) in qualitative terms as social forces that are determined by characteristics of individuals in the environment generating affective, informational, and evaluative meanings; and (b) in quantitative terms as in social network and boundary, which are related to frequency and extent of affiliation, contact, and influence. As for the first conceptualization, such phenomena as social support, expectation congruency, competition, social control, etc., are but a few aspects of social environment that have been found to have influence on health status and health behaviors. For example, social control that exists in work situations has been found to contribute to the occurrence of coronary heart diseases (Garfield, 1979), and Bruhn and Wolf (1979) attributed changes in social integration to increased rate of heart attack. Social support also has been shown to influence the occurrence of mental disorders, to modify illness responses to life's stresses, and to affect the rate and quality of health services utilization (Cassel, 1976; Cobb, 1976; Cohen & Sokolovsky, 1979; Gore, 1978). Social contamination theory has been proposed recently by many social scientists regarding the relationship between social network and human experiences such as loneliness and obesity.

The social sciences literature during the past three decades has been burgeoning with works that relate social environment to health, health-related behaviors, and health services. Many authors have documented various ways the concept of "social capital" has been applied in the study of health and health-related behaviors (for example, Baum & Ziersch, 2003; Berkman & Glass, 2000; Hawe & Shiell, 2000; Kawachi, 1999; Veenstra, 2002). Social capital has in general replaced specific concepts referring to social environment in this literature, and is used to represent relational concepts such as social networks and social support at the micro-level as well as to social resources concepts at macro levels such as social integration or resources-oriented social capital at community level (Brunie, 2009). From perspectives advanced by Bourdieu (1986, 1990), Coleman (1988), and Putnam (1993, 1995), social capital has been examined in relation both to individual health and to macrolevel health status and health practices. However, because social capital can refer to any or all aspects of social environment, it has been difficult to consolidate theoretical ideas undergirding the relationship between social capital and health at individual and collective levels (Kritsotakis & Gamarnikow, 2004).

In a related way, social environment has been conceptualized as "place" or "locality" from a social perspective, and the effects of place on individual health independent of the individual characteristics have been documented (Hawe, 1998; Kaplan, 1996; MacIntyre, Maciver, & Sooman, 1993; Sooman & MacIntyre, 1995).

As for the second conceptualization, marginality, social isolation, and disengagement have been found to have relationships to emotional distress and early death. Social environment as socio-spatial knowledge networks has been studied in relation to communities' understanding of chronic illnesses, suggesting the role of community-wide information networks in affecting health and health practices (Cravey, Washburn, Gesler, Arcury, & Skelly, 2001).

Within the social context of nursing practice, it is clear that the environment of health care produces specific meanings and contents for a client who is advertently or inadvertently affected by individuals in the situation. Nurses, as social objects, are the sources of affection, information, and appraisal to the client. Nurses provide a client with warmth, personal attachment, or emotional neutrality; impart new knowledge about health and health care; and appraise the client's behaviors as appropriate or inappropriate, dispensing approval/disapproval or rewards/punishments.

Clients, especially in nurse-controlled settings such as hospitals, are vulnerable to nurses' decisions to be an immediate part of their social environments, for clients are potential or sometimes unavoidable social objects of a nurse's environment. Nurses may use distancing, avoiding, and several forms of social interaction to control clients' behaviors in hospital settings. In addition, nurses are also frequently in a position to control the makeup of the client's social environment, by limiting visiting hours, allowing rooming-in of family members for hospital care, or by placing the client in hospice care. The social environment of dying patients in our society has been studied and criticized for its impersonality and deception. Such a context seems to prescribe social interactions between professionals, family members, and patients that are psychologically destructive and detrimental to patients. The early work by Fagerhaugh and Strauss (1977) also provides a theoretical insight into the effects of social setting on the way patients respond to pain experiences. Lauzon Clabo (2008) has shown the effects of organizational *habitus* on mode of nurses' pain assessment, suggesting the effects of social environment on nursing practice as proposed by Bourdieu.

Thus, considerations of social environment for human health and health behaviors from the nursing perspective need to be made in two ways: as that influencing the health status of individuals through direct or intervening processes, and as that contributing to the process of health care and nursing practice. The knowledge regarding the social environmental influences on human health and health practices has been translated into health care programs and interventions at individual, group, community, and societal levels.

Symbolic Environment

The meaning of symbolic environment is closely connected with the "sociality" of human history and concomitantly with social environment. It is also closely tied to a human's ability to use language. It is not possible to imagine symbolic environment without people or language and historical accumulation of our thoughts, emotions, and acts. Elements of symbolic environment, if we can call them elements, are bound to human histories and human minds. Symbolic environment is composed of shared ideas on various levels: cultural values, scientific knowledge, social norms, and role expectations, among others. Analytically, an individual's ideas, attitudes, feelings, and knowledge belong to the individual as inherent parts of the individual; hence such elements become intrinsic parts of the individual as a social object. In contrast, "shared ideas" are considered to represent the symbolic environment. In a strict sense, "shared ideas" belong to no one and to everyone. Symbolic environment has meaning for human life to the extent that our behaviors and human happenings are modified and patterned by them, and insofar as the person is able to take in the meanings of symbols. Therefore, for instance, an infant three days old has a symbolic environment that has limited meaning, whereas an adult's symbolic environment would project many and various meanings. In addition, the extent of the symbolic environment is irrelevant to the physical proximity of physical and social objects. Hence, the astronauts on the surface of the moon can be presumed to have had as extensive a symbolic environment as when they were on earth.

Sociologists consider such shared ideas to be functional to societies and social life. Cultural and social values and rules curtail human actions and control the fierce competition and conflict possible among individuals left alone to act according to their personal needs. Symbolic environment allows a client to behave in the "right" ways, while permitting a nurse to provide reinforcements for "right" behaviors. Symbolic environment provides a common reference point from which individuals in social as well as in solitary circumstances recognize and perform valued actions.

Viewed from the nursing perspective, symbolic environment has three specific components: (a) those elements that define "what health and illness are" and "what one 'should' do about one's health and illness"; (b) those elements that define available resources in dealing with health issues; and (c) those elements that prescribe role relationships in health care and nursing practice.

The first component refers to cultural values and social norms regarding health and health behaviors. Cultural definitions of mental illness and controversial "deviance" are good examples of how individuals in a given culture interpret behaviors such as depression and suicide. Social norms exert pressures on individuals to behave in certain ways, as evidenced in fertility rates in societies, or in health care-seeking behaviors for certain kinds of symptoms. Thus, symbolic environments in the form of cultural values and social norms exist for individuals, exerting influences of many sorts on their behaviors. In addition, culture as a value and language system exerts systematic effects on how we interpret human experiences, including disease and illness. Good (1994) states that "culture is not only a means of representing disease, but is essential to its very constitution as a human reality" (p. 53). In this tradition of medical anthropology, culture is viewed as the basis for ontological understanding of disease and illness, and this perspective has led to various interpretivists' studies of disease/illness (for example, Kleinmen, 1973, 1988; Mishler, 1984), and later to critical, postmodernist critiques such as those by Foucault (1965, 1975, 1980) and Waitzkin (1991).

Durkheim's study (1951) of societal differences in suicide rates of 19th-century Europe provides an important background from which the proposition regarding symbolic environments can be reaffirmed. Ills of societies can be examined and explained to a great extent by what Durkheim called "collective tendencies," that is, social conscience. The effects of symbolic environment on an individual's behaviors may be summarized as was done by Durkheim in relation to suicide rates:

> At any given moment the moral constitution of society establishes of contingent of voluntary deaths. There is, therefore, for each people a collective force of a definite amount of energy, impelling men to self-destruction. The victim's acts which at first seem to express only his personal temperament are really the supplement and prolongation of a social condition which they express externally.[5]

Social conscience as a form of symbolic environment provides a context in which members of a society evaluate the quality of life and behavioral consequences. Thus, the occurrence of actual illness conditions and labeling of them are influenced by moral forces in societies.

The second component of the symbolic environment encompasses elements of social institutions, such as science, education, and polity. Scientific knowledge and technology are the major institutional elements that constitute a set of shared ideas in this sense. Fabrega (1974) contends that both health care-seeking behaviors and health care-providing behaviors are determined by theories of illness that are present and shared in a given society. This component of symbolic environment provides a general frame of reference from which a certain level of expectations for control and recovery from illness is formulated in individuals. In primitive societies, this component was mainly made up of notions about supernatural (demonic or godly) influences on human existence. In addition, this component encompasses those symbolic aspects of a society that are defined by structures of institutions such as political, economic, labor, and health care systems. Renaud (1975) argues that capitalist societies are constrained in their problem-solving endeavor relative to health by their economic structure. Health care-providing behaviors appear to differ according to institutionalized structures of health care in different societies.[6] Social institutions thus may be considered strictly as social environment as well as representing value and ideological structures, history, and knowledge. It is necessary, then, to tease out these two different dimensions when considering social institutions as environment.

The third component is more closely tied to social situations and refers to rules of behavior for social roles. Individuals who come together in a social situation assume certain social roles that are congruent with the situation, and behave in accordance with mutual expectations and rules that have been socially learned. Parsons (1951) describes the sick-role expectations in modern Western societies as follows: (a) the person recognizing his or her state of illness considers this state undesirable and wants to get better, (b) the person is not considered to be responsible for his or her condition, (c) the person is excused from ordinary social role obligations, and (d) the person seeks professional help and cooperates with the health care givers. The role expectations of helper and helped are also socially derived and usually known to client and practitioner, who come together in service settings. Because such expectations do not belong to persons, although they are held by them and internalized by them, such elements are part of the symbolic environment.

Important questions regarding the symbolic environment from the nursing perspective should deal with the nature of shared ideas, the extent to which such shared ideas govern behaviors, and characteristics of sharing among individuals in a given society with respect to health, health behavior, and nurse–client relations. When a society goes through disintegration, or when a persisting conflict exists among individuals having different vested interests, one might experience a lack of consensus in behavioral expectations, thus creating chaotic actions. In such cases, the symbolic environment is not enhancing of individuals' behaviors.

HEALTH CARE ENVIRONMENT

When one becomes designated as a client of health care, that person's environment comes to have a rather special meaning, both in an empirical and a symbolic sense. A health care environment evolves around this client who is the recipient of health care services from other persons who have been designated as health care providers. Health care environment of a client can exist for a short duration (such as for a patient in a hospital for an episode of acute illness or in a physician's office for a visit) or for a long, extended duration (such as for a patient in a nursing home or in a long-term care institution).

A health care environment constitutes spatial and qualitative characteristics that are different from the person's ordinary and usual environment, even when the health care or nursing service takes place in the client's home. Physically, the health care environment may include elements that are only present in specialized situations and may not be present in ordinary environments such as home or office. Especially, when the client is in a health care institution such as a hospital or a nursing home, the environment contains many physical objects not found in ordinary living situations, such as various types of health care equipment, and is quite different spatially from the ordinary environment. Socially, it consists of individuals who are not usually present in the ordinary environment, and it may be lacking the usual social constituents such as family members and friends in the immediate part of the environment. Symbolically, the environment encompasses role expectations that are specific to clients, subcultural values and ideas specific to that institution, and specialized knowledge systems of health and health care. Thus, the contents of an environment hold specialized meanings and generate different kinds of influences on clients as well as on health care practices.

Although a health care environment is a somewhat specialized type of environment, an individual can be viewed to be in the core of an environmental field, moving from one form of specialized environment to another throughout the life cycle. Thus, a person gets positioned in different sorts of specialized forms of environment for certain durations through humans' self-determination and mobility as well as through universal, social, and institutional forces of living. A person is specifically in a health care environment when one is in need of health care services and assumes the role of a health care client. The concepts of therapeutic environment and healing environment relate to the qualitative aspect of health care environment, and have been studied in relation to dementia care, psychiatric mental health care, and hospice.

From the nursing perspective, health care environment is an important concept to consider in understanding and explaining clients' health care experiences. Insofar as the health care experiential phenomena of clients require special attention from nursing as suggested especially in chapter 5, the study of such phenomena must be made through the specification and understanding of the health care environment. Often, a health care environment is the source for problematic experiences for clients, such as nosocomial infection, withdrawal, and confusion. For example, Kazanjian, Green, Wong, and Reid (2005) found, in their review of the literature, an association between environmental attributes of hospital nursing practice and patient mortality. On the other hand, a health care environment also may be the source of positive influences on clients' recovery and illness experiences.

Health care environment also is the context in which client–nurse interaction takes place. Various elements (physical, social, or symbolic) of the health care environment may influence the duration, nature, and quality of client–nurse interaction positively or negatively. In addition, nursing practice takes place in a health care environment. Nurses must practice in concert with other nurses and health care providers, under the given organizational, institutional constraints and prescriptions, and in the context of a cultural, professional, and social symbolic system. A great deal of work is ongoing regarding the effects of nursing practice environment on patient outcomes and nursing practice behaviors (Aiken & Patrician, 2000; Boyle, 2004; Heath, Johanson, & Blake, 2004; Lake, 2007; Sochalski, Estabrooks, & Humphrey, 2009).

Health care environment thus needs to be specifically conceptualized in the nursing perspective for knowledge development about phenomena in the client, client–nurse, and practice domains. Understanding and explanation of selected phenomena from the health care environmental perspective would be useful in developing nursing strategies that involve the management of environmental forces. A concept that can be posed opposite to health care environment is "home." There has been some interest shown regarding the concept of home in general and in relation to clients' health and living experiences (Abraham et al., 1991; Doyle, 1992; Moloney, 1997; Rowles, 1987). The concept of home is treated somewhat differently from the concept of family, and encompasses physical, social, and symbolic elements.

ENVIRONMENT IN DIFFERENT THEORETICAL PERSPECTIVES

With the view that environment affects and shapes human conditions, experiences, and living, human civilization has striven to control and manipulate environment so that its effects may be curtailed or directed for positive consequences. Many approaches and theories have also been developed and tried in dealing with illness, including approaches that consider various aspects of environment as key facets influencing the occurrence of disease/illness or supporting healing and recovery. Even in the times when we did not have many causal theories regarding health and disease, manipulation of environment or providing supportive environment was thought critical in nursing, as espoused by Florence Nightingale.

Environment perspectives for nursing knowledge development, as suggested by the exposition in the preceding section, are neither united around a singular conceptualization of environment nor based on one specific explanatory orientation. There are multiple and diverse approaches, rooted in such paradigmatic orientations as multicause models, systems perspectives, holism, ecological or cultural determinism, cultural relativism, multiculturalism, and postmodernism. Within these diverse orientations, environment is viewed differently with respect to how environment relates to the human condition: (a) as causal factors or major determining forces for the human condition, (b) in an exchange framework or interactive/interpenetrating relations, (c) as contexts that determine interpretive frames, (d) in establishing differences, and (e) as conditions of constraints.

Accordingly, environment in nursing is conceptualized in various ways. For example, a cursory review of the literature suggests that environment is described in conjunction with such adjectives as physical, multisensory, psychological, social, cultural, learning, healing, health care, managed-care, work, organizational, global, unitary, and so on. In addition, the term "environment" is used interchangeably or in relation to such concepts as ecosystem, field, context, structure, microcosmos, or cosmos. This means that environment as the context of human existence has varied meanings. Within the conceptualization of environment discussed in the preceding sections, one can delineate several approaches to nursing knowledge development by focusing on environment. The following four approaches as relevant to nursing knowledge development will be discussed:

- Effects approaches
- Interdependence approaches
- Environment-as-context approaches
- Postmodern approaches

Effects Approaches

In these approaches, which have been the dominant ways of treating environment in relation to health, illness, and nursing practice, certain aspects of environment are viewed as having influences on human experience. Many of the causal models introduce environmental factors as one of the components explaining human states and behaviors. Physical as well as social and symbolic aspects of environment have been introduced in such models as causal, influencing, or contributing factors that bring about changes in human behaviors, human experiences, or the human condition. In such models, an environmental aspect is one of many clusters of those explaining the changes. Most commonly extracted aspects of physical environment introduced in such models relevant to nursing are related to the quality of physical environment, such as sound, air quality, crowding, and stability, although social support and family environment have been introduced quite often in such models within the social components of environment. For example, models addressing developmental trajectory of preterm infants include the physical conditions of incubators as well as the work of parents and practitioners as stimuli for maturation and development. Such models have also been used often to develop interventions and strategies in nursing, as it is quite possible to manipulate environmental factors to avert or reduce negative effects on the human condition. Especially in nursing, social support has been considered an important contributing factor that influences health behaviors, such as health promotion, as well as health care behaviors such as compliance or participation in rehabilitation.

The debates in nursing and psychology regarding nature versus nurture involve the controversy over the role of environment, in the form of family, for example, as the source of parenting, or the school environment for socialization, pitted against genetic make-up and other endowments viewed as "nature." The theoretical camp for "nurture" stresses the role of environmental stimuli rather than natural endowment as the key factor in shaping and molding personality, habits, attitudes, and so forth.

Another theoretical approach having its origin in sociology asserts social structural effects on human behaviors. In nursing, this has been adopted to explain health/illness behaviors in relation to social structural conditions and nurses' practice behaviors specifically with respect to structural conditions of health care organization. This structuralism posits the effects of socialization, enculturation, and integration as having a greater impact on human behaviors than individual differences.

The major task facing nursing knowledge development in this approach is clearly related to refining our knowledge about the causal processes with which environmental factors influence the human condition. Unfortunately, models developed from this approach often give superficial explanations, without specifying exact causal processes.

Interdependence Approaches

During the past three decades many theorists and researchers in nursing have adopted human–environment interdependence approaches. There are three distinct approaches that are relevant to nursing knowledge development: those oriented to cosmic holism, those within the systems perspective, and those that are oriented to human/environment interaction.

Rogers's science of unitary humans is most noteworthy: an approach within a holistic tradition that specifies human and environment energy fields from the perspective of mutuality and interpenetration. Rogers identifies three principles of homeodynamics to depict human/environment interaction: integrality, resonancy, and helicy. Human and environmental energy fields are viewed to be in constant, mutual interaction, interpenetrating each other through mutual and simultaneous changes that are dynamic and rhythmic as well as innovative, unpredictable, and moving toward increasing complexity and diversity (Rogers, 1992). Parse (1997a), in her human becoming theory, also supposes constant interrelationships of humans with the universe in humanity's evolving, negentropic "unfolding" that is characterized by meaning, rhythmicity and cotranscendence. To Parse, the universe is the totality of environment. These two theoretical positions are oriented to cosmic holism, in which humans and their environment form interrelated and integrated wholes. In a somewhat different orientation, Kleffel (1996) suggests that the shift in nursing to study environment from the ecocentric paradigm may be in line with the changing concept of the world as a global community.

Theorists such as Imogine King and Betty Neuman, operating from the systems perspective, consider environment in supersystem and subsystem relations. King (1981) presents a system-oriented conceptual framework for nursing and specifies the personal, the interpersonal, and the social systems as three interacting systems, in which goal, structure, function, resources, and decision making are the major orientations that determine the nature of interaction. Clients and nurses as human systems are viewed by King to be in interaction not only with each other but also with the environment. To King, the environment is the social system that is defined as "an organized boundary system of social roles, behaviors, and practices developed to maintain values and the mechanisms to regulate practice and rules" (1981, p. 115). Neuman, on the other hand, considers environment as the major source of stressors that impinge on clients as open systems. To Neuman (1998), environment consists of internal, external, and created environments.

The third approach encompasses several positions in which person–environment fit is viewed to be essential in describing and explaining human conditions and experiences. For example, a person–environment congruence model focuses on the nature of fit between a person and his/her environment as the source for negative experiences, whereas a person–environment interaction model views interaction between a person and his/her environment in a given situation as producing differences in the person's responses in situations. This means that a person does not just locate oneself in an environment (a specific situation or field), but becomes engaged with the environment and exhibits behaviors, actions, and feelings accordingly. This notion has been examined extensively in psychology, in which persons are observed to behave and act differently according to test situations (see, for example, Mortensen, 2000). In a somewhat different perspective, Gadow (1992) proposes a dialectical approach in ecology, describing ways of knowing the world and of being in the world. Person–environment relation is viewed as existential engagement of "homing," in which nature as "an irreducible web of relations" is lived and experienced locally rather than colonially. To Gadow, "living reciprocally within nature makes it a home, the fundamental form of human culture" (1992, p. 601). Nature is a home, particularized and local to a specific person, lived reciprocally, which is tied inseparably with that life. Hence, the knowledge from this perspective is local and can be expressed as nongeneralizable narratives of human experiences of homing.

In these approaches, it is clear that environment is viewed as infused within the person who carries on living. Several different methods are appropriate in developing knowledge with these approaches. Nursing scholars have been struggling to come up with appropriate methods, however there still is a great need to refine methods in this regard.

Environment-as-Context Approaches

The view of environment as context refers to the notion that humans' lives are shaped by the context that provides conceptual/linguistic, ideational, cultural, and historical frames of reference. The locality of our being, not as a temporary situation but as an enduring context, provides us with orientations necessary to form patterns of our behaviors. Hence, within this notion, people's behaviors are viewed to be more bound to culture than to individual differences. From this perspective, several different approaches to studying environment as culture are found in the literature. There has been much debate in the literature regarding cultural relativism and its relation to multiculturalism, cross-culturalism, and transculturalism, all of which consider culture as the major contextual feature that determines human lives and behaviors in an enduring way. In addition, cultural hermeneutics has been espoused as a way to move our knowledge of illness and practice to a new level.

Cultural relativism posits the supremacy of cultural determination as a legitimating process for social relations and people's behaviors, accentuating the need for acceptance and tolerance of differences that are based on culture. Culture-bound syndromes, cultural definitions of human body, culture-specific conceptions of mental illness, and cultural healing practices are examples of ways in which the origins of differences are rooted in cultural beliefs and practices and become adopted and internalized to serve as guides for people's behaviors. Cultural relativism not only refers to differences in relation to culture in general, but also has been espoused by a branch of feminist philosophy aligned with Gilligan's work of gender differences. As Baker (1997) states, cultural relativism presents dilemmas for nursing, especially in making cross-cultural judgments regarding people's health-related behaviors.

Much work in nursing in relation to cultural relativism has appeared as multiculturalism, cross-culturalism, and transculturalism, seeking to address both the dangers of normative application of the dominant cultural orientations and the difficulties associated with acknowledging, accepting, and working with differences stemming from cultural orientations. Uzarewicz defines transculturality and transcultural nursing based on "knowledge of one's own cultural foundations, the knowledge of other cultural phenomena, and the synthesis of both in a particular context of human action" (1999, p. 82). The major epistemological question in this regard has to do with the relationships between human universals (espoused by foundationalism) and differences (espoused by cultural relativism). On the other hand, political and moral implications of cultural relativism raise the dangers of accentuating stereotyping, promoting ethnic labels and segregation, and blaming, especially within professional practice.

Culture as context is also related to hermeneutic philosophy, in which all human actions are considered to be constructed with meanings originating in the context (i.e., culture), having specific history, language, and meaning systems. From this tradition, the study of health/illness and health-related practices focuses on interpretation of meaning. A Gadamerian perspective of hermeneutic philosophy points first to the context-dependent nature of meaning and second to the possibility of understanding of meanings through fusion of horizons. From this tradition, Kleinman (1973, 1977) and Good and Good (1981) proposed a "meaning-centered" or cultural hermeneutic tradition for the study of illness in anthropology, placing "the relation of culture and illness at the center of analytic interest" (Good, 1994, p. 52). Good and Good state that "a meaning-centered or interpretive medical anthropology approaches sickness not as a reflection or causal product of somatic processes but as a meaningful human reality. It views healing as transactions across meaning systems—popular, religious, folk, professional—that result in the construction of culturally specific illness realities' and as therapeutic efforts to transform those realities" (1981, p. 174). Purkis (1994) also urges nursing to include "the social" in the study of nursing practice. Understanding of illness and healing practices as well as professional practice is gained through interpretation of meanings constructed within cultural context. For nursing, such understanding can provide the foundation for practice that is not solely entrenched within the empirical outlook.

Another development in nursing that considers environment as context comes from Im and Meleis's proposal for situation-specific nursing theories. Situation-specific theories are defined as: (a) "theories that focus on specific nursing phenomena that reflect clinical practice and that are limited to specific populations or to particular fields of practice," (b) are considered in "social and historical context," and (c) are "not developed to transcend time, a socially constraining structure, or a politically limiting situation" (Im & Meleis, 1999, p. 13). This approach introduces situation-specific explanations when dealing with theories developed within the larger philosophical foundation of "contemporary empiricism," in which explanation and prediction are the major goals of theory. The span of explanation and prediction by such theories is viewed to be limited within the contextual boundaries for which the theories are developed. Situation-specific theories begin at a low level of abstraction for the phenomena of concern, build theories for nursing phenomena limited to a specific population or to a particular field of practice, and are intended for limited generalizations rather than universal generalization. Limiting generalization results from the orientation of situation-specific theories in social, cultural, and historical contexts. Hence, the foundation for this proposal is cultural relativism in a broad sense. Here, culture is considered a constraint on people's experiences, with respect not only to value systems, but also to enduring situational characteristics, such as religion, beliefs, language, customs, collective histories, and sociopolitics. As many situation-specific theories are generated, it may be possible to delineate the limits of universality and the nature of diversity and develop a base for linking generality at a broad level to contextual differences and to individual uniqueness.

Another recent development in sociology comes from Pierre Bourdieu, who considers human practice as a function of *habitus* and fields of practice. To Bourdieu, individuals act in specific social contexts or settings (that is, fields) and produce "practice" through the coordination between the *habitus* and the field within which the specific act takes place. Fields, as social contexts, are seen as "a structured space of positions in which the positions and their interrelations are determined by the distribution of different kinds of resources or 'capital' " (Bourdieu, 1990, p. 14). Practice seen in this way thus needs to be examined in relation to what the nature of *habitus* is and how it is brought to bear within a specific field as a multidimensional space of relations among relevant resources (such as cultural capital, economic capital, symbolic capital, or power). Hence, the context is not just an unorganized situation but a space with inherent rules that determine relations among actors. In nursing, it is possible to consider clients' and nurses' actions as practices that are evident in situations as the productions of coordination between a given *habitus* and its fields of actions. This perspective leads us to an understanding of the generative and transposable nature of *habitus*, and the specific forms of relations among key resources that make up the field of practice (Lauzon Clabo, 2008).

Nursing knowledge development with a view of environment as context is faced with a great challenge, as context is "so to speak" everywhere constraining clients' experiences and lives, client–nurse interaction, and nursing practice.

Postmodern Approaches

Postmodern approaches in treating environment as social context put human existence and experience as fundamentally and thoroughly constrained by language (i.e., discursive practices) and power entrenched within the historic context. The focus, however, in postmodern approaches to the human condition is collective rather than individual, with subjective experiences analyzed vis-à-vis their relation to power processes. Foucault, for example, in conjunction with his "genealogy" of power, analyzed the politics of sexuality, madness, medical practice, and hospitals via discursive practices and offered a basis for representing illness as mystification based on relations of power, specifically viewing medical practice in relation to disciplinary power (Foucault, 1965, 1973, 1980). Deleuze, in analyzing current social conditions, suggests that we "are in control societies that no longer function by internment but rather by constant control and direct communication" (as quoted by Balke, 1999, p. 178). Balke (1999), following Deleuze's analysis, suggests that the transition to control from disciplinary societies has turned around an individual's lot from that of confinement to one of indebtedness. It requires individuals to be responsible not only for self-surveillance but also for surveillance of others with respect to health and illness. Postmodern approaches direct our attention to broad social discursive practices through which power processes that govern the contextual landscape of individual acts are revealed and dissected. For nursing, investigation of power processes is vital with respect not only to an individual's illness experience but also to a nurse's practice experience.

Environment as discussed in this exposition can be brought into the study of nursing from various perspectives and approaches. Environment is not a simple milieu of our existence, but is a source for various heuristic, explanatory, and enlightening understanding about human experiences and conditions. Not only are phenomena in the client, client–nurse, and practice domains influenced by environment; the client, client–nurse, and practice domains also are entities of experience embedded in environment in concrete and symbolic ways.

SELECTED CONCEPTUAL ANALYSES

Among many possible concepts within the domain of environment appropriate for studying from the nursing perspective are sensory deprivation, social support, and sick-role expectation, as shown in Table 8.1. This table presents examples of concepts in the domain of environment that are thought to be appropriate for theoretical considerations from the nursing perspective.

Sensory deprivation is considered as an example of physical environment phenomena; social support as that of social environment phenomena; and sick-role expectation as an example of symbolic environment phenomena. The main purpose of this section is to show how a first-level analytical approach is used to gain conceptual and empirical understanding of phenomena within the domain of environment. Each concept is analyzed

Table 8.1

EXAMPLES OF CONCEPTS IN THE DOMAIN OF ENVIRONMENT FOR STUDY IN THE NURSING PERSPECTIVE

ENVIRONMENTAL COMPONENT	CONCEPT
Physical environment	■ Crowding ■ Ecosystem ■ Energy ■ Heat ■ Noise ■ Pathogens ■ Sensory deprivation ■ Sensory overload ■ Space, territory, proxemics ■ Time
Social environment	■ Affective milieu ■ Competition ■ Family ■ Marginality ■ Significant others ■ Social capital ■ Social control ■ Social isolation ■ Social proximity ■ Social support
Symbolic environment	■ Ethical standards ■ Institutional history ■ Metanarratives ■ Morality ■ Norm ■ Positivism ■ Power structure (authority) ■ Rationality ■ Role expectations ■ Scientific knowledge ■ Sick-role expectations
Holistic concepts	■ Energy field ■ Health care environment ■ Home ■ Place ■ Universe

with respect to (a) definitional clarification and conceptual meanings as reflected in the literature, (b) essential descriptive features and characteristics as a step toward an empirical analysis, and (c) the concept's relationships with other concepts that are important in nursing. The strategy and rationale for the conceptual analysis were discussed in detail in chapter 2, and that rationale is adopted in this section for the analyses of sensory deprivation, social support, and sick-role expectation. These three concepts are well established, with a long history of exposition in the literature. Most of the recent works on these concepts tend to be oriented to empirical examinations in relation to health and health behaviors rather than refinement of conceptualization. The literature base for these concepts regarding conceptualization goes back several decades.

SENSORY DEPRIVATION

Definition

Environment is the source of sensory inputs for human perceptions: sound, color, form, texture, temperature, and many other physical characteristics are perceived and sensed for a person to make assessments about the world around him or her and gauge his or her position in relation to them. A person recognizes familiar objects and persons, learns about new objects, and guards against unfamiliar objects that are judged to be potentially threatening. A person's life in a vacuum, if that is at all possible, may represent an ultimate state of absence of sensory input to the person. Persons placed in solitary confinements in jail or hospitals have been found to create sensory inputs by banging their heads on walls, scratching, or screaming. Lack of sensory input is threatening to adults who have learned to perceive the world through the senses. Thus, it tends to create a sense of disconnectedness with the world in persons when they are placed in a sensory-deprived environment. People receiving no sensory input may begin to doubt their own existence. Infants who are placed in a deprived (sensory) environment have also been found to assume the condition of "deprivation dwarfism" (Gardner, 1972).

The basic premises for the occurrence of such phenomena are that the human brain matures and develops through sensory stimulation, and that human behavior is shaped by functional and structural organization of information that occurs in the brain. Hebb's attempt (1949) to explain perceptual behavior in relation to the function of the central nervous system was the first link made between behavior and sensory experience. He postulated that perceptual behavior is influenced by early experience with deprivation of vision and other sense modalities and that monotonous, unchanging stimulation resulted in a disorganization of the ability and capacity to think. In more recent times sophisticated neuropsychological and neurobehavioral models have been advanced through testing in both animal models and humans to link sensory input with neurophysiological alteration and behaviors (see, for example, Neville & Bavelier, 2002).

By definition, then, sensory deprivation is a lack or reduction of sensory stimulation in several different forms, varying in intensity, duration, and characteristics. As early as 1949, Bakan described sensory deprivation as a state in which an organism is deprived of normal, complex sensory stimulation from the external environment for a specified period (Brownfield, 1972). Yet, there has been little agreement in the use and definition of the term describing the phenomenon. Rossi (1969) cites 25 different terms used more or less interchangeably with sensory deprivation in the literature. The problem of definition has been complicated because of the nature of research being done in the field. Many research studies adopt experimental conditions to "induce" the phenomenon of sensory deprivation artificially, and such procedural terms have been used interchangeably to denote the phenomenon in a limited sense.

In general, there are two broadly and distinctly different conceptualizations of sensory deprivation: (a) a state in which the focus is the environment and (b) a state in which the focus is the individual organism experiencing the deprivation. The first conceptualization considers the phenomenon strictly in relation to the environmental characteristics, as a lack, reduction, or monotonicity of sensory stimulation in the environment. The second conceptualization, on the other hand, refers either to the condition of the person being in a "deprived" state or to a process in which a phenomenological experience of deprivation takes place in the person (Rossi, 1969). Black, McKenna, and Deeny (1997) suggest a new term, *sensoristrain*, to describe such deprived states seen in patients, as often there is no clear demarcation between a "deprived" state and an "overload" state. This second conceptualization refers to phenomena in clients, and thus would be appropriate to study in the context of the client domain. It appears however that there is an analytical value in considering the phenomenon in two such separate ways. Our interest in the conceptualization of sensory deprivation is in line with the first type, in which the environmental characteristics are the focus.

Suedfeld (1969) categorizes sensory deprivation as exhibiting three major characteristics: the reduction of stimulus-input levels, the reduction of stimulus-variability, and sensory-social isolation and confinement. Although these three characteristics have somewhat distinct meanings, there is a circularity in meaning relationships among them. Invariably, in nonexperimental situations, a reduction of stimulus variability that is produced by monotonous stimulation will result in a reduction of stimulus-input levels, and vice versa. In addition, sensory-social isolation and confinement frequently accompany both a reduction of stimulus variability and a reduction of stimulus-input levels.

Descriptive Features and Characteristics

The phenomenal features of sensory deprivation have been described in research in two specific ways: as an environment in which there is a reduction in intensity of sensory inputs, and as an environment in which there is homogeneous and unpatterned input. Both of these features have been used to create an experimental environment in research.

The first type of operationalization generally refers to an experimental condition deliberately lacking in sensory stimulation, such as silence and darkness, as used by Myers and his colleagues (1963). The second type of operationalization refers to an experimental environment in which there is a limitation in the variability of sensory input, such as constant masking of sensory input via white noise and diffused light, as used in McGill studies (Scott, Bexton, Heron, & Doane, 1959). Operationalizations used in such experimental conditions create conceptual complications in that, when an environment has been manipulated to reduce sensory input, the remaining sensory elements in the environment take on different perceptual meanings for the person exposed to such an environment.

In addition, in most research studies, sensory deprivation has been operationalized to include the aspects of visual and auditory stimuli, with little emphasis on tactile, olfactory, kinesthetic, gustatory, and proprioceptive sense modalities. However, sensory deprivation operationalized in developmental research, in many cases, includes the concept of multisensory deprivation. Deprivation of visual, auditory, tactile, and movement stimulation has been used specifically to indicate the deprivation of novelty in stimulation in those developmental studies. Stimulation for new learning is absent as a result of such deprivation (Riesen & Zilbert, 1975).

Descriptive features of sensory deprivation referring to naturally occurring environmental conditions have been limited to hospital and nursing-home settings (Worrell, 1971). The most commonly studied settings of sensory deprivation in the health care situation are: private room for a coronary patient; private room for a surgical patient, especially a patient with cardiac surgery; elderly patient, especially the elder who has decreased sensory abilities such as blindness, hearing loss, or other perceptual loss; "isolation" or "seclusion" room (Meehan, Vermeer, & Windsor, 2000); hospital settings for immobilized patients, such as those with stroke, in traction, or with spinal cord injury; and private room for a patient with eye surgery. These kinds of nursing care situations have a reduced input of (rather than a complete lack of) sensory stimulation and usually provide monotonous or unchanging stimulations of sounds and visual objects. Monotonous sensory input of a mute nature has been defined as perceptual deprivation, differentiating it from the general concept of sensory deprivation.

Perceptual deprivation, defined as such, is more commonly detectable in clinical, practice settings. Newman (1981) studied the isolette environment of preterm infants, in which the isolette environment is perceived as an auditory environment of high ground noise and intrusive sound of a disturbing nature. This isolette environment was conceived to provide infants with a situation in which human sounds are filtered by such ground noises. It is thus seen as producing perceptual deprivation in infants.

Social isolation, confinement, withdrawal, and neglect have also been used to denote sensory deprivation in sociological and psychological studies. In particular, the isolation and confinement of the elderly in single-occupancy hotel rooms in which variation in sensory input is lacking for an extended period of time have been considered as an environment of sensory deprivation for the elderly.

It appears that how the descriptive features and characteristics of sensory deprivation are specified depends on one's definition of the term and can vary from deprivation of one sensory modality to a complete deprivation of sensory input as well as monotonization of sensory input.

Differentiation of the Concept of Sensory Deprivation From Isolation

The phenomenon of isolation encompasses a broader conceptual meaning than that of sensory deprivation. Isolation suggests removing a person to a confined area without allowing normal contacts with the external world. Brownfield (1972) suggests four kinds of isolation: (a) *confinement*, in which a person is placed in a limited space, restraining the freedom of movement and in which sensory deprivation may vary according to the nature of the space; (b) *separation*, in which a person is placed in an environment where personal contacts with particular persons, places, or things are not allowed, and which brings about deprivation of special kinds of sensory inputs; (c) *removal* from the total environment, in which a person is placed in an environment of reduced normal stimulation or no stimulation, such as solitary confinement; and (d) *monotony* of stimulation, in which a person is exposed to unchanging, invariable, and boring sensory inputs that eventually lose their ability to elicit responses.

Thus, the phenomenon of isolation may be induced by unconscious or conscious acts by a person (i.e., psychologically based), such as voluntary deprivation, self-punishment, or social isolation because of fear, religious beliefs, or conscience, but also may be imposed by external forces, such as immobility, old age, loss of sensory ability, or impoverished early experience. Of course, isolation also occurs by external force such as imprisonment and solitary confinement in hospitals for various reasons.

In general, isolation encompasses the aspects of social and psychological separation, whereas sensory deprivation is associated with the characteristics of the environment with respect to its sensory stimulation. Of course, isolation is a situation in which sensory deprivation is likely to occur. In differentiating the phenomena of isolation and sensory deprivation, one source of confusion has been in the use of experimental "isolation" techniques in sensory deprivation research. Such techniques invariably combine reduction and monotonization of stimulation in isolating experimental subjects for purposes of manipulating sensory inputs.

Relationship to Other Concepts

Most of the studies in the field of sensory deprivation may be categorized into those relating sensory deprivation to developmental consequences and those relating sensory deprivation to other behavioral responses such as hallucination and confusion.

There are many studies in the first category, emphasizing the maturational effects on specific senses and the general behavioral and developmental consequences. Animal and human studies found relationships between early visual experience (or the lack of it) and visual preference, indicating the influence of early sensory stimulation on sensory maturation (Annis & Frost, 1973; Tees, Midgley, & Bruinsma, 1980). Bingham (2009) suggests that oral sensory deprivation in premature infants during tube feeding may have effects on later swallowing competence. In addition, Prescott (1980) suggests that sensory deprivation during early development leads to stimulus-seeking behaviors relative to the deprived sensory systems, and further that somatosensory, affectional deprivation from isolation rearing may be responsible for violent behaviors toward self and others. Deprivation dwarfism has also been suggested as a secondary effect of hypopituitarism produced by sensory deprivation in animals and humans. Alcoholism and drug abuse as stimulus-seeking behaviors have been postulated to be the results of such deprivation. Thus, the individual is assumed to be attempting to gain the sensory stimulation that was deprived early in life.

One of the major variables identified as a consequence of sensory deprivation in the second category of studies is hallucinatory activity such as visual imagery and test performance found in McGill studies (Bexton, Heron, & Scott, 1954). Zuckerman (1969) explains the phenomenon of hallucination as a self-aroused imagery perceived by a person because of a lack of competing sensory inputs. A person in an environment without patterned and changing stimulation eventually may become sensitized to more organized images whose site of origin lies higher in the nervous system and may be intensified by a high state of arousal or by reduction in competing stimuli, thus appearing as visual images localized in space in front of the person.

It also has been shown that visual deprivation is associated with an increased tactual acuity, pain sensitivity, auditory discrimination, and olfactory and gustatory sensitivity. In addition, other single-modality deprivation can also produce behavioral changes (Zubek, 1969). Biochemical changes, especially those produced by steroids and endorphins, have been the concerns of many current studies, suggesting a linkage between sensory deprivation and behavioral changes mediated by internal processes of biochemical synthesis (Prescott, 1980; Zubek, 1969).

The effects of sensory deprivation associated with specific health care settings such as hospitals have been documented in relation to chronic pain experiences (Schofield & Davis, 1998), in high-risk antepartum patients' experiences (Stainton, Lohan, Fethney, Woodhart, & Islam, 2006), and in relation to functional decline and confusion in hospitalized older adults (Graf, 2006; Tullmann & Dracup, 2000).

Suedfeld (1969) and Zuckerman (1969) have examined various theoretical approaches used in studies of sensory deprivation and found diversity both in the explanations and in inclusion of various types of dependent variables in the explanations.

In the nursing literature, sensory deprivation has been handled in a casual, cursory manner. Theoretical or empirical writings are rarely found on this subject, although sensory deprivation in practice settings is often seen in hospitalized and nursing home patients, and nurses have observed its deleterious effect on patients. Many nurses in clinical case studies and at clinical conferences have reported complaints of hallucination and confusion by post-surgical patients, trauma patients, elderly patients, and immobilized patients. The importance of sensory deprivation for a nursing study is apparent, in view of the fact that most of the naturally occurring sensory deprivations are present in health care environments and also that effects of sensory deprivation are general and nonspecific to the person and his or her development. Furthermore, sensory deprivation as a phenomenon of the client's environment may complicate the client's recovery from illness in a rather complex manner. The environment of nursing care may inadvertently be the source of sensory deprivation to the client, thus becoming a deleterious rather than an enhancing environment for health recovery and health maintenance.

SOCIAL SUPPORT

Definition

In general, social support refers to positive, reinforcing attitudes generated by individuals in social relation to each other. Although it is this "supportiveness" that is central to the concept, it has been used in research synonymously with social network, social bond, and social integration. This has created some confusion in the theoretical formulation of the concept.

The main confusion is embedded in viewing the *source* of "support" (i.e., social relation and social network) interchangeably with the *nature* of "support." For example, Antonovsky (1979) states that social support is the extent to which a person is lodged in social networks to which the person is committed; yet social support is also conceptualized as the extensiveness of social relationships (Eaton, 1978). In addition, "meaningful social contact" (Cassel, 1976), availability of confidants (Miller & Ingham, 1976), human companionship (Lynch, 1977), social bond (Henderson, 1980), and social network (Mueller, 1980; Norbeck, 1981) all have been used to make inferences about social support. Although the assumption is that social relationships and networks provide support, evidence indicates that the relationship between the intensity, size, and extensity of a social network and social support is not linear.

Cobb (1976) and Turner (1981) consider social support on the basis of three types of information:

- Affective information—information suggestive of being loved and cared for
- Information of worthiness—information suggestive of being valued and esteemed
- Information of partisanship—information suggestive of belonging to mutually influencing social relations.

In similar fashion, Kaplan, Cassell, and Gore (1977) define social support as the degree to which an individual's needs for affection, security, approval, belongingness, and identity are "met" through social interaction. This definition also assumes that the person's perception is an integral part of social support.

What does not emerge from these definitions is the suggestion of different kinds of support that are possible in social relations. Linking the conceptualization of social network as the source of social support and the reference-group theory proposed by Merton (1968) could raise this question. The reference-group theory suggests that individuals use their social contacts as the framework for receiving reinforcement, support, and evaluations when making behavioral choices and in expressing ideas and attitudes. Hence, the information one receives from relationships with others may be both emotional (affective) and cognitive (evaluative), and both types of information may be "supportive" to the person in general or in specific situations. Therefore, it is possible to conceptualize social support as information generated to a person in social relations, information that has either a general affective or specific instrumental meaning of support.

Descriptive Features and Characteristics

Different definitions of social support used in the field have resulted in a confusing picture regarding the descriptive features and attributes of the concept. In defining social support as more "affective" than "instrumental" information, Turner (1981) used self-evaluation of the perceived level of information generated by others to indicate the level of social support. LaRocco, House, and French (1980) also defined social support as perceived psychological and tangible support from supervisors, coworkers, spouse, family, and friends. They specifically defined social support as "emotional supportiveness." A limitation in this kind of operationalization is the lack of objective criteria to attest to the fit between perceived information and actual supportiveness present in social relations.

It is problematic to assume that "perceived" support equals "real" support present in the social environment. This difficulty stems from two issues: (a) perception can be influenced by a person's interpretation of meanings attached to self, others, situation, and happenings; and (b) supportiveness may not be apparent until actual "incidents" or occasions call for mobilization of support being offered or already given by others. The first problem points up the need for objective criteria for interpretations; the second issue raises a further question regarding the need for differentiating generalized versus contextual or specialized support.

A more inclusive operationalization of the concept of social support is found in several studies. Gore (1978) operationalizes social support on three dimensions: (a) a person's perception of supportiveness of significant others; (b) frequency of activity outside the home with significant others that indicates amount of social interaction; and (c) perceived opportunity for engaging in supportive and satisfying social activities. Similarly, Lin, Simeone, Ensel, and Kuo (1979) define social support as support accessible to an individual through social ties to other individuals, groups, and the larger community. They measure the concept by the degree of social interaction and involvement and the level of social adjustment. Other researchers also have operationalized social support on multidimensional levels, including social relations, perceptions, and type of support.

In nursing, based on the works of Cobb (1976), Hinson and associates (1997) and House (1981) extracted four defining attributes of social support as: emotional, instrumental, informational, and appraisal, viewed as helpful and protective forces to persons receiving the support; these attributes were also identified in the study by Murray (2000). On the other hand, Finfgeld-Connett (2005) in a metasynthesis study states that social support is composed of emotional and instrumental support, suggesting different meanings and utilities social support has for individuals.

Although the concept of social support has become a rather standard concept applied to study the effects of social environment in nursing as well as in health-related fields, including medical sociology, across 4 decades, there is no consensus regarding specific attributes for the concept. Furthermore, operational difficulties in differentiating the nature of affective and instrumental support and in attaining consensus regarding perceived support vis-à-vis "apparent" support need to be addressed. Although most researchers readily associate "sources of support" with significant others and social networks, there has been a complicating development in the literature during the past 10 years with the introduction of the concept of social capital, which has become an umbrella concept for both social network and social support.

Differentiation of the Concept of Social Support From Social Capital

As mentioned earlier in this chapter, the concept of social capital emerged in the social science literature since the early 1990s, overshadowing various conceptualizations of social environment. The theoretical proposals by Bourdieu (1986, 1990), Coleman (1988), and Putnam (1993, 1995) stimulated examinations of social capital in various sociological studies as well as in nursing, studying individual behaviors such as health as well as community-level activities. The concept of social capital subsumes social networks, social support, social cohesion, and sometimes includes material as well as social resources. The definitions offered by the pioneer researchers differ somewhat, especially those by Bourdieu and Putnam, so there are various conceptualizations of the social capital in play. Bourdieu (1986) defined it as "the aggregate of actual or potential resources linked to possession of a durable network" and as that to be used by those in power to maintain their power. On the other hand, Putnam (1993, 2000) defined the concept as norms of reciprocity, social networks/voluntary associations, and generalized trust facilitating cooperation for mutual benefit, and further specified it as consisting of "bonding" and "bridging" social capital. And finally, Portes (1998) states that social capital has come to mean "the ability to secure benefits through membership in networks and other social structures."

These definitions have gone through various changes and revisions in the literature during the past two decades, and social capital has been defined as social relations and networks and as resources at individual and collective levels. Thus, Brunie (2009) specifies three characteristics of the concept used in the literature: (a) relational social capital, that is, networks in the dimensions of network resources and network structure encompassing social support; (b) collective social capital, a collective resource that facilitates cooperation at the small group level; and (c) generalized social capital, a subjective property of individuals in interrelationships such as trust. On the other hand, Hawe and Shiell (2000) differentiate the concept at the micro level to mean integrated local networks and individuals' linkages to outside groups, and at the macro level to mean the synergy between society and individuals and the autonomy for institutions and organizations, thus having relational, material, and political meanings.

However, the overall inclination has been to treat the concept of social support as a part of social capital in connection with social networks and network relationships. Thus, there has been a trend to apply the concept of social support as a study in social capital. There is a growing tension in the literature regarding the complexity, multiplicity, and lack of clarity in both the conceptual and the theoretical approaches to social capital (Ferlander, 2007; Smart, 2008; Svendsen, 2006), which has a ripple effect on the concept of social support.

Relationship to Other Concepts

Social support has been used to explain various phenomena in individuals' lives. The basic notion is that an individual's behaviors may be explained by factors in his or her social environment such as social network, interaction patterns, or structures of social institutions. This notion extends the expla nation of human behavior beyond the attributes of individuals themselves. Social support has been applied in many studies to explain the relationships among social environment, occurrence and management of stress, health status, and other social behaviors. Social support has been viewed to have mediating or buffering effects on the way individuals handle stress, modify illness responses associated with life's stresses, and affect the rate and quality of health-services utilization.

In her study of the effects of social support in moderating the health consequences of unemployment, Gore (1978) suggested that the loss of self-worth through unemployment, confounded by the lack of social support, contributed to negative health consequences. Myers, Lindenthal, and Pepper (1975) also concluded that persons with high social integration scores seem better able to cope with the impact of life's stresses, alluding to the idea that access to social support and integration contribute to better coping with stress. Many other researchers have also proposed the same mechanism.

Evidence of the effects of social support on health behaviors and health care utilization behaviors has been reported in the literature since the concept was introduced in the 1970s along with the introduction of social capital to study human behaviors. The review of the literature by Callaghan and Morrissey (1993) shows some indications of the impact of social support on illness experiences, mental health experiences, and bonding, although Pahl (2003) finds methodological and explanatory issues in making connections between social support and well-being. The studies utilizing the concept of social capital have shown positive impacts on health both at the micro level in relation to health-promoting behaviors and at the macro level for public health. However, Kritsotakis and Gamarnikow (2004) suggest that the relationships are tentative, and Ferlander (2007) suggests that there is a need to study the effects on health of bridging social capital.

Effects of social support on a client's compliance with health care practices and therapies have also been frequently documented in the nursing literature. It appears that clients who have support in their daily life are more likely to adhere to many unfavored and/or unpleasant regimens, as compared with those individuals who are lacking in social reinforcement.

From the nursing perspective, three major phenomena seem important to study in relation to social support:

- The individual's patterns of coping with stress
- The individual's reactions and behaviors related to illness experiences
- The individual's compliance behaviors with regard to health care regimens

SICK-ROLE EXPECTATION

Definition

Parsons (1951) defines illness as a state of disturbance in the "normal" functioning of the total human individual, including both the state of the organism as a biological being, and the state of his or her personal and social adjustments. It is therefore viewed as a form of "social" deviance that requires management by mechanisms of social control. Hence, the sick role as "the institutionalized expectation system" is conceptualized by Parsons as the mechanism of social control for an individual's illness.

Parsons (1951) proposed that the institutionalized expectation system of the sick role is composed of four aspects:

- A sick person expects an exemption from normal social role responsibilities, an exemption of varying extent according to the nature and severity of the illness, and expects the exemption to be legitimatized by someone and to members of immediate support groups.
- A sick person is absolved of "being responsible" for his or her illness.
- A sick person is expected to want to get well, since the state of being ill is viewed as undesirable.
- A sick person is expected—and compelled—to submit to technically competent help.

Twaddle (1979) suggests that the conceptualization of the sick role is specifically tied to the view that "sickness" is a social label for the state of being unwell or "unhealthy." He also differentiates three states that comprise "nonhealth": disease, referring to biological capacities; illness, encompassing subjective or psychological meanings; and sickness, referring to a social aspect. Thus, to be sick is to have certain rights and obligations ascribed by social role expectations, to be diseased means to have signs and symptoms of disturbance, and to be ill is to feel deviated from well feelings.

Much of the debate regarding the concept of the sick role has centered on the four components identified by Parsons as the universal construct of the sick role. Freidson (1970a) especially argues that the expectation of the exemption from social role obligations may be limited to certain types of disease; that societies attribute the causes of some illnesses to sick persons themselves; that the expectation to seek and cooperate with professional help can be universal neither for all types of illness nor for all societies; and that the basic constructs of Parsons are rooted in the value structures and institutional development of Western, modernized societies, and are thus not applicable to nonwestern societies.

Parsons proposed the sick role as containing symbolic properties of a society, especially those of American society. This role is an institutionalized basis of social control for illness in a society. Contents of the sick role reflect the major value structures of a given society. Therefore, it may be more useful to define the sick role as a system of expectations that are institutionalized and accepted as the general "guidelines" for defining the meanings of sickness and for model behaviors of the person who is sick. This goes along with Twaddle's notion that the sick role is an "effect variable," to be explained on a global scale with respect to societal differences (1979). The sick role, then, is a system of general norms and expectations that provide a context for "rightful" behaviors on the part of sick individuals in a given society or culture. Although the concept of sick role has been viewed to be too structurally oriented to provide in-depth understandings about illness behaviors and people's experiences in illness (Lawton, 2003), the concept at the symbolic level as structured attitudes and social expectations is still relevant in the study of patients' experiences. As Shilling (2002) states, there is a need to re-examine Parsons' concept of sick role, especially at the general cultural level, informing health care and the patient's role.

Descriptive Features and Characteristics

The operational definition of the sick role has suffered from the confusion that occurred when researchers applied the concept in research. Many researchers included both "expectations" and "behaviors" to indicate the sick role. For example, Twaddle (1969) included both stated expectations for behaviors and the actual behaviors to indicate the sick-role formulation, confounding the role expectations that are tied to the role behaviors.

Gordon's study of a large population sample in New York City (1966) is probably the only one that operationalized the sick-role concept as the generally held set of expectations for persons who are sick. As a system of value consensus and expectations for role behaviors, the concept needs to be operationalized on a general level, that is, at a societal level or for subsectors of a given society. For it to have any conceptual meaning as a concept representing phenomena in the symbolic environment, it needs to be operationalized vis-à-vis "generally" held expectations, that is, consensus, rather than as an individual's convictions.

Relationship to Other Concepts

There are three distinct theoretical and empirical questions related to the sick-role concept that appear to be relevant to the nursing perspective.[7]

- What are the contents of the sick role, and what are the variations of such contents?
- In what ways are variations explained? What are the relationships between the sick-role expectations and the individual's sickness behaviors?
- To what extent does the "sharedness" of the sick-role expectations between the professionals and the clients influence health care behaviors?

The first question is concerned with the descriptive validation of the sick role and focuses on the nature of institutionalization of role expectations. As indicated earlier, very little work has been done to examine the universality of the four aspects of the sick role formulated by Parsons. Segall (1976) explored the sick-role expectations held by hospitalized female patients, and found that only (a) the dimension of undesirability of illness and (b) the expectation of striving to get well were agreed upon as sick-role expectations held in common by patients. This calls into question the validity of the four dimensions as universally held expectations of the sick role.

Several researchers also suggested that the four dimensions of the sick role do not apply to all types of illness. For example, Kosa and Robertson (1969) suggest that the sick role only applies to chronic illness. In contrast, Freidson (1970a) argues that the sick role is most appropriate in considering nontrivial, acute illnesses. Furthermore, the legitimacy and social definition of certain illnesses, such as mental illness, alcoholism, or drug addiction, confound the sick-role concept whenever a society holds the individual personally responsible for the illness and its consequences. It is also apparent that the prevailing philosophy and knowledge that exist in a given society regarding health, disease, and health care practices influence the way a system of value expectations becomes institutionalized in a society.

Additionally, since in an earlier section of this chapter it was proposed that the symbolic environment be considered a function of proximity to individuals, it is necessary to question whether or not the sick-role expectations are different on a subcultural level or in social stratification sectors. Although some variations in sick-role expectation are found among different socioeconomic status groups (Berkanovic, 1972; Gordon, 1966; Twaddle, 1969), the question raised by Segall (1976) is still appropriate: Are the dimensions and contents of the sick role similar among people from different segments of society or different population groups?

The second question poses relationships between the sick role as independent variable and individuals' behaviors as dependent variables.

The basic assumption stems from Parsons' formulation of the theory of action, in which individuals' actions are explained by the actors' motivations, values, and orientations to the situations. Thus, individuals are expected to behave in ways that are in agreement with sick-role expectations. However, evidence indicates that the relationship between sick-role expectations and actual behaviors reflecting such expectations seem modified by many factors. The nature of the illness appears to have a highly modifying effect on whether or not the sick person will assume the sick-role behaviors. A person's other role obligations, specified by what Merton calls "role-set" (1968), also seem to influence the behaviors related to assuming the sick role. A person's position in the social stratification system may also determine the presence or absence of opportunities for behaving in accordance with sick-role expectations (Twaddle, 1979).

Furthermore, the degree to which an individual adheres to social norms and identifies with the value structure of society, that is, the degree of social "belongingness" or the level of social assimilation, may influence the way one behaves when sick. This may result from either the presence or the lack of validation and reinforcement offered to individuals who are behaving in a certain fashion. This would be more apparent in cases of socially stigmatized illnesses or of ambiguously defined illnesses such as depression, anorexia nervosa, or essential hypertension. On the other hand, the empowerment perspective points to the need to examine how people may reject sick-role in the context of disability or chronic illness (Hayes & Hannold, 2007; Kwan & Friel, 2002; Pearce, 2002). Wade and Halligan (2007) also suggest that sick-role behaviors may not necessarily be influenced by the belief system of sick role, as there are many other factors that force people to remain in sick role. In addition, negative impacts of sick-role behaviors on patients' recovery have been raised, especially in relation to patients' participating in decision making (Faulkner & Aveyard, 2002).

The question of alignment in sick-role expectations and behaviors between professionals and clients has direct implications for nursing. Nurses' behaviors as well as their beliefs about the sick role certainly influence the approaches nurses take toward clients. Since an assumption of the sick role requires validation of the role by others, especially by the professional, this process of validation requires empirical attention. Wolinsky and Wolinsky (1981) found that physicians do not necessarily legitimatize the sick role for everyone who assumes this role. Legitimization is offered more often to those clients who come from a lower socioeconomic background, who are seeking validation from a regular source of professional contact, and who have more frequent contact with medical care. There may be two distinct mechanisms that influence the process of validation and alignment of evaluations: (a) the systems of the sick-role expectations are, in fact, different according to the nature of illness, to the extent that professionals and laypeople define illness differently; and (b) the systems of sick-role expectations vary greatly according to substrata and segments of society, to the extent that a majority of the professionals belong to a specific subculture or substrata that is quite different from that of the general population. Consequences to the clients of such disparity and disalignment in the validation of the sick role have not been adequately studied in the field.

It is possible to imagine a case in which a person who considers himself to be sick is turned away by a physician or a nurse. The person may be thought of as a malingerer or as not being "ill enough." As a consequence, the person may experience frustration, stress, distrust, or even relief in an immediate sense, and the person furthermore learns a new normative basis for symptom evaluation that may influence his or her future behaviors. Fredericks, Odiet, Miller, and Fredericks (2006) suggest a re-examination of sick-role expectations in light of professional and patient relationships in the context of empathy.

As pointed out by Twaddle (1979), conversion of sick-role expectations into behaviors on an individual level hinges on "decisions" made by the person to classify him or herself as sick. Because all two-category decisions of this kind (e.g., sick versus not sick, or hungry versus not hungry) require a criterion of threshold, the problem rests critically on the decision rules used by individuals. Thus, as the primary validators of the sick role, nurses are frequently exposed to situations of disparity. Or, as participants in the provision of health care, nurses are in situations where legitimation has already occurred that may or may not align with the nurses' own validation rules. Conflicts of this type may result in negative behaviors toward clients.

SUMMARY

The purpose of this chapter has been to offer conceptualization of environment as a separate entity from that of client. This is done to sharpen the distinction between phenomena within the domain of client and those phenomena within the domain of environment. Consideration of environmental phenomena in a separate context should also highlight the integration between humanity and the environment. The basic premise of this chapter is the notion that environment is the source of forces exerting influences on a person and his or her existence, and that it is also a context in which living (many facets of it) takes place. Therefore, environment, either taken as a whole or as having many distinct classes of phenomena, is an essential component for theoretical thinking in nursing.

Even though environment as a unity is considered to have specific meanings when taken as a whole, it is also proposed in this exposition that there are specific benefits in considering the domain of environment as composed of separate components.

The typology of environment used here includes three qualitative components, of a physical, a social, and a symbolic nature, combined with the two dimensions of space and time. Variability of environment can thus be considered in these terms. The most elementary proposition regarding space might be that the more immediate environmental elements are likely to produce a greater impact on a person than the more remote environmental forces. This proposition of proximity requires both theoretical and empirical examinations, first in a holistic sense, then on a compartmentalized level. Specification of dependent phenomena, that is, aspects of a person on which the impact of the environment is inferred, depends on the scientific perspective of the study. Hence, from the nursing perspective, we would be mostly interested in explaining certain aspects of health-related states and health-related behaviors as affected by environment.

Time dimension in relation to environment poses two types of variability. Duration of environmental presence is the first variability. Some environmental elements are with us continuously, intermittently, or only fleetingly. Rhythmicity of the presence of environmental elements (that is, regularly appearing or randomly present) is the second variability. In many ways, the temporal aspects of one's environment are closely related to the person's habits and patterns of behavior. Continuous exposure to polluted air has a great impact on the human respiratory system, and at the same time an exposure to a highly potent radioactive substance for a fleeting moment can be fatal.

The aspect of quality is inherent in three components of environment, since these components are thought to be characteristically different. Sensory deprivation, social support, and the system of sick role as differently conceived characteristics of environment have been considered as independent variables impinging on various dependent phenomena in the domain of client as well as in the practice domain. Biological and chemical aspects of environment have been linked to many disease conditions, ranging from smallpox to cancer. Relationships between health and social and symbolic elements of environment are beginning to be explored. Rheumatoid arthritis, coronary heart disease, hypertension, as well as many psychological stress syndromes and mental illnesses have been linked to unfavorable aspects of environment.

In addition, a person's behaviors in seeking health care, responding to diseases, forming habits of everyday life, as well as gaining patterns of growth and development, and learning and unlearning behaviors and knowledge, also have been found to be related to environmental phenomena of various kinds.

Another important consideration of environment within the nursing frame of reference concerns the environment in which nursing care takes place. The environment of nursing care raises quite different kinds of theoretical and empirical questions for nursing scientists. Elements of such an environment (i.e., physical, social, and symbolic) affect not only clients who are placed in it but also the ways in which nursing care is provided. Nurses' actions are to some extent created, developed, modified, and constrained within the given environmental contexts. Studying phenomena of the environment from the nursing perspective, then, requires focusing on relationships between nursing-care variations and environment as well as those between a person's health and health-related behaviors and environment.

Four theoretical perspectives for the study of environment in nursing are offered: (a) effects approaches, (b) interdependence approaches, (c) environment-as-context approaches, and (d) postmodern approaches. These approaches to relating environment with phenomena in the client, client–nurse, and practice domain will lead to knowledge that is critical to nursing.

NOTES

1. Feibelman, J. K. (1978). The artificial environment. In J. Lenihan & W. Fletcher (Eds.), *The built environment: Environment and man* (Vol. 8, p. 161). New York: Academic Press.
2. Dubos, R. (1965). *Man adapting* (p. xvii). New Haven, CT: Yale University Press.
3. Dubos, R. (1965). *Man adapting* (p. 261). New Haven, CT: Yale University Press.
4. Dreitzel, H. P. (Ed.). (1971). *The social organization of health* (p. 3). New York: Macmillan.
5. Durkheim, E. (1951). *Suicide: A study in sociology* (J. A. Spaulding & G. Simpson, Trans.) (p. 299). New York: Free Press.
6. See, for example, Alexander Solzhenitsyn's *Cancer Ward* for an illuminating insight into the health care practices in the Gulag.
7. Twaddle compiled a set of propositions related to sickness behavior and the sick role. See: Twaddle, A. (1979). *Sickness behavior and the sick role* (Appendix B, pp. 199–206). Cambridge, MA: Schenkman Publishing.

Theory Development in Nursing

Theories are the key to the scientific understanding of empirical phenomena, and they are normally developed only when previous research has yielded a body of information, including empirical generalizations about the phenomena in question. A theory is then intended to provide deeper understanding by presenting those phenomena as manifestations of certain underlying processes, governed by characteristic laws which account for, and usually correct and refine, the previously established generalizations.

—Carl G. Hempel

OVERVIEW

This chapter aims to show the nature of the theoretical study of phenomena in the proposed four domains of nursing. Whereas the previous chapters are more strictly concerned with the nature of concepts within each domain, this chapter is concerned with the nature of theories as they emerge from relevant concepts. Attempts are made to show how concepts delineated within the four domains can be developed into systems of theoretical statements. Here the purpose is not to propose theories, but rather to point to theoretically descriptive and explanatory ideas possible for each domain. The idea is to lead to thinking about developing theoretical systems through a systematic and logical linking of concepts that compose nursing's relevance structure.

Concepts about the characteristics of scientific theories have changed significantly, especially since the demise of logical positivism in the 1970s (Suppe, 1977). Both the structure and purpose of scientific theories have been defined distinctly, distancing them from various philosophical affiliations such as positivism, scientific realism, antirealism, pragmatism, and relativism (Laudan, 1990). Theories within the human sciences also have been characterized distinctly, differentiating them from the natural sciences, with human science viewed as one of interpretation (Rabinow & Sullivan, 1987; Taylor, 1985). Of course, various authors have proposed different conceptions of scientific theories in human sciences (see, for example, Cleland, 2001; Hatch, 1997; as well as Taylor, 1985). Such philosophical debates complicate our approach to theory development, as the scientist must clarify what her or his position is and what philosophical perspective on scientific theory she or he takes.

However, in the main, scientists are engaged in their theoretical work with a general understanding about the characteristics of scientific theory, often overlooking the strict requirements of logical positivism, scientific realism, or other philosophies of science. As it is not the intention of this book to debate such philosophical questions on the nature of scientific theory, I regard scientific theory with an open mind but also on the premise that scientific theories must provide knowledge about the empirical world in a systematic, coherent, and logical manner.

At this point, it is necessary to discuss general ideas regarding theoretical development appropriate for nursing. In chapter 3, an epistemological framework for nursing was presented. In the nursing epistemology proposed, I identified five spheres of knowledge for nursing: generalized, situated hermeneutic, critical hermeneutic, ethical, and aesthetic knowledge. In each of these knowledge spheres there are specific types of theories that are appropriate to address the cognitive need identified therein, as discussed earlier (Kim, 2001) and shown in Table 9.1.

For example, in the sphere of generalized knowledge, Hempel's "comprehensive theories," which provide "an understanding of large classes of empirical phenomena and enable us to predict, to retrodict, and to explain them" (1988, p. 147), is prototypical for inferential purposes. Because the ultimate goal for the knowledge here is inference, there is a need to develop inferential theories of description, explanation, prediction, and prescription. As discussed earlier, the scope of generalization may differ according to types of phenomena and the level of contextualization used in theories. Methods such as induction, deduction and model building, abduction and retroduction, as well as phenomenological description for essences, are mostly used for developing these types of theories for inference.

Table 9.1

TYPES OF THEORIES FOR FIVE KNOWLEDGE SPHERES OF NURSING

KNOWLEDGE SPHERE	COGNITIVE NEEDS	TYPES OF THEORIES	METHODS OF THEORY DEVELOPMENT
Generalized knowledge	Inferential need	Inferential theories of description, explanation, prediction, and prescription	Induction Deduction and model building Retroduction Phenomenological description of essences
Situated hermeneutic knowledge	Referential need	Theory of heuristic	Heuristic research Thick description Discourse analysis of story Case study
Critical hermeneutic knowledge	Transformative need	Theories of interpretation, critique, transformation and change	Hermeneutic methods Critical methods Deconstruction Genealogy
Ethical knowledge	Normative need	Normative theory	Dialectics Normative model building Model-case description
Aesthetic knowledge	Desiderative need	Normative theory	Dialectics Normative model building Model-case description

Since the sphere of situated hermeneutic knowledge is based on referential cognitive need, it is oriented to developing theories for understanding. For this sphere, the most typical theory would be heuristic in the
sense that Moustakas (1990) used the term, drawing from Aristotle's theory
of rhetoric. Heuristic theories for this sphere are theories of uniqueness,
of difference, of meaning, and of context, which provide in-depth understanding about phenomena as experienced by uniquely situated human
beings. Heuristic theories for this sphere of knowledge are different from
descriptive theories for the generalized sphere, as the latter provide generalized understandings about phenomena whereas heuristic theories, al-

though descriptive, reveal stories and their meanings regarding situationally embedded and subjectively experienced phenomena. Methods such as Moustakas' heuristic research (1990), Geertz's "thick description" (1973), discourse analysis of stories, and case studies are used to develop heuristic theories for this sphere.

The sphere of critical hermeneutic knowledge—with its cognitive need for transformation—calls for theories of interpretation, of critique, and of transformation. The focus is on dissecting aspects of social life (in the nursing context, experiences of clients and nursing practice as social forms of life) to gain not only in-depth understandings about them and different meanings possible with them but also knowledge about critical features of social life that may require transformation. For theories of this sphere, various methods of interpretation (from Heidegger, Gadamer, Dithey, Rorty, and Ricoeur), critical theory building methods (for example, from Habermas and Friere), deconstruction (in line with Derrida), and genealogy (via Foucault) may be applied.

Knowledge for the spheres of the ethical and aesthetic are normative in nature, thus calling for normative theories that are based on *teleos* or *desiderata*. Such theories are developed from premises that identify what is good and desirable in practice. For developing normative theories of the ethical and aesthetic spheres, logically oriented normative constructions, dialectics, and model-case description are applicable.

This formulation regarding different types of theories for the five knowledge spheres of nursing can be overlaid on the four domains of the typology to show the relationship between the types of knowledge and the knowledge content for nursing (Figure 9.1).

This figure shows the multiple types of knowledge that are necessary and possible for nursing for each of the domains. For example, knowledge about pain, which refers to phenomena in the client domain, needs to include: (a) general descriptive and explanatory theories of pain and pain process; (b) heuristic theories of how pain is experienced uniquely and especially by people in different situations and contexts; (c) transformative theories of pain that are oriented to correcting or dismantling various misunderstandings and misrepresentations regarding pain; (d) ethical theories of pain management, especially regarding how the threshold of pain and suffering should be tolerated (for example, with cancer pain); and (e) aesthetic theories of pain management that point to various creative approaches in nurses' approaches to care. By building knowledge in all of these five spheres of knowledge in nursing for any content area specified in the four domains, it is possible to gain a comprehensive knowledge base for nursing practice.

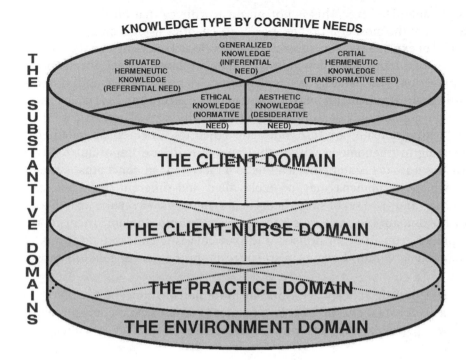

Figure 9.1. Knowledge types and the substantive domains.

Since the different types of theories identified above for the five knowledge spheres are undergirded by specific and different sets of philosophical and methodological premises, there are varying methods of theory development appropriate for different types. For this reason, and because guidelines for theory development for the generalized sphere have been well established in the literature, I will focus my exposition on theory development for the generalized sphere. It would take another book or two to address theory development issues covering all of the knowledge spheres for nursing. Thus, the following presentation will be based on prevailing notions about the characteristics of scientific theory, including abstract conceptualization of phenomena, identification of empirical referents, and selection of a theoretical form.

Presented for each domain are general models of explanation, which may guide theory development for that domain. Such models also can be used as generic guides in developing theories at various levels. The models proposed for the three domains (the client, client–nurse, and practice domains) are primarily founded on the assumption that a theory, at the most comprehensive level, must account for as complete an explanation as possible. However, this is not meant to convey that *all* theories must be built at the most comprehensive level. Theories using a comprehensive model of explanation as a guide may be developed selecting certain aspects of the total framework, depending on their explanatory foci, the scope of explanation, and paradigmatic orientation. Hence, theories and systems of theoretical statements may bring together concepts and variables from a single domain only or from across different domains. Theories may then be "within-domain" or "cross-domain" theories. Theoretical statements referring to phenomena within the same domain are important for two reasons: (a) such statements lead us to a more refined conceptual system, by which phenomena may be reclassified and differentiated from one another; and (b) a set of such theoretical statements may make up a theory for the domain (i.e., a more comprehensive "within-domain" theory). My approach, consisting of holistic and particularistic conceptualizations of phenomena within domains, also suggests three levels of relationships:

- A holistic concept with one or more holistic concept(s)
- A holistic concept with one or more particularistic concept(s)
- A particularistic concept with one or more particularistic concept(s)

On the other hand, theoretical statements among concepts drawing from two or more domains are oriented to developing "cross-domain" theories. The latter often bring in concepts from the domain of environment as the explanatory factors, in addition to two other domains. Such theories may contain different types of theoretical statements, as shown in Table 9.2. Types of theoretical statements with the explanatory focus on the client, client–nurse, and practice domains are given in this table.

Ideas with the explanatory focus on the environment domain are not included in this table, because theoretical development with an explanatory focus on environmental phenomena is not relevant to nursing, except in the case regarding the health care environment. It certainly is necessary to have knowledge about environmental phenomena from the nursing perspective, however. Theories for environment–domain phenomena are not useful for nursing in the same way that theories from biology, chemistry, or physics are not. However, as discussed in chapter 8, theories regarding environment can be developed from the four theoretical perspectives therein identified in relation to phenomena in the client, client–nurse, and practice domains. This will be discussed in a later section.

Theoretical statements linking concepts and phenomena within each domain and across domains are examined to indicate that relevant and critical relationships may be brought together both in "theories *in* nursing"

Table 9.2

TYPES OF CROSS-DOMAIN THEORETICAL STATEMENTS

| | EXPLANATORY FOCUS OF DOMAIN | |
CLIENT DOMAIN	CLIENT–NURSE DOMAIN	PRACTICE DOMAIN
Client Domain Concept(s) With:	Client–Nurse Domain Concept(s) With:	Practice Domain Concept(s) With:
Client–nurse domain concept(s)	Client domain concept(s)	Client domain concept(s)
Practice domain concept(s)	Practice domain concept(s)	Client–nurse domain concept(s)
Environment domain concept(s)	Environment domain concept(s)	Environment domain concept(s)
Client–nurse and practice domain concepts	Client and practice domain concepts	Client and client–nurse domain concepts
Client–nurse and environment domain concepts	Client and environment domain concepts	Client and environment domain concepts
Practice and environment domain concepts	Practice and environment domain concepts	Client–nurse and environment domain concepts
Client–nurse, practice, and environment domain concepts	Client, practice, and environment domain concepts	Client, client–nurse, and environment domain concepts

and in "theories *of* nursing." For each domain, I present general models of explanation and proceed to examine different theoretical systems that deal with phenomena of the domain at various levels.

In chapter 2, the major terms of importance in theory development were defined. A theoretical statement may be descriptive or explanatory. A descriptive statement provides specifications regarding the nature of concepts with respect to existence, variability, quality, and essential features, whereas an explanatory statement is a proposition that links two or more concepts in one of basically three relational forms—associational (i.e., covariance), causal, and dynamic. This means that a theoretical statement of a propositional type specifies the relationship of at least one class of phenomena to another class of phenomena to elucidate an explanation of one set of the two. An explanatory statement can be simple or complex, in that it may link two concepts in a simple association, or it may link several concepts in a set of dynamic relationships. In the following exposition, this definition primarily illustrates the types of theoretical statements examined for our purpose.

Explanatory theories are often recast into predictive and prescriptive theories. Whereas predictive theories pose what would naturally occur according to theoretical formulations, prescriptive theories designate specific controls as prescriptions or interventions that then are posed for effects on dependent variable(s). In this sense, whereas predictive theories need not be causal in their structures, prescriptive theories are invariably causal.

In nursing, during the past two decades, the development of middle-range theories constitutes the major theoretical development since the early grand theory proposals of the 1970s and early 1980s (Liehr & Smith, 1999; Smith & Liehr, 2003, 2008). Liehr and Smith (1999) identified 22 middle-range theories in nursing, adding 14 more theories in their 2003 edition and 19 additional theories in their 2008 edition. Kim and Kollak (2006) identified 38 middle-range theories reported in the literature from the 1980s to 2004. My review of MEDLINE for author-designated middle-range theories in nursing extracted nine additional theories from 2004 to 2009. There are a total of 73 middle-range theories in the two sets by Smith and Liehr and my work, some of which were duplicates whereas others were listed in only one of the sets. Of these, there are 51 theories in the client domain, 10 theories in the client–nurse domain, 10 in the practice domain, one in the environment domain, and one theory dealing with nurses' problems. Table 9.3 presents theory titles (72 theories, excluding one dealing with nurses' nonclinical problems) in the four domains.

Theory development in nursing is more active for phenomena in the client domain than in the other two domains. Some theories in the client domain are prescriptive theories.

THEORETICAL IDEAS FOR THE DOMAIN OF CLIENT

In chapter 5, several conceptualizations regarding phenomena in the client domain were presented. Such conceptualizations appear to be related to theoretical models and were, in most instances, developed in a deductive fashion. In addition, the use of the inductive method, and a combined inductive and deductive method for conceptual clarification, were evident in nursing research literature.

A review of three nursing journals (*Nursing Research, Research in Nursing and Health,* and *Advances in Nursing Science*) in 1982 revealed that 51 out of a total of 316 articles dealt with conceptualization of client

Table 9.3

MIDDLE-RANGE THEORIES IN NURSING BY DOMAIN: 1980–2009*

THE CLIENT DOMAIN	THE CLIENT–NURSE DOMAIN	THE PRACTICE DOMAIN
Acute pain (Good & Moore, 1996)	Attentively embracing story (Smith & Liehr, 1999)	Caregiving effectiveness (Smith et al., 2002)
Acute pain management in infants and children (Huth & Moore, 1998)	Caring (Swanson, 1991)	Conflict resolution through culture brokering (Jezewski, 1995)
Adaptation as a mediator of intimate abuse and traumatic stress in battered women (Woods & Isenberg, 2001)	Caring and comfort metaphors (Jenny & Logan, 1996)	Cultural negotiation (Engerbretson & Littleton, 2001)
Adaptation to chronic pain (Dunn, 2004)	Caring through relation and dialogue (Sanford, 2000)	Figuring it out in the moment (Janes, Sidani, Cott, & Rappolt, 2008)
Adapting to diabetes mellitus (Whittemore & Roy, 2002)	Collaborative decision making in nursing practice (Kim, 1983)	Nurse midwifery care (Thompson, Oakley, Burke, Tay, & Konklin, 1989)
Agitation (Acton, 1997)		
Attachment and coping with chronic illness (Schmidt, Nachtigall, Wuethrich-Martone, & Strauss, 2002)	Interpersonal perceptual awareness (Brooks & Thomas, 1997)	Nursing art (Chinn, 2001)
Becoming a success story (Lawson, 2003)	Negotiating partnership (Powell-Copp, 1994)	Nursing intellectual capital (Covell, 2008)
Caregiver stress (Tsai, 2003)	Nurse-expressed empathy (Olson & Hanchett, 1997)	Patient advocacy (Bu & Jezewski, 2007)
Chronic pain (Tsai, Tak, Moore, & Palencia, 2003)	The comforting interaction (Morse, Havens, & Wilson, 1997)	Person-centered nursing care for person with dementia (Penrod et al., 2007)
Chronic sorrow (Eakes, Burke, & Hainsworth, 1998)		
Chronic stress emotions (Peters, 2006)		Prevention (August-Brady, 2000)
Chronotherapeutic intervention for postsurgical pain (Auvil-Novak, 1997)	Touch (Estabrooks & Morse, 1992)	
Cognition-sensitive approach to dementia (Barnes & Adair, 2002)		
Comfort (Kolcaba, 2001)		

(continued)

Table 9.3 *(continued)*

THE CLIENT DOMAIN	THE CLIENT– NURSE DOMAIN	THE PRACTICE DOMAIN
Commitment to health (Kelly, 2008)		
Coping among relatives of patients in intensive care units (Johansson, Hildingh, Wenneberg, Fridlund, & Ahlström, 2006)		
Courage as a process of pushing beyond the struggle (Finfgeld, 1999)		
Enduring love: women's experience of domestic violence (Kearney, 2001)		
Enlightenment (Hills & Hanchett, 2001)		
Epileptic stigma (Scambler & Hopkins, 1990)		
Experiencing transitions (Meleis, Sawyer, Im, Messias, & Schumacher, 2000)		
Facilitating growth and development (Kinney, 1990)		
Family health (Doornbos, 2000)		
Generative quality of life for the elderly (Register & Herman, 2006)		
Hazardous secrets and reluctantly taking charge (Burke, Kauffman, Costello, & Dillon, 1991)		
Health promotion for preterm infants (Mefford, 2004)		
Homelessness/helplessness (Tollett & Thomas, 1995)		
Inner strength in women (Roux, Dingley, & Bush, 2002)		
Intergenerational solidarity in aging families (Bengton & Roberts, 1991)		
Investing in self-care (Leenerts & Magilvy, 2000)		

Table 9.3 (continued)

THE CLIENT DOMAIN	THE CLIENT–NURSE DOMAIN	THE PRACTICE DOMAIN
Learned resourcefulness (Bekhet & Zauszniewski, 2008)		
Passive behaviors in people with Alzheimer's disease (Colling, 2003)		
Peaceful end of life (Ruland & Moore, 1998)		
Perceived family dynamics of persons with chronic pain (Smith & Friedemann, 1999)		
Precarious ordering: women's caring (Wuest, 2001)		
Psychological adaptation (Levesque, Ricard, Ducharme, Duquette, & Bonin, 1998)		
Reconciling the good patient persona with humor (McCreaddie & Wiggins, 2009)		
Recovery in schizophrenia (Noiseux & Ricard, 2008)		
Resilience (Polk, 1997)		
Self-care management for vulnerable populations (Dorsey & Murdaugh, 2003)		
Self-transcendence (Reed, 1991)		
Spirituality (Walton & Sullivan, 2004)		
Suffering (Morse, 2001)		
Teetering on the edge: postpartum depression (Beck, 1993)		
Trajectory of chronic illness management (Cooley, 1999)		
Uncertainty in illness (Mishel, 1988, 1990)		

(continued)

Table 9.3 *(continued)*

THE CLIENT DOMAIN	THE CLIENT–NURSE DOMAIN	THE PRACTICE DOMAIN
Unpleasant symptoms (Lenz, Pugh, Milligan, Gift, & Suppe, 1995, 1997)		
Urine control (Jirovex, Jenkins, Isenberg, & Baiardi, 1999)		
Women's anger (Thomas, 1991)		

Environment Domain: Violence prevention (Johnson & Delaney, 2006)

*For complete references, see: Kim, H. S., & Kollak, I. (Eds.). (2006). *Nursing theories: Conceptual and philosophical foundations* (2nd ed., pp. 302–304). New York: Sage; Liehr, P., & Smith, J. J. (1999). Middle range theory: Spinning research and practice to create knowledge for the new millennium. *Advances in Nursing Science, 21,* 81–91; Smith, M. J., & Liehr, P. R. (Eds.). (2003). *Middle range theory for nursing* (pp. 1–23). New York: Springer Publishing; and Smith, M. J., & Liehr, P. R. (Eds.). (2008). *Middle range theory for nursing* (Appendix) (2nd ed.). New York: Springer Publishing Company.

domain phenomena: some were holistic concepts, such as adaptation, health, and recovery; whereas others were particularistic, such as anxiety, fatigue, obesity, and self-esteem. This picture changed dramatically during the ensuing period, up to the present. We now see often two or three articles in a given nursing journal dealing with concept development, concept clarification, or concept analysis. We now have conceptualizations of phenomena in the client domain that range from transcendence, self-efficacy, chronic sorrow, suffering, fatigue, restlessness, confusion, homelessness, and energy use to many nursing-diagnosis concepts developed within the NANDA-I system. Concept development associated with the nomenclature of nursing diagnoses proposed by NANDA-I has been very active during the past two decades. Mostly, nursing diagnoses, as problematic concepts within this typology, have been identified descriptively through empirical generalizations for identification purposes in nursing practice, without much effort devoted to developing explanatory theories for them.

In addition to the conceptual work, there are mainly three types of theoretical efforts for knowledge generation for this domain: (a) grand-level theory formulation and refinement of general nursing theories having their focus on the client domain; (b) development and refinement of middle-range theories ; and (c) empirical testing of theories (mostly from other disciplines) for specification, reformulation, and adaptation from the nursing perspective. The first type of effort has been evident in the works associated with nursing's grand theories and theoretical models, which are oriented to providing explanatory frameworks for client phenomena, such as those advanced by Rogers, Roy, Orem, Neuman, and Parse. The second type of effort is evident in the works using the framework of grounded theory in nursing, as summarized by Benoliel (1996), as well as in middle-range theory development and theoretical modeling work, such as those in the areas of women's health (Voda & George, 1986; Woods, 1993), fatigue (Lenz, et al., 1995, 1997), self-transcendence (Reed, 1991), uncertainty in illness (Mishel, 1988, 1990), elderly health, chronic sorrow, suffering, and confusion. The third type of effort has been summarized partly by Barnard (1983), Denyes (1983), and Flemming (1986) for work in the area of child phenomena, by Stevenson (1983) for those in adult phenomena, and by Adams (1986) for works in aging phenomena.

Kirkevold (1994) has also shown that there have been numerous works that present theoretical development with a focus on phenomena in the client domain. She found in her review of the nursing literature from 1983 to 1993 that about 32% of the articles dealt with client domain phenomena, ranging from 16 thematic areas pertaining to essentialistic phenomena, 9 areas pertaining to developmental phenomena, 12 areas pertaining to problematic phenomena, and two health care experiential phenomena. She suggests that cumulative knowledge development leading to theoretical ideas is evident in the following areas[1]:

- Patterns of stress-coping
- Mothering/parenting role enactment and decision making
- Explanation of fatigue
- Caregiver burden
- Patient falls
- Elderly care

Kirkevold (1994) also found that much of the empirical research is carried out within common theoretical frameworks, such as the Lazarus stress-coping model and the theory of rational decision making. This review suggests that nursing scholars are moving forward to codifying their work with a view toward theoretical development. With this type of effort, diverse theoretical models in physiology, psychology, anthropology, and sociology have been empirically tested in an effort to reformulate and redefine theories within the nursing context.

The major thrusts for knowledge development in this domain should be oriented toward the development of nursing theories of human phenomena dealing with general and holistic phenomena as well as the development and testing of middle-range theories that deal with particularistic phenomena. To provide a starting point for further analysis and additional expansion of theoretical knowledge for the client domain, three generic models of explanation are presented in the following section. The three explanatory models presented below are the generic prototypes for thinking theoretically about phenomena in the client domain.

Explanatory Model 1—"Within-Domain" Formula

An explanation of phenomena in the client domain may be offered, eliciting other phenomena in the client, as has occurred in many theories in physiology, psychology, and nursing. This model focuses on seeking explanatory factors or processes by looking into those aspects that are intrinsic and internal to humans and human conditions. In this model, selected human phenomena are thought to be providing associational, processual, or causal influences on the other human phenomena that are the focus of attention for a given theory.

For example, the theory of self-transcendence advanced by Reed (1991) proposes a relationship between transcendence and developmental level in the aging. In the theory of parenting, parental self-esteem is proposed to have influence on parenting efficacy. Many psychological and cognitive theories being examined in the nursing literature, such as the theory of reasoned action, self-efficacy theory, and theory of learning, adopt this model of explanation. Many biobehavioral theories, including the genetic theory of disease and structural theory of functioning, are also examples adopting this model.

In addition, this model is also applicable in delineating conceptual categories among closely related, often coexisting phenomena through the Concept Differentiation Model (Kim, 1992). For example, conceptual differentiation between pain and suffering would be an important beginning for a theoretical development regarding human experiences associated with pain, as would be the differentiation between anxiety and stress.

Explanatory Model 2—Additive Model ("Cross-Domain" Formula)

The second explanatory model refers to the thinking that a given set of client domain phenomena are associated with factors and conditions that exist not just in the client domain but also in different domains and other

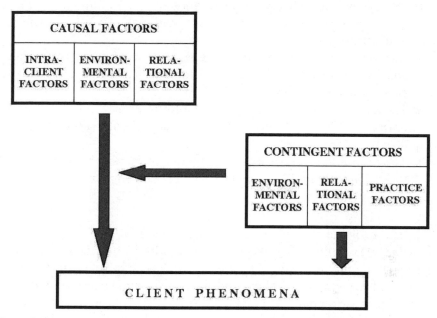

Figure 9.2. Example of an additive model of explanation for client domain phenomena.

phenomenal spheres, producing additive, nonintersecting influences. This is depicted in Figure 9.2.

Roy's propositions in her adaptation model (Roy & Andrews, 1991) explain a person's adaptation in relation to the person's existing adaptation level, with the environment being the source of external stimuli. The Roy adaptation model includes propositions that pose relationships among particularistic phenomena in the self-concept, role-function, and interdependence modes of adaptation, as well as those in the physiological needs mode (Roy & Andrews, 1991; Roy & Roberts, 1981). The major propositions in the model are concerned with certain concepts in the domain of client in relation to other concepts in the domain of client and those in the domain of environment. For example, the following selected propositions[2] from the theory considered together illustrate an adoption of this additive model of explanation in her theory:

- Characteristics of internal and external stimuli a person receives influence his or her adaptive responses (a cross-domain proposition).
- Structural and functional integrities of a subsystem of a person influence his or her adaptive responses (a within-domain proposition).

- Mastery with which a person responds to stimuli influences consequent processing of internal and external stimuli (a within-domain proposition).
- The positive quality of social experience in the form of others' approval positively influences the level of feelings of adequacy (a cross-domain proposition).
- The amount of clarity of input in the form of role cues and cultural norms positively influences the adequacy of role taking (a cross-domain proposition).
- The optimum level of environmental changes positively influences the adequacy of seeking nurturance and nurturing (a cross-domain proposition).

In the evolving theory of unpleasant symptoms, Lenz and her colleagues (1995) identify three sets of variables for the explanation of unpleasant symptoms, adopting the additive model of explanation. However, in their subsequent work, they revised the theory, structuring it in a dynamic, feedback model (Lenz et al., 1997). Many of the theories developed within the framework of grounded theory have adopted this model of explanation, including as antecedent variables those factors present in the person, in the environment, and in interactive patterns. Orem's statements (1991) that "universal self-care requisites and ways of meeting them may be modified by the age, sex, or developmental or health state of individuals" and "some self-care requisites have their origins in the environment" are also depicted within this model of explanation. This form of explanation is multifactorial and additive.

Explanatory Model 3—Dynamic, Comprehensive Model

This model of explanation of a theory for the domain of client brings in various factors and aspects in a dynamic, interactive fashion, to provide a comprehensive, total explanation of a given phenomenon. Nursing theories of the client domain adopting this model invariably include factors from the individual (the client domain), the nurse (the practice domain), client–nurse interaction (the domain of client–nurse), and the environment. Whereas in Model 2 explanatory variables are viewed to have additive influence, in this model the influences of the variables in a given theory are interactive, modifying, and dynamic.

For example, Rogers (1970, 1980, 1992) proposes as the main thrust in her theory of unitary humans the synergistic, evolutionary repatterning of human energy field in relation to environmental energy field. The

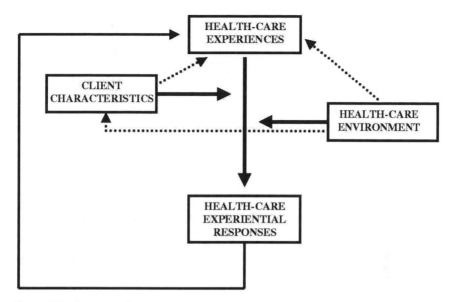

Figure 9.3. Example of an explanatory model for health care experiential phenomena.

three theoretical principles in this theory consider the existing pattern characteristics of the human energy field with its creative, evolutionary potential to move unidirectionally toward greater complexity in concert with the environmental energy field. The relationships between the human and environment energy fields are interactive, interpenetrating, and dynamic. Cartwright, Archbold, Stewart, and Limandri (1994) propose a theory regarding enrichment processes of family caregiving developed through the grounded theory approach that includes factors in the caregiver and care receiver, and dyadic relations in a dynamic relationship.

Theories for health-care experiential phenomena may be developed from this explanatory model. In the literature, there is little evidence of theory development for health care experiential phenomena. Health care experiential phenomena arise from a person's experiences in receiving health care. Such phenomena are byproducts of a person's involvement in the health care system and are not necessarily germane to the problems that bring the individual to the attention of health care professionals. Although they are experiential, they may be influenced by the person's health problems; but, more important, they may impact on the processes of health care, such as recovery. A generic theoretical model adopting this form (Model 3) of explanation is proposed as an overall framework for theoretical and empirical considerations for studying health care experiential phenomena, as shown in Figure 9.3.

Theoretical development for the domain of client, therefore, may be oriented to any of these three models. Of course, there are many other types of explanatory models that are possible, for example a complex process model. Various theory construction methods, inductive, deductive, and retroductive, may be applied to develop theories for the domain of client. The form of a theory may be identified to hold any explanatory model; whether a theorist begins with a mental picture of a specific explanatory model prior to the development of a theory, or whether a theory as a product assumes a specific explanatory model may not be an important question.

THEORETICAL IDEAS FOR THE CLIENT–NURSE DOMAIN

Theory development for the client–nurse domain has been rather limiting in nursing. In the 1960s, there were several nurse scholars who paid attention to client–nurse interaction as an important aspect of nursing work, as discussed in chapter 6. For example, both Orlando (1961) and Wiedenbach (1964) considered client–nurse interaction as a helping process that is dynamic in nature, affecting the way clients cope with the demands of a healthy life. Peplau (1952) defined nursing as a therapeutic, interpersonal process that helps the client solve problems and likewise moves the client in the direction of creative, constructive, productive, personal, and community living. After a hiatus of nearly 2 decades, during which little theoretical attention was given to client–nurse interaction, King (1981) proposed a theory of goal attainment, in which transaction between a client and a nurse is considered the major factor influencing goal attainment in the client. Cox's theory of client–nurse interaction (1982) and the theory of collaborative decision making in nursing practice (Kim, 1983) are middle-range theories proposed in the 1980s that focus on explaining client–nurse phenomena.

There have also been some theoretical works oriented to reformulating sociological theories to explain client–nurse phenomena, such as Riehl's work in symbolic interactionism in nursing (1980) and Leininger's transcultural nursing (1995). Garvin and Kennedy (1990), in their review of the state of knowledge regarding communication between nurses and patients, found four areas of study pertaining to the client–nurse domain: empathy, self-disclosure, interpersonal support, and confirming communication. However, theory development in nursing with a focus on the client–nurse domain still remains at a beginning stage. Although Shattell (2004) identified an increased number of studies addressing nurse–patient interaction and communication in recent decades, most of these studies applied sociological theories to examine the client–nurse phenomena. The middle-range theories developed in the client–nurse domain, as shown in Table 9.3, focus on collaboration, negotiation, caring relations, and empathy.

Two generic explanatory models for theory development in the client–nurse domain are proposed. An essential point in developing theories for the client–nurse domain is inclusion of client phenomena for either a manifest or a latent focus of explanation. This does not mean that a client phenomenon must be a component of a client–nurse theory, but that, if one is not identified as such, a theoretical assumption should specify the theory's connection to client phenomena.

Explanatory Model 1—"Within-Domain" Formula

Theories that link the properties and processes of client–nurse interaction must be developed as the first-level theoretical work for understanding and explaining client–nurse domain phenomena. Such theories may be developed adopting this model of explanation. This model of explanation appeals to an elaboration and understanding of the nature of client–nurse relations by making theoretical connections among different aspects of relationship between a client and a nurse. For example, client–nurse negotiation may be elaborated by considering interpersonal understanding or client–nurse mutuality.

Some of the studies of client–professional encounters using narrative analysis are oriented to developing theories of client–professional communication from this explanatory model. Language use and the construction of talk is investigated to understand the process of communication.

Explanatory Model 2—Comprehensive Model

As suggested earlier, many theories of human interaction require reformulation within the nursing perspective to the extent that the ultimate concepts for explanation of significance in this perspective have to reside in the client. Since client–nurse phenomena with any of the three orientations of client–nurse relation (i.e., the medium therapy, and care orientations) have either vicarious or intentional impact on clients, it is necessary to develop nursing theories adopting an explanatory model that include client phenomena as the final explanatory component.

There is a need to develop and refine theories of client–nurse relations that can be applied to examine influences on client outcomes of nursing's

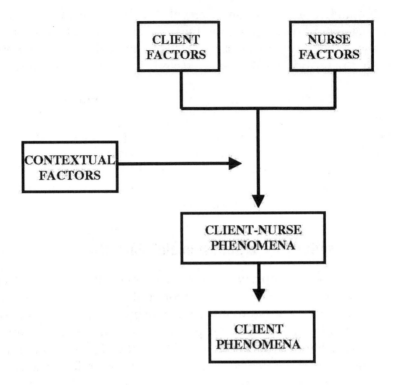

Figure 9.4. Example of an explanatory model for client–nurse phenomena.

interactive therapies, from the process of mediation, and as a result of the process of care. There are at least four sets of variables identified as components of this explanatory model: (a) individual actors (client and nurse); (b) context of interaction; (c) nature of interaction (process and property); and (d) client-health-related phenomena. Theoretical linkages among the four components are specified in Figure 9.4 regarding this model of explanation for the client–nurse domain.

The first component includes aspects of the individual actors who are participants in an interaction, namely the client and the nurse within the client–nurse domain conceptualization. The "participant set" may not be limited to just client and nurse, but may refer to parents (parents of a child patient) and nurse, or caregiver and nurse. Individual actors bring with them physical, psychological, cognitive, social, and ethical character-istics, including abilities, values, attitudes, behaviors, and interactive patterning developed through past social experiences. Such attributes may be considered predisposing, enabling, or hindering factors for the process and property of interaction. Garvin and Kennedy (1990) found that most of the studies in the literature focused on patient-communicative elements and nurse-communicative elements as the major factors included in the explanation of client–nurse communication. Shattell (2004) also identified studies in which the effects of nurses' backgrounds were examined in relation to the quality of nurse–patient interaction.

The interactive encounters between client and nurse may be initiated, developed, or terminated in various forms and contents according to individual orientations the participants bring with them to interactive situations. Theoretical work in therapeutic touch and empathy suggests the influence of nurses' abilities, attitudes, and orientations on the nature of client–nurse interactive process. The literature in the area of stigmatization and labeling suggests also that socially undesirable facets of personal characteristics tend to affect the ways in which people maintain social distance from each other (see Goffman, 1963; Scheff, 1966). From the critical, hermeneutic perspective, Mishler (1984) proposes that interactional processes proceed (and encounters are shaped) based on the "voices" (or perspectives) with which the participants carry on the conversation in client–professional encounters. Participants' perspectives/"voices" orient their aims and experiences in client–provider encounters. These and other studies point to a need for in-depth understanding and reformulation regarding the effects of participants' attributes on the client–nurse relation.

The second component refers to the context of client–nurse relation. The context of relation includes all aspects of environment—physical, social, and symbolic—that exist in the situation of client–nurse relation. Social aspects of the context have been studied a great deal in sociology. The social context of interaction may not only be influential as a prerequisite condition for interactional encounters in nursing, but may actually become a significant aspect of therapeutic communication. Several studies of social interaction from the perspective of symbolic interactionism, such as the study of pain management by Fagerhaugh and Strauss (1977), suggest that the context of interaction influences the ways in which clients' experiences and patterns of interaction are developed according to the established rules of behavior, the meanings of specific communicative symbols, and the structural orientations of the context. Client–nurse interactions take place in somewhat specialized social contexts in which the power distribution is unequal among the participants, role prescriptions are socially institutionalized, instrumental requirements vary, and the system of control is often preestablished. The major theoretical focus of interest for nursing is in gaining understanding about how different aspects of the interactional context influence the interactive processes between client and nurse. Recently, in a number of studies on home visiting and home care, there has been an increasing interest in the context of home having a great effect on how client–nurse interaction is shaped and how it continues.

The third component pertains to the client–nurse relation itself. Client–nurse relation is considered along two dimensions: (a) the process of relation, and (b) the property, form, or quality of relation. The process of relation refers to the relational sequence, trajectories, progression, and patterning. On the other hand, the property of relation refers to the form and quality of relation with respect to the elements of exchange, such as information, affection, energy, support, resources, and communication types. This component, as the middle component, is essential both for understanding the nature of client–nurse relation and for explaining client phenomena as influenced by phenomena in the client–nurse relation.

The fourth component pertains to client phenomena, especially those related to clients' health and health care outcomes. All major explanatory and predictive models in nursing ultimately have to deal with clients' well-being or client outcomes as the main explanatory focus and, in so doing, place theories within the nursing framework. Client phenomena in relation to client–nurse relation reported in the literature are recovery, compliance, coping, information retention, relief of pain, satisfaction, goal-attainment, and sense of control. Although many studies suggest a beginning for an emergence of important theoretical ideas, there still exists a paucity of theories for phenomena in the client–nurse domain.

Although there has been a great deal of rhetorical emphasis on the importance of client–nurse relation in the delivery of nursing care, very little real work has been done either in theory development or in empirical testing of theories. There is a rich array of theoretical and empirical work accomplished in sociology, social psychology, and medicine that is adaptable to the study of this domain. However, there is a critical need for understanding of how the *special* nature of client–nurse relation modifies sociological, social psychological, and communication theories for explanation of client–nurse domain phenomena and client outcomes.

THEORETICAL IDEAS FOR THE DOMAIN OF PRACTICE

Theories for phenomena in the practice domain are essential for understanding what goes on in practice situations as well as for developing ways to normatively influence the way nurses practice, that is, shape their work. My review of the literature on the practice domain in 1994 revealed the beginning development of theories for this domain related to intuitive knowing in nursing, clinical decision making, ethical decision making, and knowledge utilization in nursing (Kim, 1994). However, much of the work is at the concept development or descriptive level, pointing to the need to move toward developing explanatory theories. The review results shown in Table 9.3 show the paucity of theory development in the practice domain. Two explanatory models are proposed also for this domain.

Model of Explanation 1—"Within-Domain" Formula

As presented in chapter 7, the phenomena in the practice domain are conceptualized as two processes: the deliberation phase and the enactment phase. The "within-domain" formula for theory development for phenomena in this domain leads to several areas of emphasis. Theories need to be developed that examine (a) relationships among phenomena within each of the two processes of nursing practice, (b) critical linkages between the deliberation phenomena and the enactment phenomena, and (c) relationships among many different aspects of nursing practice (see Figure 7.1). For example, the works by Benner and her associates (Benner, 1984, 1996b, 2009; Benner & Tanner, 1987; Benner, Tanner, & Chesla, 1992) are oriented to developing a theory of expertise in nursing in relation to intuitive process. Also, the refinement of various theoretical formulations regarding clinical decision making, such as the information-processing theory and the prospect theory, is a movement toward developing descriptive theories of nurses' diagnosing and clinical decision making in practice.

Theories adopting this explanatory model are oriented to understanding and explaining the nature of nursing practice in relation to various aspects of practice itself or from what nurses bring to practice. Figure 9.5 shows three sets of theoretical formulations possible as "within-domain" theories in the practice domain.

Model of Explanation 2—Comprehensive Formula

This model of explanation for phenomena in the practice domain encompasses four components: (a) exogenous component, (b) nurse component, (c) practice domain phenomena component, and (d) client phenomena component. Two components are primarily linked to the phenomena of the practice domain: One set refers to the exogenous aspects of the nurse in practice and the other is inherent in the nurse in practice. Secondarily, phenomena in the practice domain are theoretically linked to client phe-

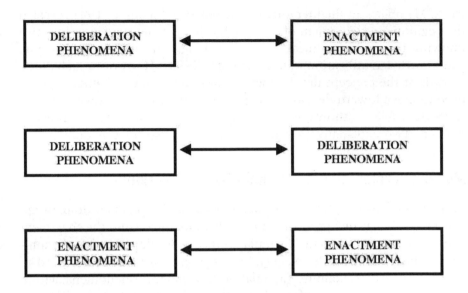

Figure 9.5. Within-domain explanations in the practice domain.

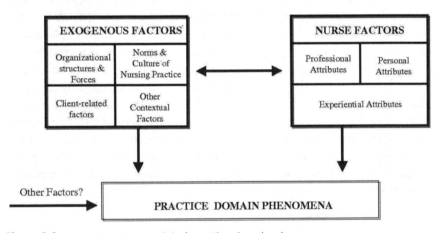

Figure 9.6. An explanatory model of practice domain phenomena.

nomena, as both nurses' deliberations and nurses' enactment are viewed as influencing clients in various ways. This generic model is shown in Figure 9.6.

The sources for the exogenous component are the structural elements outside of the nurse-agent, as specified in the preceding section for the deliberation and enactment dimensions. These include attributes within the structures of client and situation of nursing practice and some areas of the structures of nursing goals and nursing means, which reside externally to the practicing nurse. Aspects of the exogenous component that may provide explanation about practice phenomena include organizational structures and forces that exist in the clinical situation, nursing service structure, the client's nursing care requirements, peer support, climate of nursing care, the culture of nursing, etc. For example, a theory may be proposed to suggest that the quality of nursing process is influenced by the normative expectations apparent in the nursing service setting, the amount of actual as well as perceived time available to nurses to systematize nursing care, and the complexity of nursing care requirements presented to nurses by clients. Lauzon Clabo's study of pain assessment specifically addresses the effects of organizational *habitus* on the individual nurse's pain-assessment behaviors (2008). Organizational and external stresses have been attributed to less-than-ideal provisions of nursing care and to the phenomenon of "reality shock" in new graduates. The atmosphere of practice and its meanings to the nurse, contextual changes that occur within the nursing situation, and the complexity of a situation that requires complicated management skills are some of the external forces that may influence the nature of nursing practice and nursing-practice outcomes.

The intrinsic component refers to various aspects of the nurse in practice. It includes characteristics, attributes, and experiences intrinsic to the nurse as a person. Nurses' deliberations and enactment are affected by many factors inherent in the nurse. The nurse's knowledge level, educational preparation, intellectual skill, personality, past experiences, worldview, ethical and moral commitments, and physical and feeling states may affect the "quality" and process of nursing practice. For example, as Fagermoen (1997) suggests, the nature of nursing practice may be influenced by nurses' value commitments. Wrong clinical decisions may result from the way a nurse evaluates the situation in light of her or his limited knowledge base, or because the nurse has limited experience with specific life and nursing situations with which he or she can develop evaluative frameworks. The model of learning adopted by a nurse may also influence the way a nurse practices, as suggested by Argyris, Putnam, and Smith (1985).

The third component refers to phenomena of the practice domain, treated as the primary level of focus for explanation. It is essential and critical to understand and have explanations about how differences in the quality of deliberation and enactment and the structure and patterns of deliberative and enactment processes are brought about through both exogenous and intrinsic components. For example, theoretical questions pertaining to these would be: What influences the way nurses make individualized nursing care planning? (or) How are nursing care strategies modified to meet patients' needs and the demands of the situation? These are important theoretical questions.

The fourth component pertains to client phenomena. Theories of the practice domain must consider directly or indirectly the impact of nursing practice on clients. Clients' experiences through their involvement in nursing practice and client outcomes of care must be linked to the ways nursing is practiced in relation to clients.

There are several areas of importance in the domain of practice that require rigorous theoretical work. One such area is the uncertainty that is inherent in nursing practice. The uncertainty in nursing practice is parallel to that found in medical practice (Coser, 1978; Fox, 1957; Merton, 1976) and refers especially to uncertain outcomes of nursing interventions. However, uncertainty in nursing practice can also occur in making assessments about a client's presenting problems. Apparent interactions among physiological, psychological, and cognitive aspects of human responses produce complex phenomena in the client, making it rather difficult to make cause–effect linkages in a nursing assessment.

Even though the prescriptiveness in the way nursing interventions are recommended for different client problems in several nursing models is suggestive of the deterministic nature of nursing practice, the practice implications of any prescription remain uncertain in judgment as well as in outcome. Thus, actual and potential uncertainty in nursing practice may influence the behavioral patterns of the nurse. Grier and Schnitzler (1979), examining the nurse's risk-taking behaviors in decision making, found that a nurse's propensity to take risk is related to the nature of the decision-making situation as well as the nurse's educational level. Nursing decisions are uncertain to the extent that the outcomes of decisions are probabilistic or multifactorially complicated and to the extent that the decisions themselves are based on incomplete information. Such uncertainty will, in turn, influence the nurse's actual decision-making and practice behaviors. The phenomena of uncertainty in practice may need to be examined from a comprehensive framework that brings in both the exogenous and intrinsic components.

Another area of importance is knowledge utilization in nursing practice, especially in this era of evidence-based practice. Quality of nursing practice essentially depends upon the richness and rigor of scientific knowledge from which the prescriptions of nursing activities are derived. Practice without a scientific foundation will flounder because of the inadequacy of trial-and-error by itself. However, the fact that nursing practitioners are educated to use systematic knowledge for practice, and that nursing practice is based on prescriptive theories, is no guarantee that nursing practice in reality will be implemented accordingly (Kim, 1993b).

The issue is how nursing knowledge that is internalized and learned by an individual nurse as a system of individualized knowledge becomes transformed into nursing actions, that is, into knowledge-in-use. Another related issue is how nurses can obtain and internalize available knowledge in the public domain so that it is used in practice. What prompts the nurse to behave in a specific way? Is there a mental or psychological explanation for why one nurse might behave differently from another in a given nursing situation, provided that there is a standardized level of knowledge? A nurse's perception of the world and situation, value structures used to evaluate the situation, personal relationships, psychomotor and cognitive skills of generalized and specialized types that are acquired from experience, and the ability to focus have all been found to influence the degree of congruency between knowledge and knowledge use in practice. Intuition has also been proposed as one of the major explanatory concepts that influence nursing practice.

Thus, theories for the practice domain should aim to apply various aspects of nursing practice and their relationships to client outcomes. The aim of such theories inherently would be to produce "better" nursing practice, and "better" outcomes and experiences in clients.

THEORETICAL IDEAS FOR THE DOMAIN OF ENVIRONMENT

Theory development for the domain of environment is not central to nursing in general. However, nursing may need to pay attention to developing theories about phenomena of the environment domain, to the extent that explanation about such phenomena illuminates and provides deeper understanding about clients, client–nurse phenomena, and nursing practice. Especially important areas for theory development are those pertaining to phenomena in the health care environment, such as institutionalized form of nursing practice, professional standards of nursing care, structural patterns within nursing service organizations, and the nature of public knowledge in nursing.

Theories regarding how the character of a given nursing-care environment (e.g., the structure of routinization) is brought about through interactive processes of the setting or how the service practice models are adopted through political processes are important for understanding nurses' practice behaviors (Esposito, 1998). Theoretical explanations about such phenomena are essential, as they impact nursing practice and client outcomes.

SUMMARY

This provisional look suggests a need to develop systems of theories and theoretical statements dealing with phenomena appropriate for nursing attention at several different levels and with different focuses. Indeed, theoretical questions for the domains of client, client–nurse, practice, and environment can be appropriately addressed on three levels of theory: grand theories, meso- and middle-range theories, and micro-theories.

Grand Theories

The nursing models by Rogers, Roy, and Orem, among others, may be extended to include propositions that link client phenomena of holistic and particularistic types with client–nurse interaction and nursing practice. Grand theories contain propositions dealing with nursing problems that may exist in various types of clients and nursing-care situations. Thus, grand theories should be comprehensive in their explanations of nursing phenomena. A grand theory of nursing should contain a complex system of propositions, based on assumptions about human nature. So far, with the exception of Rogers's theory of unitary humans, nursing's grand theories tend to focus on the domain of client.

I believe it is necessary that grand theories focus specifically on each domain rather than try to deal with all relevant phenomena in nursing. This is because both the ontological and epistemological orientations must be delineated with a different focus for each domain. It is also critical that the existing grand theories of nursing be further developed to include systematic formulations of theoretical propositions based on their assumptions and conceptualizations. In the last two decades, there has been a growing interest in middle-range theories and work to develop middle-range theories deduced from the grand theories has been undertaken, especially with the theories of Neuman, Orem, Rogers, and Roy (see, for instance, Barrett, 2000; Dobratz, 2008; Dobratz & Pilkington, 2004; Fawcett, 2004, 2005; Gigliotti, 2003; Kim, 2008; Skalski, DiGerolamo, & Gigliotti, 2006; Wright, 2007). This certainly is a critical development that needs to be more rigorous.

Meso- and Middle-Range Theories

Although theory development at the middle-range level has been active during the last two decades, as shown earlier, there has been less focus on developing mesotheories. Although there is a continuing need to develop middle-range theories, it is becoming necessary also to examine ways to develop mesotheories. For example, the literature shows a great deal of knowledge regarding various aspects of women's health with some middle-range theories for specific phenomena such as perimenstural syndrome. A mesotheory for women's health would make it possible to view women's experiences in a more integrated way. Similarly, there are possibilities for mesolevel theory development in such broad areas as chronic illness, symptom experiences, disability, and the experiences of older adults.

Microtheories

Many microtheory developments are in progress. Theoretical efforts dealing with a limited range of application, such as maternal attachment, pressure sores, wound healing, and positioning, have culminated in microtheories. In many instances, as theoretical development becomes enriched, several microtheories together may become a middle-range theory. Microtheories provide the backbone for more general, complex theories. Efforts in microtheory development are also closely related to efforts in empirical generalization, which some scientists value as the first step in theory development.

Our efforts in theoretical developments should continue on all three levels if we are to develop a knowledge system that offers comprehensive "answers" to nursing questions that are posed for different domains.

Theory development for one type of theory that is not addressed in this exposition is for theory of process. Theories of process take a special form, for which the theoretical articulation is to identify the structure, characteristics, and workings of processes. The specific nature of process theories depend upon the nature of process to be examined in a given theory. Thus, there could not be a standard model for process theories.

My review of the literature presented in this chapter is by no means comprehensive, but is used to illustrate the usefulness of the theoretical approaches presented here. The examples shown in this chapter are indeed only examples of (a) what might be appropriate questions for nursing study, (b) what might be necessary for explanations, and (c) how phenomena might be approached for different kinds of explanations. The nursing perspective, the nursing way of viewing the "reality," comes out more clearly in these examples, even if the examples are only selective. By no means are the examples noted in this chapter intended to be taken as representative or comprehensive. Yet they tell the story about the status of nursing in relation to subject matter and theoretical concerns. The burden, then, is on the systematic thinkers who must strive to define, classify, codify, and explain whatever is essential for what we are all about—nursing.

NOTES

1. Kirkevold, M. (1994). The contribution of nursing research—Knowledge about client. In *The Proceeding of 7th Biennial Conference of the Workgroup of European Nurse Researchers: The contribution of nursing research: Past–present–future* (p. 9). Oslo, Norway.
2. Roy, S. C., & Roberts, S. L. (1981). *Theory construction in nursing: An adaptation model.* Englewood Cliffs, NJ: Prentice-Hall.

10 Concluding Remarks: Issues in Theoretical Development in Nursing

There must be a clear and distinct separation of the subjective and objective components in any situation in order for us to take rational hold of the problem. The objective problem, thus isolated, is to be dealt with by a logical procedure that seeks to resolve it into a finite number of steps or operations.

—William Barrett

Modern developments and philosophies within the scientific world have subjected nursing to some grand and to some stifling effects. By arriving late at the scene of 20th-century scientific development, nursing had to quickly adopt prevailing modes of how scientific theories develop and what structure they take. In a sense, nursing science behaved as if it were a "developing country" in its effort to catch up with accomplishments in "developed countries." In another sense, nursing had to scramble, leap, and make far-reaching connections to catch up with developments in many scientific fields. Now we have reached a stage where our development of scientific knowledge must reach beyond "what nursing is all about" to "what problems nursing knowledge can 'take on' as its subject matter."

The discipline of nursing has approached the development of scientific knowledge in a multifaceted fashion. On the one hand, during the 1970s and 1980s, a prevailing (if unwitting) commitment to logical positivism encouraged and stimulated nursing scientists to consider theory building in a dogmatic fashion or to follow the route of empirical generalizations. Of course, although theory development is certainly possible through the use of deductive logic, there is no evidence that any nursing scientist is seriously committed to this method in a strict sense. Yet, as the preceding chapter shows, there has been some effort to systematize nursing knowledge into various levels of theories by imaginative and quasi-deductive forms of theoretical thinking.

Nursing has also used empirical generalization in theory development. However, because nursing has presented so little systematically found empirical evidence, theories based on inductive generalizations have suffered. Isolated cases of empirical generalizations have not reached the level of inductive hypotheses (either deterministic or probabilistic) that are required for the development of theories. Lately, nursing scientists have rediscovered this inductive method of generating knowledge, especially adopting the position taken by Glaser and Strauss (1967) for "discovering grounded theories."

On the other hand, several nursing theorists and researchers have been engaged in theory development in the spirit of Toulmin. Toulmin (1972, 1977) suggests that the function of science is to build up systems of explanatory techniques and that theories in science are devices used to describe and explain phenomena in a scientific field. To Toulmin, it is proper or even preferable in science to introduce "theories, techniques of representation, and terminologies together, at one swoop" (1953, p. 146). Toulmin further suggests that scientific problems that face a discipline at any given time are the result of differences that may exist between the intellectual explanatory ideals of that discipline and its capacity to account for phenomena scientifically (1972).

In general, nursing scientists appear to be working within Toulmin's characterizations with respect to scientific development in nursing. Thus, the maturity of a scientific discipline is evident in the way rational objectivity is adopted by the scientific community to select and maintain those conceptual schemes that have a relatively higher capacity to resolve conceptual problems in the discipline.

Furthermore, there has been a growing mistrust and disalignment with the positivist or realist ideals of science. Many researchers and scholars have flocked to the notion of human science, rooted in hermeneutics, as the correct epistemological attitude for nursing. Indeed, over the past 2 decades the literature has seen a great deal of work from the viewpoints of phenomenology and hermeneutic philosophy; as the proper means to study phenomena in the domains of client, client–nurse interaction, and practice. In addition, nursing has engaged various postmodern perspectives, including critical philosophy and poststructuralism (Omery, Kasper, & Page, 1995).

In my view, adopting an interpretive perspective is appropriate to the extent that it is used to study those aspects of nursing requiring interpretive understanding and explanation. But there remains a need to carve out the exact nature of nursing as a scientific discipline, as a distinct human practice science that differs from the general notion of human sciences designated as "interpretive."

Given these needs, and the continuing influx of many types and levels of understanding about the problems that nursing faces, it may be useful to file a "status report" on scientific advancement here, which includes (in summary form) the following: (a) identification of subject matter, (b) conceptual clarification, (c) nursing orientations or philosophies, (d) theory development, (e) the theory–practice–research link, and (f) methodology.

IDENTIFICATION OF SUBJECT MATTER

Donaldson and Crowley (1978) summarized three themes as the essence of nursing that recur in the literature: (a) concern with principles and laws that govern the life processes, well-being, and optimum functioning of a human being, sick or well; (b) concern with the patterning of human behavior in interaction with the environment in critical life situations; and (c) concern with the processes by which positive changes in health status are effected. These three themes point to the domains of client, client–nurse interaction, practice, and environment proposed in this book as the fundamental categorization schema for phenomena essential to nursing studies.

Fawcett (1984) also categorizes essential phenomena in nursing theory as man, health, environment, and nursing. Even though there is general agreement on the typology of nursing's subject matter, the actual delineation of subject matter within that typology is still tentative (see chapters 5, 6, 7, and 8). Elasticity in identifying disciplinary boundaries thus remains for us a basic premise.

At the same time, identifying subject matter for nursing must come from within the discipline. This can be accomplished by adopting a nursing perspective when conceiving of, and analyzing phenomena in the four domains. Pain as a phenomenon, for example, becomes an appropriate subject matter for nursing by conceptualizing it from a specific nursing perspective that is different from a medical, biological, or psychological perspective. Thus, identification of subject matter is a definitional issue that must be performed with a clear idea of what nursing's perspective consists of. Nursing's subject matter, especially in relation to what aspects of the human condition nursing is primarily concerned with, also requires re-thinking vis-à-vis the changing characteristics of 21st-century health care needs. As presented in chapter 5, the focus of nursing may need to expand, from mere "states" or "responses" to health problems, to how such "states" and "responses" affect the ways people manage their living in their life situations. This means that we need to re-specify nursing phenomena in relation to "living," so that nursing is oriented not only to responding to health problems, but also to addressing problems of living associated with health and health problems. The change will require that nursing expand its ontological and epistemological commitments.

CONCEPTUAL CLARIFICATION

Activities in conceptual clarification are the first-level scientific work that culminates in theories. This phase of theoretical work is especially important when a scientific discipline is striving to develop theories and theoretical systems, transplanting many concepts from other scientific fields. Conceptual clarification requires analytic and empirical identification of definitional terms.

The phases of conceptual clarification involve the following:

- A concept is selected as appropriate subject matter for a scientific explanation from the nursing perspective.
- The level of abstraction for conceptual analysis is defined.
- Definitional terms for the concept are organized into an interlinked system so as to have a theoretically appropriate meaning.
- Descriptive features of empirical referents are identified.
- Empirical inquiry is made of the definitional meanings, and the definitional terms are reaffirmed, refined, and revised.

Conceptual clarification has been fervently pursued in nursing during the past decades in preparation for development of theories, as shown in the preceding chapters. Conceptual clarification may also serve to redefine, narrow, or broaden concepts that have already been used in theoretical systems. Rodgers and Knafl (2000) have identified several different methods for concept development for nursing. Concepts become more clearly and rigorously defined and differentiated from similar concepts by applying various concept development methods. My recent review of the literature through MEDLINE, for the period 1995 to 2009 with keywords for concept analysis, concept development, and nursing, revealed 200 concepts in 252 articles published in refereed journals in English. Of these, 122 concepts were in the client domain, 18 concepts in the client–nurse domain, 56 concepts in the practice domain, and 4 concepts in the environment domain. Even though this is a remarkable increase in concept development in nursing, it also points to the need to consolidate and review for further clarification of meanings of concepts in nursing.

NURSING ORIENTATIONS OR PHILOSOPHIES

Orientations in and philosophies of nursing influence the way nursing's subject matter is viewed, and provide the general frameworks within which theories and research methodologies are developed. General worldviews held by nursing scientists also influence the way nursing theories are developed. Currently, such philosophical strands as realism, pragmatism, relativism, and postmodernism (as epistemological philosophies) and holism, humanism, existentialism, phenomenology, general systems philosophy, and material dialectics (as ontological philosophies) are found in nursing theorists' writings. Such orientations push the theoretical formulations of each theorist in somewhat different directions when it comes to the kinds of phenomena selected for study and the approaches developed for nursing strategies.

Nursing scholars often hold these orientations concurrently with philosophies of scientific inquiry. Empirical positivism, physicalism, rationalism, and logical positivism, for example, are held in combination with specific philosophies regarding humanity, life, and the world to produce a specific set of nursing knowledge. Such philosophical commitments influence the way scientific knowledge is generated. In nursing, the level of sophistication regarding the philosophy of scientific inquiry is maturing. The number of books and articles espousing specific philosophical approaches is growing, indicating a need for awareness and greater examination of the impact of philosophy on scientific development.

My position on these philosophies is clear: nursing needs to develop an epistemological framework that ties together multifaceted aspects of its subject matter in a comprehensive framework. Nursing, we must remember, is a system of knowledge within the context of a human practice science. Its epistemological framework must be built on specific ontologies of human nature, human living, and human practice that are fundamentally appropriate for nursing. Toward this end, I refer the reader to my framework for nursing epistemology (chapter 3).

THEORY DEVELOPMENT

Throughout this book, the level of theory development has been explicitly and implicitly expressed. Major theoretical work in nursing is still at the level of theoretical orientations, consisting of major assumptions about the way essential concepts are identified and developed. Theoretical propositions are very seldom stated in explanatory or predictive terms. In general, nursing's grand theories are mostly descriptive, with some evidence of development toward explanatory frameworks.

The testability of statements in nursing theories (especially of grand nursing theories) tends to be limited because of a deficiency in precise designations of empirical referents in those theories. Formalization of theoretical statements has not been attempted, and may be premature in the current state of affairs. A need exists for extensive conceptual clarification of essential phenomena in nursing so as to develop testable theories. However, an active middle-range theory development in nursing, as evidenced by the literature, does indicate that theories grow more relevant to practice as their levels of abstraction decrease.

THEORY–RESEARCH–PRACTICE LINKAGE

Although there is evidence to suggest a narrowing of gaps among theory, research, and practice, real and "artificial" gaps still exist. Real gaps result from a paucity of dialogue among practitioners in the three areas, and from a structural arrangement that segregates practitioners into different organizational settings. Artificial gaps result from discontent, power struggles, and competition among practitioners, which usually end in mutual accusation. In earlier decades, professional concerns focused on economic security, public image, and recognition. In recent decades, the profession has emerged with a new spirit of scientific discipline. This is especially true since the idea of evidence-based practice became a gold standard for professional practice in health care, including nursing. Since its introduction in the 1990s in a medical context, nursing's scientific orientation has become firmly established. This, along with the burgeoning amount of scientific output in the literature, points to the critical need for theory–research–practice linkages.

Since theory development and research in nursing exist to improve nursing practice, I have proposed *knowledge-based practice* instead of the narrow-sounding evidence-based practice (Kim, 2006). This proposal contains three key assumptions: (a) knowledge for nursing practice refers to a body of specialized knowledge that is multidimensional, complex in its configuration, and derived from multiple sources; (b) the processes by which individual practitioners use or apply knowledge in practice are context-specific, situated, and individualistic in the sense that each practice instance is unique in its presentation of a patient's conditions, problems, trajectory, history, and context; and (c) the practitioner is the user of knowledge who must adopt certain cognitive, strategic, and action processes (Kim, 2006).

Massive and continuing output of theoretical and empirical work in the literature requires that nursing scientists engage not only in producing such work, but also in reviewing and evaluating the literature so as to systematize the knowledge base for practitioners. This, it seems, is the only way we can narrow the gap between theory, research, and practice. The advent of the Cochrane database for medicine and health care is one example to consider. However, since this database is guided by a narrow ideal of scientific evidence, there is a need to develop a set of specific guidelines to review advances in nursing knowledge that apply the framework for the nursing epistemology proposed in this book. This also requires intersector collaboration (among theorists, researchers, and practitioners). Only through detailed scrutiny of the influence of theory on practice and research, and of the influence of practice on theory and research, can nursing evolve into a viable science. It is by grounding theoretical formulations in practice and aligning practice problems for research that nursing can expand its rich scientific capacities. Such detailed scrutiny is needed to overcome the real gaps among the three sectors.

METHODOLOGY

It is an attractive idea to be highly competent in one or two methodologies of scientific inquiry. However, a growing scientific discipline needs to be diverse in its use of techniques of inquiry. The themes for nursing science must be "discovery" and "expansion." The diversity of subject matter for nursing science necessitates the application of various techniques and methodologies of inquiry and scientific study. This is especially appropriate if we are to accept the notion of nursing epistemology (as proposed in this book) as the general framework for developing nursing knowledge. Five epistemological spheres in nursing knowledge point to various methodological orientations not only as possibility but also as necessity.

FINAL REMARKS

In this book, I have focused on the nature of theoretical thinking rather than on the substance of theories. Since I believe that systematic formulation and reformulation are necessary in nursing for identifying subject matter and developing theories, I have suggested several different ways of viewing aspects of the world that are of interest to nursing. I have not attempted to evaluate or criticize theories in a systematic or comprehensive manner. I thus have included those appropriate aspects of nursing and other theories mainly to illustrate, expand on, and apply the ideas discussed. As suggested in chapter 1, both theories *of* nursing and theories *in* nursing need to be developed, tested, and refined if we are to develop a codified body of scientific knowledge that is ultimately required for the responsible practice of nursing.

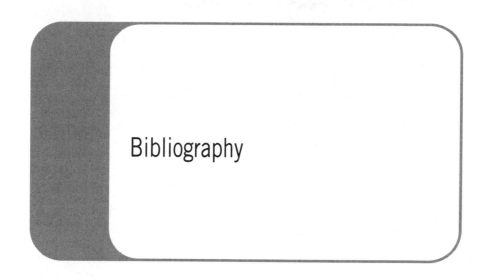

Bibliography

Abdellah, F. G., Beland, I. L., Martin, A., & Matheney, R. V. (1960). *Patient-centered approaches to nursing*. New York: Macmillan.

Abell, P. (1971). *Model building in sociology*. New York: Schochen Books.

Abraham, L., Danielson, M. B., Eberle, N., Green, L., Rosenberg, J., & Stoner, C. (1991). *Reinventing home*. New York: Plume.

Adams, A., Pelletier, D., Duffield, C., Nagy, S., Crisp, J., & Mitten-Lewis, S. (1997). Determining and discerning expert practice: A review of the literature. *Clinical Nurse Specialist, 11*, 217–222.

Adams, M. (1986). Aging: Gerontological nursing research. In J. J. Fitzpatrick, H. H. Werley, & R. Taunton (Eds.), *Annual review of nursing research* (Vol. 4, pp. 77–103). New York: Springer Publishing Company.

Ader, R., & Cohen, N. (1975). Behaviorally conditioned immunosuppression. *Psychosomatic Medicine, 37*, 333–340.

Ader, R., Felten, D. L., & Cohen, N. (2006). *Psychoneuroimmunology* (4th ed.). New York: Academic Press.

Aiken, L., & Patrician, P. (2000). Measuring organizational traits of hospitals: The Revised Nursing Work Index. *Nursing Research, 49*, 146–153.

Alexander, T. M. (1987). *John Dewey's theory of art, experience, and nature: The horizons of feeling*. Albany, NY: State University of New York Press.

Allen, D. (1985). Nursing research and social control: Alternative models of science that emphasize understanding and emancipation. *Journal of Nursing Scholarship, 17*, 59–64.

Allen, D. (2007). What do you do at work? Profession building and doing nursing. *International Nursing Review, 54*, 41–48.

Allen, D. G. (1995). Hermeneutics: Philosophical traditions and nursing practice research. *Nursing Science Quarterly, 8*, 174–182.

Allen, D., Benner, P., & Diekelmann, N. L. (1983). Three paradigms for nursing research: Methodological implications. In P. Chinn (Ed.), *Nursing research methodology* (pp. 23–38). Washington, DC: Aspen Systems.

Allmark, P. (1995). A classical view of the theory–practice gap in nursing. *Journal of Advanced Nursing, 22,* 18–23.

American Nurses Association. (1965). American Nurses Association first position on education for nursing. *American Journal of Nursing, 65,* 106–111.

American Nurses Association. (1995). *Nursing: A social policy statement.* Washington, DC: Author.

American Psychiatric Association. (1994). *Diagnostic and statistical manual of mental disorders* (4th ed.). Washington, DC: American Psychiatric Press.

Anderson, R. M., & Funnell, M. M. (2008). The art and science of diabetes education: A culture out of balance. *Diabetes Educator, 34,* 109–117.

Annis, R. C., & Frost, B. (1973). Human visual ecology and orientation anisopropics in acuity. *Science, 182,* 729–231.

Antonovsky, A. (1979). *Health, stress, and coping.* San Francisco: Jossey-Bass.

Appleton, C. (1993). The art of nursing: The experience of patients and nurses. *Journal of Advanced Nursing, 18,* 892–899.

Appleton, C. (1994). The gift of self: A paradigm for originating nursing as art. In P. L. Chinn & J. Watson (Eds.), *Art & aesthetic in nursing* (pp. 91–114). New York: National League for Nursing.

Argyris, C., Putnam, R., & Smith, D. (1985). *Action science.* San Francisco: Jossey-Bass.

Argyris, C., & Schön, D. (1976). *Theory in practice: Increasing professional effectiveness.* San Francisco: Jossey-Bass.

Aristotle. (1980). *The Nicomachean ethics* (Trans. by D. Ross). Oxford, UK: Oxford University Press.

Aspinall, M. J., Jambruno, N., & Phoenix, B. S. (1977). The why and how of nursing diagnosis. *MCN: American Journal of Maternal and Child Nursing, 2,* 354–358.

Austgard, K. (2006). The aesthetic experience of nursing. *Nursing Philosophy: An International Journal for Healthcare Professionals, 7,* 11–19.

Avant, K. (1979). Nursing diagnosis: Maternal attachment. *Advances in Nursing Science, 2,* 45–55.

Avery, J. A. (2003). *Assessment and treatment of end stage restlessness and agitation.* Unpublished manuscript. Largo, FL: Hospice of the Florida Suncoast.

Babrow, A. S., & Mattson, M. (2003). Theorizing about health communication. In T. L. Thompson, A. M. Dorsey, K. I. Miller, & R. Parrott (Eds.), *Handbook of health communication* (pp. 35–61). Mahwah, NJ: Lawrence Erlbaum.

Baker, C. (1997). Cultural relativism and cultural diversity: Implications for nursing practice. *Advances in Nursing Science, 20,* 3–11.

Baldwin, S. A., Wampold, B. E., & Imel, Z. E. (2007). Untangling the alliance-outcome correlation: Exploring the relative importance of therapist and patient variability in the alliance. *Journal of Consulting and Clinical Psychology, 75,* 842–852.

Balke, F. (1999). The health/illness continuum. In H. S. Kim & I. Kollak (Eds.), *Nursing theories: Conceptual and philosophical foundations* (pp. 161–188). New York: Springer Publishing Company.

Bandura, A. (1969). *Principles of behavior modification.* New York: Holt, Rinehart, and Winston.

Bandura, A. (1997). *Self-efficacy: The exercise of control.* New York: Freeman.

Barnard, C. (1957). *An introduction to the study of experimental medicine* (H. C. Greene, Trans.). New York: Dover Publications. (Originally published in 1865; original translation published 1927)

Barnard, K. (1973). The effect of stimulation on the sleep behavior of the premature infant. *Communicating Nursing Research, 6,* 12–33.

Barnard, K. E. (1983). Nursing research related to infants and young children. *Annual Review of Nursing Research, 1,* 3–25.

Barnes, J. (Ed.). (1984). *The complete works of Aristotle: The revised Oxford translation* (Vol. 2, p. 802). Princeton, NJ: Princeton University Press.

Barnes, R., & Raskin, M. (1980). Strategies for diagnosing and treating agitation in the aging. *Geriatrics, 35,* 111–119.

Barnum, B. J. S. (1994). *Nursing theory: Analysis, application, evaluation* (4th ed.). Philadelphia: J. B. Lippincott.

Barofsky, I. (1978). Compliance, adherence, and the therapeutic alliance: Steps in the development of self-care. *Social Science and Medicine, 12A,* 369–376.

Barrett, E. (2000). The theoretical matrix for a Rogerian nursing practice. *Theoria: Journal of Nursing Theory, 9*(4), 3–7.

Barrett, E. A. M. (2002). What is nursing science? *Nursing Science Quarterly, 15,* 51–60.

Barrett, W. (1978). *The illusion of technique.* Garden City, NY: Anchor Press.

Baum, F. E., & Ziersch, A. M. (2003). Social capital. *Journal of Epidemiology and Community Health, 57,* 320–323.

Baumann, S. L. (1999). Art as a path of inquiry. *Nursing Science Quarterly, 12,* 106–110.

Becker, M. H. (1974). The health belief model and personal health behavior. *Health Education Monogram, 2,* 326–473.

Becker, M. H. (1976). Sociobehavioral determinants of compliance. In D. L. Sackett & R. B. Haynes (Eds.), *Compliance with therapeutic regimens* (pp. 40–50). Baltimore, MD: Johns Hopkins University Press.

Beckstrand, J. (1978a). The notion of a practice theory and the relationships of scientific and ethical knowledge to practice. *Research in Nursing and Health, 1,* 131–136.

Beckstrand, J. (1978b). The need for a practice theory as indicated by the knowledge used in the conduct of practice. *Research in Nursing and Health, 1,* 175–179.

Benne, K. D., Chin, R., & Bennis, W. G. (1976). Science and practice. In W. G. Bennis, K. D. Benne, R. Chin, & K. E. Corey (Eds.), *The planning of change* (3rd ed., pp. 128–137). New York: Holt, Rinehart, and Winston.

Benner, P. (1984). *From novice to expert: Excellence and power in clinical nursing practice.* Menlo Park, CA: Addison-Wesley.

Benner, P. (1991). The role of experience, narrative, and community in skilled ethical comportment. *Advances in Nursing Science, 14,* 1–21.

Benner, P. (1996a). A response by P. Benner to K. Cash, "Benner and expertise in nursing: A critique." *International Journal of Nursing Studies, 33,* 669–674.

Benner, P. (1996b). *Expertise in nursing practice.* New York: Springer Publishing Company.

Benner, P. (2000). The role of embodiment, emotion and lifeworld for rationality and agency in nursing practice. *Nursing Philosophy, 1,* 5–19.

Benner, P. (2001). *From novice to expert: Excellence and power in clinical nursing practice* (Commemorative ed.). Englewood Cliffs, NJ: Prentice-Hall.

Benner, P. (2009). *Expertise in nursing practice: Caring, clinical judgment, and ethics* (2nd ed.). New York: Springer Publishing Company.

Benner, P., & Tanner, C. (1987). Clinical judgment: How expert nurses use intuition. *American Journal of Nursing, 87,* 23–31.

Benner, P., & Wrubel, J. (1989). *The primacy of caring: Stress and coping in health and illness.* Reading, MA: Addison-Wesley.

Benner, P., Tanner, C., & Chesla, C. (1992). From beginner to expert: Gaining a differentiated clinical world in critical care nursing. *Advances in Nursing Science, 14,* 13–28.

Benoist, J., & Cathebras, P. (1993). The body: From an immateriality to another. *Social Science and Medicine, 36,* 857–865.

Benoliel, J. Q. (1977). Conceptual precision and research about human dying. *Communicating Nursing Research, 9,* 237–243.

Benoliel, J. Q. (1985). Loss and terminal illness. *Nursing Clinics of North America, 20,* 439–448.

Benoliel, J. Q. (1996). Grounded theory and nursing knowledge. *Qualitative Health Research, 6,* 406–428.

Berger, P. L. (1963). *Invitation to sociology: A humanistic perspective.* Garden City, NY: Doubleday.

Berger, P. L., & Kellner, H. (1981). *Sociology reinterpreted.* Garden City, NY: Anchor Books.

Berkanovic, E. (1972). Lay conceptions of the sick role. *Social Forces, 51,* 53–64.

Berkman, L. F., & Glass, T. (2000). Social integration, social networks, social support and health. In L. F. Berkman & I. Kawachi (Eds.), *Social epidemiology* (pp. 137–173). Oxford: Oxford University Press.

Bernstein, R. J. (1971). *Praxis and action: Contemporary philosophies of human activity.* Philadelphia: University of Philadelphia Press.

Bexton, W. H., Heron, W., & Scott, T. H. (1954). Effects of decreased variation in the sensory environment. *Canadian Journal of Psychology, 8,* 70–76.

Bhaskar, R. (1986). *Scientific realism and human emancipation.* London: Verso.

Bhaskar, R. (1991). *Philosophy and the idea of freedom.* Oxford, UK: Blackwell.

Biley, F. C. (1996). Rogerian science, phantoms, and therapeutic touch: Exploring potentials. *Nursing Science Quarterly, 9,* 165–169.

Bingham, P. M. (2009). Deprivation and dysphagia in premature infants. *Journal of Child Neurology, 24,* 743–749.

Bishop, A. H., & Scudder, J. R., Jr. (1990). *The practical, moral, and personal sense of nursing: A phenomenological philosophy of practice.* Albany, NY: State University of New York Press.

Bissonnette, J. M. (2008). Adherence: A concept analysis. *Journal of Advanced Nursing, 63,* 634–643.

Black, P., McKenna, H., & Deeny, P. (1997). A concept analysis of the sensoristrain experienced by intensive care patients. *Intensive & Critical Care Nursing: The Official Journal of the British Association of Critical Care Nurses, 13,* 209–215.

Blalock, H. M., Jr. (1969). *Theory construction: From verbal to mathematical formulations.* Englewood Cliffs, NJ: Prentice-Hall.

Blalock, H. M., Jr. (1979). Measurement and conceptualization problems: The major obstacles to integrating theory and research. *American Sociological Review, 44,* 881–884.

Blanchette, H. (2005). Assessment and treatment of terminal restlessness in the hospitalized adult patient with cancer. *Medsurg Nursing, 14*(1), 17–23.

Blau, P. M. (Ed.). (1975). *Approaches to the study of social structure.* New York: Free Press.

Bonner, A. (2003). Recognition of expertise: An important concept in the acquisition of nephrology nursing expertise. *Nursing & Health Science, 5,* 123–131.

Booth, K., Kenrick, M., & Woods, S. (1997). Nursing knowledge, theory and method revisited. *Journal of Advanced Nursing, 26,* 804–811.

Bourdieu, P. (1977). *Outline of a theory of practice.* Cambridge: Cambridge University Press.

Bourdieu, P. (1986). The forms of capital. In J. Richardson (Ed.), *Handbook of theory and research for the sociology of education* (pp. 241–258). Westport, CT: Greenwood Press.

Bourdieu, P. (1990). *The logic of practice* (R. Nice, Trans.). Stanford, CA: Stanford University Press.

Boyle, S. (2004). Nursing unit characteristics and patient outcomes. *Nursing Economics, 22,* 111.

Briant, S., & Freshwater, D. (1998). Exploring mutuality within the nurse-patient relationship. *British Journal of Nursing, 7,* 204–206.

Bridgman, P. W. (1927). *The logic of modern physics.* New York: Macmillan.

Brook, R. H., Ware, J. E., Davis-Avery, A., et al. (1979). Overview of adult health status measures fielded in Rand's health insurance study. *Medical Care, 17*(Suppl.), 1–131.

Brown, N. O. (1959). *Life against death: The psychoanalytical meaning of history.* Middletown, CT: Wesleyan University Press.

Brownfield, C. A. (1972). *The brain benders: A study of the effects of isolation* (2nd enlarged ed.). New York: Exposition Press.

Browning, D. S. (1973). *Generative man: Psychoanalytic perspectives.* Philadelphia: Westminster Press.

Bruhn, J. G., & Wolf, S. (1979). *The Roseto story: An anatomy of health.* Norman, OK: University of Oklahoma Press.

Brunie, A. (2009). Meaningful distinctions within a concept: Relational, collective, and generalized social capital. *Social Science Research, 38,* 251–265.

Buetow, S. (1998). Four strategies for negotiated care. *Journal of The Royal Society of Medicine, 91,* 199–201.

Bulechek, G. M., & McCloskey, J. C. (1992). Defining and validating nursing intervention. *Nursing Clinics of North America, 22,* 289–299.

Burke, A. L. (1997). Palliative care: An update on "terminal restlessness." *Medical Journal of Australia, 166,* 39–42.

Byrd, M. E. (2006). Social exchange as a framework for client-nurse interaction during public health nursing maternal-child home visits. *Public Health Nursing, 23,* 271–276.

Callaghan, P., & Morrissey, J. (1993). Social support and health: A review. *Journal of Advanced Nursing, 18,* 203–210.

Cannon, W. B. (1932). *The wisdom of the body.* New York: W.W. Norton.

Carper, B. (1978). Fundamental patterns of knowing in nursing. *Advances in Nursing Science, 1,* 13–23.

Carper, B. (1988). Response to "Perspectives on knowing: a model of nursing knowledge." *Scholarly Inquiry for Nursing Practice: An International Journal, 2,* 141–144.

Cartwright, J. C., Archbold, P. G., Stewart, B. J., & Limandri, B. (1994). Enrichment processes in family caregiving to frail elders. *Advances in Nursing Science, 17,* 31–43.

Cash, K. (1995). Benner and expertise in nursing: A critique. *International Journal of Nursing Studies, 32,* 527–534.

Cassel, J. (1976). The contribution of the social environment to host resistance. *American Journal of Epidemiology, 104,* 107–122.

Catty, J. (2004). "The vehicle of success": Theoretical and empirical perspectives on the therapeutic alliance in psychotherapy and psychiatry. *Psychology and Psychotherapy, 77*(Pt. 2), 255–272.

Chatterjee, J. S. (2006). From compliance to concordance in diabetes. *Journal of Medical Ethics, 32,* 507–510.

Chevrolet, J., & Jolliet, P. (2007). Clinical review: Agitation and delirium in the critically ill—significance and management. *Critical Care, 11,* 214–218.

Chinn P. L., Maeve, K., & Bostick, C. (1997). Aesthetic inquiry and the art of nursing. *Scholarly Inquiry for Nursing Practice, 11,* 83–95.

Chinn, P. L. (1985). Debunking myths in nursing theory and research. *Journal of Nursing Scholarship, 17,* 45–49.

Chinn, P. L. (2001). Toward a theory of nursing art. In N. Chaska (Ed.), *The nursing profession: Tomorrow and beyond* (pp. 287–298). Thousand Oaks, CA: Sage.

Chinn, P. L., & Kramer, M. K. (2003). *Integrated knowledge development in nursing* (6th ed.). St. Louis: Mosby.

Chinn, P. L., & Kramer, M. K. (2007). *Integrated theory and knowledge development in nursing* (7th ed.). St. Louis: Elsevier.

Christensen, M., & Hewitt-Taylor, J. (2006). From expert to tasks, expert nursing practice redefined? *Journal of Clinical Nursing, 15,* 1531–1539.

Cialdini, R. B., & Goldstein, N. J. (2004). Social influence: Compliance and conformity. *Annual Review of Psychology, 55,* 591–621.

Clark, J. (1998). The international classification for nursing practice project. *Online Journal of Issues in Nursing.* Retrieved November 10, 2009, from www.nursingworld.org/Main MenuCategories/ANAMarketplace/ANAPeriodicals/OJIN/TableofContents/vol31998/ No2Sept1998/TheInternationalClassificationForNursingProject.aspx

Cleland, C. E. (2001). Historical science, experimental science, and the scientific method. *Geology, 29,* 987–990.

Cobb, S. (1976). Social support as a moderator of life stress. *Psychosomatic Medicine, 38,* 300–314.

Coenen, A. (2003). The international classification for nursing practice (ICNP) programme: Advancing a unifying framework for nursing. *Online Journal of Issues in Nursing.* Retrieved November 10, 2009, from www.nursingworld.org/MainMenuCategories/ANA Marketplace/ANAPeriodicals/OJIN/TableofContents/vol82003/No2May2003/Articles PreviousTopics/TheInternationalClassificationForNursingProject.aspx

Cohen, C. I., & Sokolovsky, J. (1979). Health-seeking behavior and social network of the aged living in single-room occupancy hotels. *Journal of American Geriatrics Society, 27,* 270–278.

Cohen, S. M. (2009). Concept analysis of adherence in the context of cardiovascular risk reduction. *Nursing Forum, 44,* 25–36.

Coleman, J. (1988). Social capital in the creation of human capital. *American Journal of Sociology, 94*(Suppl.), S95–S120.

Colwell, C. (1996). The virtual body of medicine. *International Studies in Philosophy, 28,* 1–9.

Comte, A. (2009). *A general view of positivism* (J. H. Bridges, Trans.). Cambridge: Cambridge University Press. (Originally published in 1851; original translation initially published in 1865)

Connor, M. J. (2004). The practical discourse in philosophy and nursing: An exploration of linkages and shifts in the evolution of praxis. *Nursing Philosophy, 5,* 54–66.

Constantino, M., & Smith-Hansen, L. (2008). Patient interpersonal factors and the therapeutic alliance in two treatments for bulimia nervosa. *Psychotherapy Research: Journal of the Society for Psychotherapy Research, 18,* 683–698.

Coser, R. L. (1978). *Training in ambiguity: Learning through doing in a mental hospital.* New York: Free Press.

Cox, C. L. (1982). An interaction model of client health behavior: Theoretical prescription for nursing. *Advances in Nursing Science, 5,* 41–56.

Craig, R. T. (1999). Communication theory as a field. *Communication Theory, 9,* 119–161.

Cramer, J. A., Mattson, R. H., Prevey, M. L., Scheyer, R. D., & Ouellette, V. L. (1989). How often is medication taken as prescribed? *Journal of the American Medical Association, 22,* 3273–3277.

Cravey, A. J., Washburn, S. A., Gesler, W. M., Arcury, T. A., & Skelly, A. H. (2001). Developing socio-spatial knowledge networks: A qualitative methodology for chronic disease prevention. *Social Science & Medicine, 52,* 1763–1775.

Crawford, D. W. (1974). *Kant's aesthetic theory.* Madison, WI: University of Wisconsin Press.

Darbyshire, P. (1994). Skilled expert practice: Is it 'all in the mind'? A response to English's critique of Benner's novice to expert model. *Journal of Advanced Nursing, 19,* 755–761.

Darbyshire, P. (1999). Nursing, art and science: Revisiting the two cultures. *International Journal of Nursing Practice, 5,* 123–131.

De Raeve, L. (1998). The art of nursing: Aesthetics or praxis? *Nursing Ethics, 5,* 401–411.

Deering, C. G. (1987). Developing a therapeutic alliance with the anorexia nervosa client. *Journal of Psychosocial Nursing, 25,* 11–17.

Denyes, M. J. (1983). Nursing research related to school age children and adolescents. *Annual Review of Nursing Research, 1,* 27–53.

Dewey, J. (1934). Aesthetic experience. In J. A. Boydston & H. F. Simon (Eds.). (1987), *John Dewey: The later works, 1925–1953. Volume 10: 1934.* Carbondale, IL: Southern Illinois University Press.

Dickoff, J., & James, P. (1968). A theory of theories: A position paper. *Nursing Research, 17,* 197–203.

Dickoff, J., James, P., & Wiedenbach, E. (1968a). Theory in a practice discipline; Part I—Practice oriented theory. *Nursing Research, 17,* 415–435.

Dickoff, J., James, P., & Wiedenbach, E. (1968b). Theory in a practice discipline; Part II—Practice oriented research. *Nursing Research, 17,* 545–554.

Dobratz, M. C. (2008). Moving nursing science forward within the framework of the Roy adaptation model. *Nursing Science Quarterly, 21,* 255–259.

Dobratz, M. C., & Pilkington, F. B. (2004). Research issues. A dialogue about two nursing science traditions: The Roy adaptation model and the human becoming theory. *Nursing Science Quarterly, 17,* 301–307.

Dobzhansky, T. (1967). *The biology of ultimate concern.* New York: New American Library.

Donaldson, S. K., & Crowley, D. M. (1978). The discipline of nursing. *Nursing Outlook, 26,* 113–120.

Doyle, K. O. (1992). The symbolic meaning of house and home. *American Behavioral Scientist, 35,* 790–802.

Draucker, C. B. (1999). The critique of Heideggerian hermeneutical nursing research. *Journal of Advanced Nursing, 30,* 360–373.

Dreitzel, H. P. (Ed.). (1971). *The social organization of health* (p. 3). New York: Macmillan.

Dreyfus, H. L., & Dreyfus, S. E. (1986). *Mind over machine: The power of human intuition and expertise in the era of the computer.* New York: Free Press.

Dubin, R. (1978). *Theory building* (rev. ed.). New York: Free Press.

Dubos, R. (1976). The state of health and the quality of life. *Western Journal of Medicine, 125,* 8–11.

Dubos, R. (1965). *Man adapting.* New Haven, CT: Yale University Press.

Durkheim, E. (1951). *Suicide: A study in sociology* (J. A. Spaulding & G. Simpson, Trans.). New York: Free Press.

Dzik, W. H., Laposata, M., Hertl, M., Sandberg, W. C., Chatterji, M., & Misdraji, J. (2008). Case 38-2008: A 58-year-old man with hemophilia, hepatocellular carcinoma, and intractable bleeding. *New England Journal of Medicine, 359,* 2587–2597.

Eaton, W. W. (1978). Life events, social supports, and psychiatric symptoms: A reanalysis of the New Haven data. *Journal of Health and Social Behavior, 19,* 230–234.

Edwards, B. (1998). A & E nurses' constructs on the nature of nursing expertise: A repertory grid technique. *Accident and Emergency Nursing, 6,* 18–23.

Edwards, S. D. (1998). The art of nursing. *Nursing Ethics, 5,* 393–400.

Einstein, A. (1961). *Relativity: The special and general theory.* New York: Crown.

Ellefsen, B. (2004). Frames and perspectives in clinical nursing practice: A study of Norwegian nurses in acute care settings. *Research & Theory for Nursing Practice, 18,* 95–109.

Ellefsen, B., & Kim, H. S. (2004). Nurses' construction of clinical situations: A study conducted in an acute-care setting in Norway. *Canadian Journal of Nursing Research, 36,* 114–131.

Ellefsen, B., & Kim, H. S. (2005). Nurses' clinical engagement: A study from an acute-care setting in Norway. *Research and Theory for Nursing Practice, 19,* 297–313.

Ellefsen, B., Kim, H. S., & Han, K. J. (2007). Nursing gaze as framework for nursing practice: A study from acute care settings in Korea, Norway, and the USA. *Scandinavian Journal of Caring Science, 21,* 98–105.

Ellis, R. (1968). Characteristics of significant theories. *Nursing Research, 17,* 217–222.

Ellis, R. (1970). Values and vicissitudes of the scientist nurse. *American Journal of Nursing, 19,* 440–445.

Elvins, R., & Green, J. (2008). The conceptualization and measurement of therapeutic alliance: An empirical review. *Clinical Psychology Review, 28,* 1167–1187.

Emden, C. (1991). Ways of knowing in nursing. In G. Gray & R. Pratt (Eds.), *Towards a discipline of nursing* (pp. 11–30). Melbourne, Australia: Churchill Livingstone.

Engebretson, J. (1997). A multiparadigm approach to nursing. *Advances in Nursing Science, 20,* 21–33.

Engebretson, J., & Littleton, L. Y. (2001). Cultural negotiation: A constructivitst-based model for nursing practice. *Nurisng Outlook, 49,* 223–230.

Engel, G. A. (1975). A unified concept of health and disease. In T. Mullin (Ed.), *Medical behavioral science* (pp. 185–200). Philadelphia: W.B. Saunders.

Engel, G. A. (1977). The need for a new medical model: A challenge for biomedicine. *Science, 196,* 129–136.

Engel, G. L. (1970). Sudden death and the medical model in psychiatry. *Canadian Psychiatric Association Journal, 15,* 527–538.

Engelhardt, H. T., Jr. (1976). Ideology and etiology. *Journal of Medicine & Philosophy, 1,* 256–268.

English, H. B., & English, A. C. (1958). *A comprehensive dictionary of psychological and psychoanalytical terms.* New York: Longman, Green.

English, I. (1993). Intuition as a function of the expert nurse: A critique of Benner's novice to expert model. *Journal of Advanced Nursing, 18,* 387–393.

Engster, D. (2005). Rethinking care theory: The practice of caring and the obligation to care. *Hypatia, 20,* 50–74.

Eraut, M. (1994). *Developing professional knowledge and competence.* London: Falmer Press.

Erikson, E. H. (1959). *Identity and the life cycle: Selected papers* (Psychological Issues Monograph, Vol. 1, no. 1). New York: International University Press.

Erikson, E. H. (1964). *Insight and responsibility: Lectures on the ethical implications of psychoanalytic insight.* New York: W.W. Norton.

Esposito, M. B. (1998). *An exploration of the nature of nursing practice in patient-focused care.* PhD Dissertation, University of Rhode Island, Kingston, RI.

Fabrega, H., Jr. (1974). *Disease and social behavior: An interdisciplinary perspective.* Cambridge: MIT Press.

Fagerhaugh, S., & Strauss, A. (1977). *Politics of pain management.* Menlo Park, CA: Addison-Wesley.

Fagermoen, M. S. (1997). Professional identity: Values embedded in meaningful nursing practice. *Journal of Advanced Nursing, 25,* 434–441.

Faulkner, M., & Aveyard, B. (2002). Is the hospital sick role a barrier to patient participation? *Nursing Times, 98*(24), 35–36.

Fawcett, J. (1978). The "what" of theory development. In *Theory development: What, why, how?* (pp. 17–33). New York: National League for Nursing.

Fawcett, J. (1984). The metaparadigm of nursing: Present status and future refinements. *Image: Journal of Nursing Scholarship, 16,* 84–87.

Fawcett, J. (1993). From a plethora of paradigms to parsimony in worldviews. *Nursing Science Quarterly, 6,* 56–59.

Fawcett, J. (1994). *Analysis and evaluation of theoretical models of nursing.* Philadelphia: F. A. Davis.

Fawcett, J. (2000). The state of nursing science: Where is the nursing in the science? *Theoria: Journal of Nursing Theory, 9*(3), 3–10.

Fawcett, J. (2004). The theory of human becoming in action. *Nursing Science Quarterly, 17,* 226–226.

Fawcett, J. (2005). Scholarly dialogue. Using the Roy adaptation model to guide nursing research. *Nursing Science Quarterly, 18,* 320–320.

Fawcett, J., Watson, J., Neuman, B., Walker, P. H. & Fitzpatrick, J. J. (2001). On nursing theories and evidence. *Journal of Nursing Scholarship, 33,* 115–119.

Feibelman, J. K. (1978). The artificial environment. In J. Lenihan & W. Fletcher (Eds.), *The build environment: Environment and man* (Vol. 8, pp. 145–168). New York: Academic Press.

Ferlander, S. (2007). The importance of different forms of social capital for health. *Acta Sociologica, 50,* 115–128.

Finfgeld-Connett, D. (2005). Clarification of social support. *Journal of Nursing Scholarship, 37,* 4–9.

Finfgeld-Connett, D. (2008a). Concept synthesis of the art of nursing. *Journal of Advanced Nursing, 62,* 381–382.

Finfgeld-Connett, D. (2008b). Qualitative convergence of three nursing concepts: Art of nursing, presence and caring. *Journal of Advanced Nursing, 63,* 527–534.

Fitzpatrick, J. J. (1991). Taxonomy II: Definitions and development—Table I: Definitions of human response. In R. M. Carroll-Johnson (Ed.), *Classification of nursing diagnoses: Proceedings of the Ninth Conference* (p. 25). Philadelphia: Lippincott Williams & Wilkins.

Flaming, D. (2001). Using *phronesis* instead of 'research-based practice' as the guiding light for nursing practice. *Nursing Philosophy, 2,* 251–258.

Fleming, J. W. (1986). Research on nursing practice: Preschool children. *Annual Review of Nursing Research, 4,* 21–54.

Fletcher, J. (1979). *Humanhood: Essays in biomedical ethics.* Buffalo, NY: Prometheus Books.

Foucault, M. (1965). *Madness and civilization* (R. Howard, Trans.). New York: Vintage/Random House. (Originally published in 1961)

Foucault, M. (1973). *The birth of the clinic. An archeology of medical perception* (A. M. Sheridan Smith, Trans.). London: Tavistock Publications. (Originally published in 1963)

Foucault, M. (1980). *The history of sexuality* (Vol. 1–3, R. Hurley, Trans.). New York: Random House. (Original work published in 1976)

Fox, R. C. (1957). Training for uncertainty. In R. K. Merton, G. G. Reeder, & P. L. Kendall (Eds.), *The student physician.* Cambridge, MA: Harvard University Press.

Fredericks, M., Odiet, J. A., Miller, S. I., & Fredericks, J. (2006). Toward a conceptual reexamination of the patient-physician relationship in the healthcare institution for the new millennium. *Journal of the National Medical Association, 98,* 378–385.

Frege, G. (1884/1980). *The foundations of arithmetic: A logico-mathematical inquiry into the concept of number* (2nd rev. ed.). Evanston, IL: Northwestern University Press.

Freidson, E. (1970a). *Professional dominance.* New York: Atherton Press.

Freidson, E. (1970b). *Profession of medicine.* New York: Dodd, Mead.

Freire, P. (1970/1992). *Pedagogy of the oppressed.* Harmondsworth, UK: Penguin.

Freud, S. (1955a). *The interpretation of dreams. A standard edition of the complete psychological works by Sigmund Freud* (Vols. IV & V). London: Hogarth Press. (Original work published in 1900)

Freud, S. (1955b). *The ego and id. A standard edition of the complete psychological works by Sigmund Freud* (Vol. XIX). London: Hogarth Press. (Original work published in 1923)

Frieswyk, S. H., Allen, J. G., Colson, D. B., et al. (1986). Therapeutic alliance and its place as a process and outcome in dynamic psychotherapy research. *Journal of Consulting Clinical Psychology, 54,* 32–38.

Fromm, E. (1964). *The heart of man: Its genesis for good and evil.* New York: Harper & Row.

Fromm, E., & Xiran, R. (Eds.). (1968). *The nature of man: A reader.* New York: Macmillan.

Fuhrman, E., & Snizek, W. (1990). Neither proscience nor antiscience: Metasociology as dialogue. *Sociological Forum, 5,* 17–36.

Gadamer, H. (1996). *The enigma of health: The art of healing in a scientific age* (J. Gaiger & N. Walker, Trans.). Stanford: Stanford University Press.

Gadamer, H. G. (1976). *Philosophical hermeneutics.* Berkeley, CA: University of California Press.

Gadow, S. (1980). Body and self: A dialectic. *Journal of Medicine and Philosophy, 5,* 172–185.

Gadow, S. (1992). Existential ecology: The human/natural world. *Social Science and Medicine, 35,* 597–602.

Gadow, S. (1996). Ethical narratives in practice. *Nursing Science Quarterly, 9,* 8–9.

Gallant, M. H., Beaulieu, M. C., & Carnevale, F. A. (2002). Partnership: An analysis of the concept within the nurse-client relationship. *Journal of Advanced Nursing, 40,* 149–157.

Gardner, L. I. (1972). Deprivation dwarfism. *Scientific American, 227,* 76–82.

Garfield, J. (1979). Social stress and medical ideology. In C. A. Garfield (Ed.), *Stress and survival: The emotional realities of life-threatening illness.* St. Louis: C. V. Mosby.

Garvin, B. J., & Kennedy, C. W. (1990). Interpersonal communication between nurses and patients. In *Annual review of nursing research,* (Vol. 8, pp. 213–234). New York: Springer Publishing Company.

Geanellos, R. (1997). Nursing knowledge development: Where to from here? *Collegian, 4,* 13–21.

Gebbie, K. M., & Lavin, M. A. (1975). *Proceedings of the first national conference: Classification of nursing diagnoses.* St. Louis: C.V. Mosby.

Geertz, C. (1973). *The interpretation of culture* (pp. 3–30). New York: Basic Books.

Georges, J. M. (2003). An emerging discourse: Toward epistemic diversity in nursing. *Advances in Nursing Science, 26,* 44–52.

Gigliotti, E. (2003). The Neumann systems model institute: Testing middle-range theories. *Nursing Science Quarterly, 16,* 201–206.

Gillett, G. R. (1987). Concepts, structures, and meanings. *Inquiry, 30,* 101–112.

Giuliano, K. K., Tyer-Viola, L., & Lopez, R. P. (2005). Unity of knowledge in the advancement of nursing knowledge. *Nursing Science Quarterly, 18,* 243–248.

Given, C. W., Simoni, L., & Gallin, R. (1977). The design and use of a health status index for family physician. *Journal of Family Practice, 4,* 287–291.

Glaser, B. G., & Strauss, A. (1967). *The discovery of grounded theory: Strategies for qualitative research.* Chicago: Aldine.

Gobet, F., & Chassy, P. (2008). Towards an alternative to Banner's theory of expert intuition in nursing: A discussion paper. *International Journal of Nursing Studies, 45*(1), 129–139.

Goffman, E. (1963). *Stigma: Notes on the management of spoiled identity.* Englewood Cliffs, NJ: Prentice-Hall.

Good, B. J. (1994). *Medicine, rationality, and experience: An anthropological perspective.* Cambridge, UK: Cambridge University Press.

Good, B. J., & Good, M. D. (1981). The meaning of symptoms: A cultural hermeneutic model for clinical practice. In L. Eisenberg & A. Kleinman (Eds.), *The relevance of social science for medicine* (pp. 165–196). London: D. Reidel Publishing.

Goodkin, K., & Visser, A. P. (Eds.). (2000). *Psychoneuroimmunology: Stress, mental disorders, and health.* Arlington, VA: American Psychiatric Press.

Gordis, L. (1976). Methodologic issues in the measurement of patient compliance. In D. L. Sackett & R. B. Haynes (Eds.), *Compliance with therapeutic regimens* (pp. 51–66). Baltimore, MD: Johns Hopkins University Press.

Gordon, G. (1966). *Role theory and illness.* New Haven, CT: Yale University Press.

Gordon, M. (1990). Toward theory-based diagnostic categories. *Nursing Diagnosis, 1,* 5–11.

Gordon, M. (1998). Nursing nomenclature and classification system development. *Online Journal of Issues in Nursing, 3*(2). Retrieved November 9, 2009, from www.nursing world.org/MainMenuCategories/ANAMarketplace/ANAPeriodicals/OJIN/TableofContents /vol31998/No2Sept1998/NomenclatureandClassification.aspx

Gordon, M., & Sweeney, M. A. (1979). Methodological problems and issues in identifying and standardizing nursing diagnosis. *Advances in Nursing Science, 2,* 1–15.

Gore, S. (1978). The effect of social support in moderating the health consequences of unemployment. *Journal of Health and Social Behavior, 19,* 157–165.

Gortner, S. R. (1993). Nursing's syntax revisited: A critique of philosophies said to influence nursing theories. *International Journal of Nursing Studies, 30,* 477–488.

Gortner, S. R., & Schultz, P. R. (1988). Approaches to nursing science methods. *Image: Journal of Nursing Scholarship, 22,* 101–105.

Graf, C. (2006). Functional decline in hospitalized older adults. *American Journal of Nursing, 106,* 58–67.

Grier, M. R., & Schnitzler, C. P. (1979). Nurses' propensity to risk. *Nursing Research, 28,* 186–191.

Guarnaccia, P. J. (2001). Introduction: The contributions of medical anthropology to anthropology and beyond. *Medical Anthropology Quarterly, 15,* 423–427.

Gupta, A. (2008, Spring). Definitions. In E. N. Zalta (Ed.), *The Stanford encyclopedia of philosophy.* Retrieved June 10, 2009, from http://plato.stanford.edu/archives/spr2009/ entries/definitions/

Habermas, J. (1986). *Knowledge and human interests.* Cambridge, UK: Polity.

Hagerty, B. M., & Patusky, K. L. (2003). Reconceptualizing the nurse-patient relationship. *Journal of Nursing Scholarship, 35,* 145–150.

Hall, J. A., Roter, D. L., & Katz, N. R. (1988). Meta-analysis of correlates of provider behavior in medical encounters. *Medical Care, 26,* 657–675.

Hall, J. M. (2004). Marginalization and symbolic violence in a world of differences: War and parallels to nursing practice. *Nursing Philosophy, 5,* 41–53.

Hall, L. (1966). Another view of nursing care and quality. In K. M. Straub & K. S. Parker (Eds.), *Continuity of patient care: The role of nursing* (pp. 47–66). Washington, DC: Catholic University Press.

Hanson, N. R. (1958). *Patterns of discovery: An inquiry into the conceptual foundation of science.* Cambridge, UK: University Press.

Hansson, S. O. (2007). Values in pure and applied science. *Foundations of Science, 12,* 257–268.

Hardcastle, M. A., Usher, K. J., & Holmes, C. A. (2006). An overview of structuration theory and its usefulness for nursing research. *Nursing Philosophy, 7,* 175–180.

Harder, I. (1992). *The world of the hospital nurse: Nurse patient interactions—body nursing and health promotion: Illustrated by use of a combined phenomenological/grounded theory approach.* Doctoral dissertation, The Faculty of Health Sciences of the University of Aarhus.

Hardy, M. E. (1974). Theories: Components, development, evaluation. *Nursing Research, 23,* 100–107.

Hardy, M. E. (1978). Evaluating nursing theory. In *Theory development: Why, what, how?* (pp. 75–86). New York: National League for Nursing.

Hardy, S., Titchen, A., Manley, K., & McCormack, B. (2006). Re-defining nursing expertise in the United Kingdom. *Nursing Science Quarterly, 19,* 260–264.

Hartman, H. (1958). *Ego psychology and the problems of adaptation* (D. Rapaport, Trans.). New York: International Universities Press.

Hartshorne, C., Weiss, P., & Burks, A. (1935/1958). *Charles Sanders Peirce, collected papers.* Cambridge, MA: Harvard University Press.

Hatch, E. (1997). Humanistic theory of theory. *Cultural Dynamics, 9,* 301–324.

Hatcher, R. L., & Barends, A. W. (1996). Patients' view of the alliance in psychotherapy: Exploratory factor analysis of three alliance measures. *Journal of Consulting and Clinical Psychology, 64,* 1326–1336.

Hawe, P. (1998). Making sense of context-level influences on health. *Health Education Research, 13(6),* i–iv.

Hawe, P., & Shiell, A. (2000). Social capital and health promotion. *Social Science & Medicine, 51,* 871–885.

Hayes, J., & Hannold, E. L. (2007). The road to empowerment: A historical perspective on the medicalization of disability. *Journal of Health and Human Services Administration, 30,* 352–377.

Head, B., & Faul, A. (2005). Terminal restlessness as perceived by hospice professionals. *American Journal of Hospice & Palliative Care, 22,* 277–282.

Heath, J., Johanson, W., & Blake, N. (2004). Healthy work environments: A validation of the literature. *Journal of Nursing Administration, 34,* 524–530.

Hebb, D. O. (1949). *The organization of behavior.* New York: John Wiley.

Hempel, C. G. (1952). *Fundamentals of concept formation in empirical sciences.* Chicago: University of Chicago Press.

Hempel, C. G. (1965). *Aspects of scientific explanation, and other essays in the philosophy of science.* New York: Free Press.

Hempel, C. G. (1966). *Philosophy of natural science.* Englewood Cliffs, NJ: Prentice-Hall.

Hempel, C. G. (1988). Provisoes: A problem concerning the inferential functioning of scientific theories. *Erkennesi, 28,* 147–164.

Henderson, B. (1978). Nursing diagnosis: Theory and practice. *Advances in Nursing Science,* *1,* 75–83.

Henderson, S. (1980). A development in social psychiatry: The systematic study of social bonds. *Journal of Nervous and Mental Disease, 168,* 63–69.

Henderson, V. (1961). *Basic principles of nursing care.* London: International Council of Nurses.

Henderson, V. (1966). *The nature of nursing: A definition and its implications for practice, research, and education.* New York: Macmillan.

Henderson, V., & Harmer, B. (1955). *Textbook of the principles and practice of nursing.* New York: Macmillan.

Henson, R. H. (1997). Analysis of the concept of mutuality. *Image: Journal of Nursing Scholarship, 29,* 77–81.

Herdman, E. A. (2001). The illusion of progress in nursing. *Nursing Philosophy, 2,* 4–13.

Herdman, T. H. (Ed.). (2009). *NANDA International nursing diagnoses: Definitions and classification 2009–2011.* Chichester, UK: Wiley-Blackwell.

Hinkle, L. E. (1961). Ecological observations of the relation of physical illness, mental illness, and the social environment. *Psychosomatic Medicine, 23,* 289–297.

Hinson Langford, G. P., Bowsher, J., Moloney, J. P., & Lillis, P. P. (1997). Social support: A concept analysis. *Journal of Advanced Nursing, 25,* 95–100.

Hofstadter, D. R. (1979). *Gödel, Escher, Bach: An eternal golden braid.* New York: Vintage Books.

Hollis, M. (1977). *Models of man: Philosophical thoughts on social action.* Cambridge, UK: Cambridge University Press.

Holmes, C., & Warelow, P. (2000). Nursing as normative praxis. *Nursing Inquiry, 7,* 175–181.

Holmes, C. A. (1990). Alternatives to natural science foundations for nursing. *International Journal of Nursing Studies, 27,* 187–198.

Holmes, C. A. (1992). The drama of nursing. *Journal of Advanced Nursing, 17,* 941–950.

Holmes, D., & Gastaldo, D. (2004). Rhizomatic thought in nursing: An alternative path for the development of the discipline. *Nursing Philosophy, 5,* 258–267.

Homans, G. C. (1961). *Social behavior: Its elementary forms.* New York: Harcourt and Brace.

Horrocks, S. (2000). Hunting for Heidegger: Questioning the sources in the Benner/Cash debate. *International Journal of Nursing Studies, 37,* 237–243.

Hougaard, E. (1994). The therapeutic alliance—A conceptual analysis. *Scandinavian Journal of Psychology, 35,* 67–85.

House, J. S. (1981). *Work stress and social support.* Reading, MA: Addison-Wesley.

Howard, H., & Scott, R. A. (1965). Proposed framework for the analysis of stress in the human organism. *Behavioral Sciences, 10,* 141–160.

Howgego, I. M., Yellowlees, P., Owen, C., Meldrum, L., & Dark, F. (2003). The therapeutic alliance: The key to effective patient outcome? A descriptive review of the evidence in community mental health case management. *Australian and New Zealand Journal of Psychiatry, 37,* 169–183.

Hummelvoll, J. K. (1996). The nurse-client alliance model. *Perspectives in Psychiatric Care, 32,* 12–21.

Im, E. O. (2005). Development of situation-specific theories. An integrative approach. *Advances in Nursing Science, 28,* 137–151.

Im, E. O., & Meleis, A. I. (1999). Situation-specific theories: Philosophical roots, properties, and approach. *Advances in Nursing Science, 22,* 11–24.

James, W. (1955). *Pragmatism, and four essays from the meaning of truth* (pp. 22–23). New York: Meridian.

Jasper, M. A. (1994). Expert: A discussion of the implications of the concept as used in nursing. *Journal of Advanced Nursing, 20,* 769–776.

Jenney, J., & Logan, J. (1992). Knowing the patient: One aspect of clinical knowledge. *Image: Journal of Nursing Scholarship, 24,* 254–258.

Johnson, D. E. (1959). The nature of a science of nursing. *Nursing Outlook, 7,* 291–294.

Johnson, D. E. (1968). Theory in nursing: Borrowed or unique. *Nursing Research, 17,* 206–209.

Johnson, D. E. (1980). The behavioral system model for nursing. In C. Roy & J. P. Riehl (Eds.), *Conceptual models for nursing practice* (2nd ed., pp. 207–216). New York: Appleton-Century-Crofts.

Johnson, J. E., Christman, N. J., & Stitt, C. (1985). Personal control interventions: Short- and long-term effects on surgical patients. *Research in Nursing & Health, 8,* 131–145.

Johnson, J. E., & Rice, V. H. (1974). Sensory and distress components of pain: Implications for the study of clinical pain. *Nursing Research, 23,* 203–209.

Johnson, J. E., Rice, V. H., Fuller, S. S., & Endress, M. P. (1978). Sensory information, instruction in a coping strategy, and recovery from surgery. *Research in Nursing & Health, 1,* 4–17.

Johnson, J. L. (1994). A dialectical examination of nursing art. *Advances in Nursing Science, 17,* 1–14.

Johnson, M. E., & Hauser, P. M. (2001). The practices of expert psychiatric nurses: Accompanying the patient to a calmer personal space. *Issues in Mental Health Nursing, 22,* 651–668.

Johnston, B., & Smith, L. N. (2006). Nurses' and patients' perceptions of expert palliative nursing care. *Journal of Advanced Nursing, 54,* 700–709.

Jones, C. L., King, M. B., Speck, P., Krowska, A., & Tookman, A. J. (1998). Development of an instrument to measure terminal restlessness. *Palliative Medicine, 12,* 99–104.

Jones, P. E. (1979). A terminology for nursing diagnoses. *Advances in Nursing Science, 2,* 65–72.

Jonsdottir, H., Litchfield, M., & Pharris, M. D. (2003). Partnership in practice. *Research & Theory for Nursing Practice, 17,* 51–63.

Jonsdottir, H., Litchfield, M., & Pharris, M. D. (2004). The relational core of nursing practice as partnership. *Journal of Advanced Nursing, 47,* 241–250.

Jordan, J. V. (1986). *The meaning of mutuality* (Work in Progress: No. 23). Wellesley, MA: Wellesley College.

Julius, R. J., Novitsky, M. A., Jr., & Dubin, W. R. (2009). Medication adherence: A review of the literature and implications for clinical practice. *Journal of Psychiatric Practice, 15,* 34–44.

Kaplan, A. (1964). *The conduct of inquiry.* San Francisco: Chandler Publishing.

Kaplan, B. H., Cassel, J. C., & Gore, S. (1977). Social support and health. *Medical Care, 15*(Suppl.), 47–58.

Kaplan, G. A. (1996). People and places: Contrasting perspectives on the association between social class and health. *International Journal of Health Services, 26,* 507–519.

Kaplan, R. M., Bush, J. W., & Berry, C. C. (1976). Health status: Types of validity and the index of well-being. *Health Services Research, 11,* 478–507.

Katims, I. (1993). Nursing as aesthetic experience and the notion of practice. *Scholarly Inquiry for Nursing Practice: An International Journal, 7,* 269–278.

Kawachi, I. (1999). Social capital and community effects on population and individual health. In N. Adler, M. Marmot, B. McEwen, & J. Stewart (Eds.), Socioeconomic status and health in industrial nations. *Annals of the New York Academy of Sciences, 896,* 120–130.

Kazanjian, A., Green, C., Wong, J., & Reid, R. (2005). Effect of the hospital nursing environment on patient mortality: A systematic review. *Journal of Health Services Research & Policy, 10,* 111–117.

Kennedy, L. W., Northcott, H. C., & Kinzel, C. (1978). Subjective evaluation of well-being: Problems and prospects. *Social Indicators Research, 5,* 457–474.

Kim, H. S. (1983). Collaborative decision making in nursing practice: A theoretical framework. In P. Chinn (Ed.), *Advances in nursing theory development* (pp. 271–283). Washington, DC: Aspen Systems.

Kim, H. S. (1987). Structuring the nursing knowledge system: A typology of four domains. *Scholarly Inquiry for Nursing Practice: An International Journal, 1,* 99–110.

Kim, H. S. (1992). An approach to concept differentiation and theory generation in nursing. *Korean Journal of Nursing Query, 1,* 44–55.

Kim, H. S. (1993a). Identifying alternative linkages among philosophy, theory, and method in nursing science. *Journal of Advanced Nursing, 18,* 793–800.

Kim, H. S. (1993b). Putting theory into practice: Problems and prospects. *Journal of Advanced Nursing, 18,* 1632–1639.

Kim, H. S. (1993c). Response to "Nursing as aesthetic experience and the notion of practice." *Scholarly Inquiry for Nursing Practice: An International Journal, 7,* 279–282.

Kim, H. S. (1994). Practice theories in nursing and a science of nursing practice. *Scholarly Inquiry for Nursing Practice: An International Journal, 8,* 123–137.

Kim, H. S. (1996). Nursing epistemology as a human practice science. In T. Bjerkreim, J. Mathisen, & R. Nord (Eds.), *Vision, viten og virke: Festskrift til sykepleieren Kjellaug Lerheim, 70 år* (pp. 36–45). Oslo, Norway: Universitetsforlager AS.

Kim, H. S. (1997). Terminology in structuring and developing nursing knowledge. In I. M. King & J. Fawcett (Eds.), *The language of nursing theory and metatheory* (pp. 27–36). Indianapolis, IN: Sigma Theta Tau International Center Nursing Press.

Kim, H. S. (1999). Critical reflective inquiry for knowledge development in nursing practice. *Journal of Advanced Nursing, 29,* 1205–1212.

Kim, H. S. (2000). An integrative framework for conceptualizing clients: A proposal for a nursing perspective in the new century. *Nursing Science Quarterly, 13,* 37–44.

Kim, H. S. (2001). Directions for theory development in nursing. In N. Chaska (Ed.), *The nursing profession: Tomorrow and beyond* (pp. 273–285). Thousand Oaks, CA: Sage.

Kim, H. S. (2006). Knowledge synthesis and use in practice—Debunking "evidence-based." *Klinisk sygepleje, 20*(2), 24–34.

Kim, H. S. (2007). Toward an integrated epistemology for nursing. In C. Roy & D. A. Jones (Eds.), *Nursing knowledge development and clinical practice* (pp. 181–190). New York: Springer Publishing Company.

Kim, H. S., Ellefsen, B., Han, K. J., & Alves, S. L. (2008). Clinical constructions by nurses in Korea, Norway, and the United States. *Western Journal of Nursing Research, 30,* 54–72.

Kim, H. S., & Kollak, I. (Eds.). (2006). *Nursing theories: Conceptual & philosophical foundations* (2nd ed.). New York: Springer Publishing Company.

Kim, M. J., & Moritz, D. A. (Eds.). (1982). *Classification of nursing diagnoses: Proceedings of the third and fourth national conferences.* New York: McGraw-Hill.

Kim, T. S. (2008). Science of unitary human beings: An update on research. *Nursing Science Quarterly, 21,* 294–299.

King, I. M. (1971). *Toward a theory for nursing: General concepts of human behavior*. New York: John Wiley.

King, I. M. (1981). *A theory for nursing: Systems, concepts, process*. New York: John Wiley.

King, I. M. (1990). King's conceptual framework and theory of goal attainment. In M. E. Parker (Ed.), *Nursing theories in practice* (pp. 73–84). New York: National League for Nursing.

King, I. M. (1992). King's theory of goal attainment. *Nursing Science Quarterly, 5,* 19–26.

King, L., & Appleton, J. V. (1997). Intuition: A critical review of the research and rhetoric. *Journal of Advanced Nursing, 26,* 194–202.

Kirk, S. (2001). Negotiating lay and professional roles in the care of children with complex health care needs. *Journal of Advanced Nursing, 34,* 593–602.

Kirkevold, M. (1994). The contribution of nursing research—Knowledge about the patient. *Proceedings of 7th Biennial Conference of WENR: The contribution of nursing research: Past-present-future* (Vol. 1, pp. 1–16). Oslo, Norway: Workgroup of European Nurse Researchers.

Kirkham, S. R., Baumbusch, J. L., Schultz, A. S. H., & Anderson, J. M. (2007). Knowledge development and evidence-based practice: Insights and opportunities from a postcolonial feminist perspective for transformative nursing practice. *Advances in Nursing Science, 30,* 26–40.

Kitson, A. L. (1997). Johns Hopkins Address: Does nursing have a future? *Image: Journal of Nursing Scholarship, 29,* 111–115.

Kleffel, D. (1996). Environmental paradigms: Moving toward an ecocentric perspective. *Advances in Nursing Science, 18,* 1–10.

Kleinman, A. (1973). Medicine's symbolic reality: On the central problem in the philosophy of medicine. *Inquiry, 16,* 206–213.

Kleinman, A. (1977). Depression, somatization and the "new cross-cultural psychiatry." *Social Science and Medicine, 2,* 3–10.

Kleinman, A. (1988). *The illness narratives: Suffering, healing and the human condition*. New York: Basic Books.

Korzybski, A. (1921). *Manhood of humanity*. New York: E.P. Dutton.

Kosa, J., & Robertson, L. (1969). The social aspects of health and illness. In J. Kosa, A. Antonovsky, & I. Zola (Eds.), *Poverty and health*. Cambridge, MA: Harvard University Press.

Krieger, D. (1990). Therapeutic touch: Two decades of research, teaching and clinical practice. *Imprint, 37,* 83, 86–88.

Kritek, P. (1978). The generation and classification of nursing diagnoses: Toward a theory of nursing. *Image: Journal of Nursing Scholarship, 10,* 33–40.

Kritsotakis, G., & Gamarnikow, E. (2004). What is social capital and how does it relate to health? *International Journal of Nursing Studies, 41,* 43–50.

Kuhn, T. S. (1962). *The structure of scientific revolution*. Chicago: University of Chicago Press.

Kuhn, T. S. (1970). *The structure of scientific revolution* (enlarged ed.). Chicago: University of Chicago Press.

Kunkel, J., & Nagasawa, R. H. (1973). A behavioral model of man: Propositions and implications. *American Sociological Review, 38,* 530–543.

Kwan, O., & Friel, J. (2002). Clinical relevance of the sick role and secondary gain in the treatment of disability syndromes. *Medical Hypotheses, 59,* 129–134.

Kyngäs, H., Duffy, M. E., & Kroll, T. (2000). Concept analysis of compliance. *Journal of Clinical Nursing, 9,* 5–12.

Lake, E. T. (2007). The nursing practice environment: Measurement and evidence. *Medical Care Research & Review, 64*(Suppl.), 104S–122S.

Lang, N. (1988). Empower the nurse: A time for renewal. In *Nursing practice in the 21st century* (pp. 5–16). Kansas City, MO: American Nurses' Foundation.

LaRocco, J. M., House, J. S., & French, J. R. P., Jr. (1980). Social support, occupational stress, and health. *Journal of Health and Social Behavior, 21,* 202–218.

Laudan, L. (1977). *Progress and its problems.* Berkeley, CA: University of California Press.

Laudan, L. (1990). *Science and relativism: Some key controversies in the philosophy of science.* Chicago: University of Chicago Press.

Lauzon Clabo, L. M. (2008). An ethnography of pain assessment and the role of social context on two postoperative units. *Journal of Advanced Nursing, 61,* 531–549.

Lawler, J. (1991). *Behind the screens: Nursing, somology, and the problem of the body.* Melbourne: Churchill Livingstone.

Lawton, J. (2003). Lay experiences of health and illness: Past research and future agendas. *Sociology of Health & Illness, 25,* 23–40.

Lee, F., Leppa, C., & Schepp, K. (2006). Using the Minimum Data Set to determine predictors of terminal restlessness among nursing home residents. *Journal of Nursing Research, 14,* 286–295.

Leininger, M. M. (1969). Introduction: Nature of science in nursing. *Nursing Research, 18,* 388–389.

Leininger, M. M. (1995). *Transcultural nursing: Concepts, theories, research and practice* (2nd ed.). New York: McGraw-Hill.

Lenihan, J., & Fletcher, W. (Eds.). (1978). *The built environment: Environment and man* (Vol. 8, p. 161). New York: Academic Press.

Lenz, E. R., Pugh, L. C., Milligan, R. A., Gift, A., & Suppe, F. (1995). Collaborative development of middle-range nursing theories: Toward a theory of unpleasant symptoms. *Advances in Nursing Science, 17,* 1–13.

Lenz, E. R., Pugh, L. C., Milligan, R. A., Gift, A. G., & Suppe, F. (1997). The middle-range theory of unpleasant symptoms: An update. *Advances in Nursing Science, 19,* 14–27.

LeVasseur, J. J. (1999). Toward an understanding of art in nursing. *Advances in Nursing Science, 21,* 48–63.

Levin, M. E. (1966). Adaptation and assessment: A rationale for nursing intervention. *American Journal of Nursing, 66,* 2450–2454.

Liaschenko, J. (1997). Knowing the patient? In S. E. Hayes & V. E. Hayes (Eds.), *Nursing praxis: Knowledge and action* (pp. 23–38). Thousand Oaks, CA: Sage.

Liehr, P. R., & Smith, M. (1999). Middle range theory: Spinning research and practice to create knowledge for the new millennium. *Advances in Nursing Science, 21,* 81–91.

Lin, N., Simeone, R. S., Ensel, W. M., & Kuo, W. (1979). Social support, stressful life events, and illness: A model and an empirical test. *Journal of Health and Social Behavior, 20,* 108–119.

Lobkowicz, N. (1967). *Theory and practice: History of a concept from Aristotle to Marx.* Notre Dame, IN: University of Notre Dame Press.

Ludwig, T. D. (1968). Recent marine soils and resistance to dental caries. In J. B. Bresler (Ed.), *Environments of man* (pp. 45–51). Reading, MA: Addison-Wesley.

Lupton, D. (2003). *Medicine as culture: Illness, disease, and the body in western societies* (2nd ed.). London: Sage.

Lynch, J. J. (1977). *The broken heart.* New York: Basic Books.

MacIntyre, S., Maciver, S., & Sooman, A. (1993). Area, class, and health: Should we be focusing on places or people? *Journal of Social Policy, 22,* 213–234.

Mackey, S. (2005). Phenomenological nursing research: Methodological insights derived from Heidegger's interpretive phenomenology. *International Journal of Nursing Studies, 42,* 179–186.

Madden, B. P. (1990). The hybrid model for concept development: Its value for the study of therapeutic alliance. *Advances in Nursing Science, 12,* 75–87.

Malinski, V. M. (2006). Rogerian science-based nursing theories. *Nursing Science Quarterly, 19,* 7–12.

Malinski, V. M. (2009). Intentionality, consciousness, and creating community. *Nursing Science Quarterly, 22,* 13–14.

Margolis, E. (1994). A reassessment of the shift from the classical theory of concepts to prototype theory. *Cognition, 51,* 73–89.

Marinker, M. (2003). Coercion, compliance and concordance. *British Medical Journal, 327,* 858.

Martin, D. J., Garske, J. P., & Davis, M. K. (2000). Relation of the therapeutic alliance with outcome and other variables: A meta-analytic review. *Journal of Consulting and Clinical Psychology, 68,* 438–450.

Maskit, J. (2007). 'Line of wreckage': Towards a postindustrial environmental aesthetics. *Ethics, Place, and Environment, 10,* 323–337.

Maslow, A. H. (1967). A theory of metamotivation: The biological rooting of the value-life. *Journal of Humanistic Psychology, 7,* 93–127.

Maslow, A. H. (1973). Towards a humanistic biology. In J. Stulman & E. Laszlo (Eds.), *Emergent man: His chances, problems and potentials* (pp. 1–23). New York: Gordon and Breach.

McAndrew, S., & Samociuk, G. A. (2003). Reflecting together: Developing a new strategy for continuous user involvement in mental health nurse education. *Journal of Psychiatric Mental Health Nursing, 10,* 616–621.

McCann, D., Young, J., Watson, K., Ware, R. S., Pitcher, A., Bundy, R., et al. (2008). Effectiveness of a tool to improve role negotiation and communication between parents and nurses. *Paediatric Nursing, 20,* 14–19.

McCloskey-Dochterman, J., & Bulecheck, G. (2004). *Nursing interventions classification (NIC)* (4th ed.). St. Louis, MO: Mosby.

McCorkle, R. (1974). Effects of touch on seriously ill patients. *Nursing Research, 23,* 125–132.

McCorkle, R. (1976). The advanced cancer patient: How he will live—and die. *Nursing, 6*(10), 46–49.

McCorkle, R. (1981). A good death. *Cancer Nursing, 4,* 267.

Medin, D. L., & Smith, E. E. (1984). Concepts and concept formation. *Annual Review of Psychology, 35,* 113–138.

Meehan, T., Vermeer, C., & Windsor, C. (2000). Patients' perceptions of seclusion: A qualitative investigation. *Journal of Advanced Nursing, 31,* 370–377.

Meehan, T. C. (1990). *The science of unitary human beings and theory-based practice: Therapeutic touch* (NLN Publication 15-2285). New York: National League for Nursing.

Meissner, W. W. (1992). The concept of the therapeutic alliance. *Journal of American Psychoanalysis Association, 40,* 1059–1087.

Meissner, W. W. (2006). Finding and refinding the therapeutic alliance: On thinking and thirds. *Journal of the American Academy of Psychoanalysis and Dynamic Psychiatry, 34,* 651–678.

Meleis, A. I. (1997). *Theoretical nursing: Development and progress* (3rd ed.). Philadelphia: J. B. Lippincott.

Meleis, A. I. (2004). *Theoretical nursing: Development and progress* (4th ed.). Philadelphia: J.B. Lippincott.

Mercer, R. T. (1974). Mothers' responses to their infants with defects. *Nursing Research, 23,* 133–137.

Mercer, R. T. (1981). A theoretical framework for studying factors that impact on the maternal role. *Nursing Research, 30,* 73–77.

Mermin, N. D. (1992). Is the moon there when nobody looks? Reality and the quantum theory. In R. Boy, P. Casper, & J. D. Trout (Eds.), *The philosophy of science* (pp. 501–516). Cambridge, MA: MIT Press.

Merton, R. (1968). *Social theory and social structure* (Rev. ed.). New York: Free Press.

Merton, R. K. (1976). *Sociological ambivalence and other essays.* New York: Free Press.

Miller, P. M., & Ingham, J. G. (1976). Friend, confidants, and symptoms. *Social Psychiatry, 11,* 51.

Milton, C. L. (2008). Boundaries: Ethical implications for what it means to be therapeutic in the nurse-person relationship. *Nursing Science Quarterly, 21,* 18–21.

Mishel, M. H. (1988). Uncertainty in illness. *Image: Journal of Nursing Scholarship, 20,* 225–232.

Mishel, M. H. (1990). Reconceptualization of the uncertainty in illness theory. *Image: Journal of Nursing Scholarship, 22,* 256–262.

Mishel, M. H. (1997). Uncertainty in acute illness. In J. J. Fitzpatrick & J. Norbeck (Eds.), *Annual review of nursing research* (Vol. 15, pp. 57–80). New York: Springer Publishing Company.

Mishler, E. (1984). *The discourse of medicine: Dialectics of medical interviews.* Norwood, NJ: Ablex.

Mitchell, G. J. (1991). Nursing diagnosis: An ethical analysis. *Journal of Nursing Scholarship, 23,* 99–103.

Mitchell, S. J., & Cody, W. K. (2002). Ambiguous opportunity: Tolling for truth of nursing art and science. *Nursing Science Quarterly, 15,* 71–79.

Moch, S. (1990). Personal knowing: Evolving research and practice. *Scholarly Inquiry for Nursing Practice: An International Journal, 4,* 155–165.

Moloney, M. F. (1997). The meanings of home in the stories of older women. *Western Journal of Nursing Research, 19,* 166–176.

Moore, M. (1968). Nursing: A scientific discipline. *Nursing Forum, 7,* 340–347.

Moorehead, S., Johnson, M., Maas, M., & Swanson, E. (2007). *Nursing outcomes classification (NOC)* (4th ed.). St. Louis, MO: Mosby.

Morse, J. M., Havens, G. A., & Wilson, S. (1997). The comforting interaction: Developing a model of nurse-patient relationship. *Scholarly Inquiry for Nursing Practice: An International Journal,* 321–343.

Mortensen, A. (2000). *Culture and microcosmos of individuals: The idiosyncratic room of the person.* Retrieved November 16, 2009, from http://communication.ucsd.edu/MCA/Paper/Mortensen/Mortensen.html

Moustakas, C. (1990). *Heuristic research: Design, methodology, and applications.* Newbury Park, CA: Sage.

Mueller, D. P. (1980). Social networks: A promising direction for research on the relationship of the social environment to psychiatric disorder. *Social Science and Medicine, 14A,* 147–161.

Mullen, P. (1997). Compliance becomes concordance. *British Medical Journal, 314,* 691.

Mundinger, M. O., & Jauron, G. D. (1975). Developing a nursing diagnosis. *Nursing Outlook, 23,* 94–98.

Munhall, P. L. (1993). 'Unknowing': Toward another pattern of knowing in nursing. *Nursing Outlook, 41,* 125–128.

Murdock, G. P. (1980). *Theories of illness: A world survey.* Pittsburgh: University of Pittsburgh Press.

Murphy, N., & Canales, M. (2001). A critical analysis of compliance. *Nursing Inquiry, 8,* 173–181.

Murray, J. S. (2000). A concept analysis of social support as experienced by siblings of children with cancer. *Journal of Pediatric Nursing, 15,* 313–322.

Myers, J. K., Lindenthal, J. J., & Pepper, M. P. (1975). Life events, social integration and psychiatric symptomatology. *Journal of Health and Social Behavior, 16,* 421–427.

Naef, R. (2006). Bearing witness: A moral way of engaging in the nurse-person relationship. *Nursing Philosophy, 7,* 146–156.

Naegel, K. D. (1970). *Health and healing* (E. Cummings, Comp. Ed.). San Francisco: Jossey-Bass.

Neuman, B. (1974). The Betty Neuman health-care systems model: A total person approach to patient problems. In J. P. Riehl & C. Roy (Eds.), *Conceptual models for nursing practice.* New York: Appleton-Century-Crofts.

Neuman, B. (1995). *The Neuman systems model* (3rd ed.). Stamford, CT: Appleton & Lange.

Neuman, B. (1998). *The Neuman systems model* (4th ed.). Norwalk, CT: Appleton & Lange.

Neville, H., & Bavelier, D. (2002). Human brain plasticity: Evidence from sensory deprivation and altered language experience. *Progress in Brain Research, 138,* 177–188.

Newman, L. F. (1981). Social and sensory environment of low birth weight infants in a special care nursery: An anthropological investigation. *Journal of Nervous and Mental Disease, 169,* 448–455.

Newman, M. A. (1979). *Theory development in nursing.* Philadelphia: F.A. Davis.

Newman, M. A. (1992). Prevailing paradigms in nursing. *Nursing Outlook, 40,* 10–13, 32.

Newman, M. A. (1994). *Health as expanding consciousness* (2nd ed.). New York: National League for Nursing.

Newman, M. A. (2002). The pattern that connects. *Advances in Nursing Science, 24,* 1–7.

Newman, M. A., & Jones, D. A. (2007). Experiencing the whole: Health as expanding consciousness (state of the art). In C. Roy & D. A. Jones (Eds.), *Nursing knowledge development and clinical practice* (pp. 119–128). New York: Springer Publishing Company.

Newman, M. T. (1968). Ecology and nutritional stress in man. In J. B. Bresler (Ed.), *Environment of man* (pp. 104–116). Reading, MA: Addison-Wesley.

Nicoll, L. H. (Ed.). (1997). *Perspectives on nursing theory* (3rd ed.). Philadelphia: J.B. Lippincott.

Nightingale, F. (1859). *Notes on nursing: What it is and what it is not.* London: Harrison and Sons.

Nightingale, F. (1992). *Notes on nursing: What it is and what it is not.* Philadelphia: J. B. Lippincott.

Nissan, E. (2008). From embodied agents or their environments reasoning about the body, to virtual models of the human body: A quick overview. *Journal of Intelligent and Robotic Systems, 52,* 489–513.

Norbeck, J. S. (1981). Social support: A model for clinical research and application. *Advances in Nursing Science, 3,* 43–59.

Norbeck, J. S. (1987). In defense of empiricism. *Image:The Journal of Nursing Scholarship, 19,* 28–30.

Norris, C. M. (1975). Restlessness: A nursing phenomenon in search of meaning. *Nursing Outlook, 23,* 103–107.

Nortvedt, P. (2001). Needs, closeness and responsibilities: An inquiry into some rival moral considerations in nursing care. *Nursing Philosophy, 2,* 112–121.

Nortvedt, P. (2003). Immersed subjectivity and engaged narratives: Clinical epistemology and normative intricacy. *Nursing Philosophy: An International Journal for Healthcare Professionals, 4,* 129–136.

Oiler, C. (1982). The phenomenological approach in nursing research. *Nursing Research, 31,* 178–181.

Olds, J. (1976). Behavioral studies of hypothalamic functions: Drives and reinforcements. In R. G. Grennell & S. Gagay (Eds.), *Biological foundations of psychiatry.* New York: Raven Press.

Omery, A. (1983). Phenomenology: A method for nursing research. *Advances in Nursing Science, 5,* 49–63.

Omery, A., Kasper, C. E., & Page, G. G. (Eds.). (1995). *In search of nursing science.* Thousand Oaks, CA: Sage.

Orem, D. E. (1971). *Nursing: Concepts of practice.* New York: McGraw-Hill.

Orem, D. E. (1980). *Nursing: Concepts of practice* (2nd ed.). New York: McGraw-Hill.

Orem, D. E. (1991). *Nursing: Concepts of practice* (4th ed.). St. Louis, MO: Mosby.

Orem, D. E. (1995). *Nursing: Concepts of practice* (5th ed.). St Louis, MO: Mosby.

Orlando, I. J. (1961). *The dynamic nurse-patient relationship: Function, process, and principle.* New York: G. Putnam's Sons.

Pahl, R. (2003). Some sceptical comments on the relationship between social support and well-being. *Leisure Studies, 22,* 357–368.

Paley, J. (1996a). How not to clarify concepts in nursing. *Journal of Advanced Nursing, 24,* 572–578.

Paley, J. (1996b). Intuition and expertise: Comments on the Benner debate. *Journal of Advanced Nursing, 23,* 665–671.

Paley, J., Cheyne, H., Dalgleish, L., Duncan, E. A. S., & Niven, C. A. (2007). Nursing's ways of knowing and dual process theories of cognition. *Journal of Advanced Nursing, 60,* 692–701.

Parse, R. R. (1981). *Man-living-health: A theory of nursing.* New York: John Wiley.

Parse, R. R. (1987). *Nursing science: Major paradigms, theories, and critiques.* Philadelphia: W. B. Saunders.

Parse, R. R. (1992). Human becoming: Parse's theory of nursing. *Nursing Science Quarterly, 4,* 8–12.

Parse, R. R. (1997a). The human becoming theory: The was, is, and will be. *Nursing Science Quarterly, 10,* 32–38.

Parse, R. R. (1997b). Concept inventing: Unitary creations. *Nursing Science Quarterly, 10,* 63–64.

Parse, R. R. (1998). *The human becoming school of thought: A perspective for nurses and other health professionals.* Thousand Oaks, CA: Sage.

Parse, R. R. (1999). The discipline and the profession. *Nursing Science Quarterly, 12,* 275.

Parse, R. R., Barrett, E., Bourgeois, M., Dee, V., Egan, E., Germain, C., et al. (2000). Nursing theory—guided practice: A definition. *Nursing Science Quarterly, 13,* 177.

Parsons, T. (1951). *The social system.* New York: Free Press.

Parsons, T. (1958). The definitions of health and illness in the light of American values and social structure. In G. E. Jaco (Ed.), *Patients, physicians, and illness.* Glenco, IL: Free Press.

Parsons, T. (1975). The sick role and the role of the physician reconsidered. *Milbank Memorial Quarterly, 53*, 257–278.

Paterson, J. G., & Zderad, L. T. (1976). *Humanistic nursing.* New York: John Wiley.

Paterson, J. G., & Zderad, L. T. (1988). *Humanistic nursing* (NLN Publication No. 41-2218). New York: National League for Nursing.

Pearce, J. M. (2002). Psychosocial factors in chronic disability. *Medical Science Monitor: International Medical Journal of Experimental and Clinical Research, 8*, RA275–RA281.

Penny, W., & Warelow, P. J. (1999). Understanding the prattle of praxis. *Nursing Inquiry, 6*, 259–268.

Penrod, J., & Hupcey, J. E. (2005). Enhancing methodological clarity: Principle-based concept analysis. *Journal of Advanced Nursing, 50*, 403–409.

Peplau, H. E. (1952). *Interpersonal relations in nursing.* New York: G. Putnam's Sons.

Peter, E., & Liaschenko, J. (2004). Perils of proximity: A spatiotemporal analysis of moral distress and moral ambiguity. *Nursing Inquiry, 11*, 218–225.

Phillips, D. C. (1987). *Philosophy, science, and social inquiry: Contemporary methodological controversies in social science and related applied fields of research* (pp. 80–101). Oxford, UK: Pergamon Press.

Pitre, N. Y., & Myrick, F. (2007). A view of nursing epistemology through reciprocal interdependence: Towards a reflexive way of knowing. *Nursing Philosophy, 8*, 73–84.

Playle, J. F. (1995). Humanism and positivism in nursing: Contradictions and conflicts. *Journal of Advanced Nursing, 22*, 979–984.

Polakov, W. N. (1925). *Man and his affairs: From the engineering point of view.* Baltimore: Williams and Wilkins.

Polanyi, M. (1964). *Personal knowledge* (rev. ed.). New York: Harper Torchbooks.

Polaschek, N. (2003). Negotiated care: A model for nursing work in the renal setting. *Journal of Advanced Nursing, 42*, 355–363.

Pollock, J. L. (2008). What am I? Virtual machines and the mind/body problem. *Philosophy and Phenomenological Research, 76*, 237–309.

Ponsi, M. (2000). Therapeutic alliance and collaborative interactions. *The International Journal of Psycho-Analysis, 81*, 687–704.

Popper, K. R. (1959). *The logic of scientific discovery.* New York: Harper and Row.

Popper, K. R. (1985). Knowledge: Subjective versus objective. In D. Miller (Ed.), *Popper: Selections* (pp. 58–77). Princeton, NJ: Princeton University Press.

Portes, A. (1998). Social capital: Its origins and applications in modern sociology. *Annual Review of Sociology, 24*, 1–24.

Prescott, J. W. (1980). Somatosensory affectional deprivation (SAD) theory of drug and alcohol use. *National Institute Drug Abuse Research Monograph Series, 30*, 286–296.

Prochaska, J. O., & Velicer, W. F. (1997). The transtheoretical model of health behavior change. *American Journal of Health Promotion, 12*, 38–48.

Purkis, M. E. (1994). Entering the field: Intrusions of the social and its exclusion from studies of nursing practice. *International Journal of Nursing Studies, 31*, 315–336.

Purkis, M. E., & Bjornsdottir, K. (2006). Intelligent nursing: Accounting for knowledge as action in practice. *Nursing Philosophy: An International Journal for Healthcare Professionals, 7*, 247–256.

Puschner, B., Bauer, S., Horowitz, L. M., & Kordy, H. (2005). The relationship between interpersonal problems and the helping alliance. *Journal of Clinical Psychology, 61*, 415–429.

Putnam, R. (1993). *Making democracy work: Civic traditions in modern Italy.* Princeton, NJ: Princeton University Press.

Putnam, R. (2000). *Bowling alone: The collapse and revival of American community.* New York: Simon & Schuster.

Putnam, R. (1995). Bowling alone: America's declining social capital. *Journal of Democracy, 6,* 65–78.

Quan, L., Xu, Y., Luo, S. P., Wang, L., LeBland, D., & Wang, T. (2006). Negotiated care improves fluid status in diabetic peritoneal dialysis patients. *Peritoneal Dialysis International, 26,* 95–100.

Quinn, J. F. (1984). Therapeutic touch as energy exchange: Testing the theory. *Advances in Nursing Science, 6,* 42–49.

Quinn, J. F. (1989). Therapeutic touch as energy exchange: Replication and extension. *Nursing Science Quarterly, 2,* 79–87.

Rabinow, P., & Sullivan, W. M. (Eds.). (1987). *Interpretive social science: A second look.* Berkeley, CA: University of California Press.

Radwin, L. E. (1996). "Knowing the patient": A review of research on an emerging concept. *Journal of Advanced Nursing, 23,* 1142–1146.

Reach, G. (2003). Observance in diabetes: From therapeutic education to therapeutic alliance. *Annales De Medecine Interne, 154,* 117–120.

Reed, P. G. (1991). Toward a nursing theory of self-transcendence: Deductive formulation using developmental theories. *Advances in Nursing Science, 13,* 64–77.

Reed, P. G. (1995). A treatise on nursing knowledge development for the 21st century: Beyond postmodernism. *Advances in Nursing Science, 17,* 70–84.

Reed, P. G. (2000). Nursing reformation: Historical reflections and philosophic foundations. *Nursing Science Quarterly, 13,* 129–136.

Reed, P. G., & Shearer, N. B. C. (2009). *Perspectives on nursing theory* (5th ed.). Philadelphia: Lippincott Williams & Wilkins.

Renaud, M. (1975). On the structural constraints to state intervention in health. *International Journal of Health Services, 5,* 559–571.

Rew, L. (1990). Intuition in critical care nursing. *Dimensions in Critical Care Nursing, 9,* 30–38.

Reynolds, P. D. (1971). *A primer in theory construction.* Indianapolis: Bobbs-Merrill.

Rhynas, S. J. (2005). Bourdieu's theory of practice and its potential in nursing research. *Journal of Advanced Nursing, 50,* 179–186.

Rieff, P. (1966). *The triumph of the therapeutics: Uses of faith after Freud.* New York: Harper and Row.

Riehl, J. P. (1980). The Riehl interaction model. In J. P. Riehl & C. Roy (Eds.), *Conceptual models for nursing practice* (2nd ed., pp. 350–356). New York: Appleton-Century-Crofts.

Riehl, J. P, & Roy, C. (Eds.). (1980). *Conceptual models for nursing practice* (2nd ed.). New York: Appleton-Century-Crofts.

Riesen, A. H., & Zilbert, D. E. (1975). Behavioral consequences of variations in early sensory environment. In A. H. Riesen (Ed.), *The developmental neuropsychology of sensory deprivation* (pp. 211–252). New York: Academic Press.

Ritter, B. J. (2003). An analysis of expert nurse practitioners' diagnostic reasoning. *Journal of the American Academy of Nurse Practitioners, 15,* 137–141.

Ritzer, G. (Ed.). (1992). *Metatheorizing.* Newbury Park, CA: Sage.

Ritzer, G. (1988). Sociological metatheory: Defending a subfield by delineating its parameters. *Sociological Theory, 6,* 187–200.

Ritzer, G., Zhao, S., & Murphy, J. (2006). Metatheorizing in sociology: The basic parameters and the potential contributions of postmodernism. In J. H. Turner (Ed.), *Handbook of sociological theory* (pp. 113–134). New York: Springer Publishing Company.

Rodgers, B. I. (2000a). Philosophical foundations of concept development. In B. I. Rodgers & K. A. Knafl (Eds.), *Concept development in nursing: Foundations, techniques, and applications* (pp. 7–37). Philadelphia: W.B. Saunders.

Rodgers, B. I. (2000b). Concept analysis: An evolutionary view. In B. I. Rodgers & K. A. Knafl (Eds.), *Concept development in nursing: Foundations, techniques, and applications* (pp. 77–102). Philadelphia: W.B. Saunders.

Rodgers, B. L., & Knafl, K. A. (Eds.). (1993). *Concept development in nursing: Foundations, techniques, and applications*. Philadelphia: W. B. Saunders.

Rodgers, B. L., & Knafl, K. A. (Eds.). (2000). *Concept development in nursing: Foundations, techniques, and applications* (2nd ed.). Philadelphia: W. B. Saunders.

Rogers, M. E. (1963). Some comments on the theoretical basis for nursing practice. *Nursing Science, 63*(1), 11–13, 60–61.

Rogers, M. E. (1970). *An introduction to the theoretical basis of nursing*. Philadelphia: F.A. Davis.

Rogers, M. E. (1980). Nursing: A science of unitary man. In J. P. Riehl & C. Roy (Eds.), *Conceptual models for nursing practice* (2nd ed., pp. 329–337). New York: Appleton-Century-Crofts.

Rogers, M. E. (1989). Nursing: A science of unitary human beings. In J. Riehl-Sisca (Ed.), *Conceptual models for nursing practice* (3rd ed., pp. 181–188). Norwalk, CT: Appleton & Lange.

Rogers, M. E. (1990). Nursing: Science of unitary, irreducible, human beings: Update 1990. In E. A. M. Barrett (Ed.), *Visions of Rogers' science-based nursing* (pp. 5–11). New York: National League for Nursing.

Rogers, M. E. (1992). Nursing science and the space age. *Nursing Science Quarterly, 5,* 27–34.

Rogers, M. E. (1994). The science of unitary human beings. *Nursing Science Quarterly, 7,* 33–35.

Rolfe, G. (1993). Closing theory-practice gap: A model for nursing praxis. *Journal of Clinical Nursing, 2,* 173–177.

Rolfe, G. (1997a). Beyond expertise: Theory, practice and the reflexive practitioner. *Journal of Clinical Nursing, 6,* 93–97.

Rolfe, G. (1997b). Science, abduction and the fuzzy nurse: An exploration of expertise. *Journal of Advanced Nursing, 25,* 1070–1075.

Rolfe, G. (2005). The deconstructing angel: Nursing, reflection and evidence-based practice. *Nursing Inquiry, 12,* 78–86.

Rolfe, G. (2006). Nursing praxis and the science of the unique. *Nursing Science Quarterly, 19,* 39–43.

Rossi, A. M. (1969). General methodological considerations. In J. P. Zubek (Ed.), *Sensory deprivation: Fifteen years of research* (pp. 16–43). New York: Appleton-Century-Crofts.

Rothenberg, A. (1992). Form and structure and their function in psychotherapy. *American Journal of Psychotherapy, 66,* 357–382.

Rowles, G. D. (1987). A place to call home. In L. L. Carstensen & B. A. Edelstein (Eds.), *Handbook of clinical gerontology* (pp. 335–353). New York: Pergamon.

Roy, C. (1970). Adaptation: A conceptual framework for nursing. *Nursing Outlook, 18,* 42–45.

Roy, C. (1975). A diagnostic classification system for nursing. *Nursing Outlook, 23,* 90–94.

Roy, C. (1976). *Introduction to nursing: An adaptation model*. Englewood Cliffs, NJ: Prentice-Hall.

Roy, C. (2007). Knowledge as universal cosmic imperative. In C. Roy & D. A. Jones (Eds.), *Nursing knowledge development and clinical practice* (pp. 145–161). New York: Springer Publishing Company.

Roy, C., & Andrews, H. A. (1991). *The Roy adaptation model: A definitive statement.* Norwalk, CT: Appleton & Lange.

Roy, C., & Jones, D. A. (Eds.). (2007). *Nursing knowledge development and clinical practice.* New York: Springer Publishing Company.

Roy, C., & Roberts, S. L. (1981). *Theory construction in nursing: An adaptation model.* Englewood Cliffs, NJ: Prentice-Hall.

Rutherford, M. (2008). Standardized nursing language: What does it mean for nursing practice? *OJINL: The Online Journal of Issues in Nursing, 13*(1). Retrieved November 11, 2009, from www.nursingworld.org/MainMenuCategories/ANAMarketplace/ANA Periodicals/OJIN/TableofContents/vol132008/No1Jan08/ArticlePreviousTopic/Standard izedNursingLanguage.aspx

Rycroft-Malone, J., Seers, K., Titchen, A., Harvey, G., Kitson, A., & McCormack, B. (2004). What counts as evidence in evidence-based practice? *Journal of Advanced Nursing, 47,* 81–90.

Sackett, D. L. (1976). Introduction and the magnitude of compliance and noncompliance. In D. L. Sackett & R. B. Haynes (Eds.), *Compliance with therapeutic regimens* (pp. 1–25). Baltimore, MD: Johns Hopkins University Press.

Sahlsten, M. J., Larsson, I. E., Sjöström, B., Lindencrona, C. S., & Plos, K. A. (2007). Patient participation in nursing care: Towards a concept clarification from a nurse perspective. *Journal of Clinical Nursing, 16,* 630–637.

Scheel, M. E., Pedersen, B. D., & Rosenkrands, V. (2008). International nursing—A practice-theory in the dynamic field between the natural, human, and social sciences. *Scandinavian Journal of Caring Science, 22,* 629–636.

Scheff, T. J. (1966). *Being mentally ill: A sociological theory.* Chicago: Aldine.

Scheper-Hughes, N., & Lock, M. M. (1987). The mindful body: A prolegomenon to future work in medical anthropology. *Medical Anthropology Quarterly, 1,* 6041.

Schlotfeldt, R. M. (1960). Reflections on nursing research. *American Journal of Nursing, 60,* 492–494.

Schlotfeldt, R. M. (1978). The professional doctorate: Rationale & characteristics. *Nursing Outlook, 26,* 302–311.

Schlotfeldt, R. M. (1987). Resolution of issues: An imperative for creating nursing's future. *Journal of Professional Nursing, 3,* 136–142.

Schmidt, H. G., Norman, G. R., & Boshuizen, H. P. A. (1990). A cognitive perspective on medical expertise: Theory and implications. *Academic Medicine, 65,* 611–621.

Schofield, P., & Davis, B. (1998). Sensory deprivation and chronic pain: A review of the literature. *Disability and Rehabilitation, 20,* 357–366.

Schön, D. (1983). *The reflective practitioner.* New York: Basic Books.

Schön, D. (Ed.). (1991). *The reflective turn: Case studies in and on educational practice.* New York: Columbia University Teachers College Press.

Schraeder, B. D., & Fischer, D. K. (1986). Using intuitive knowledge to make clinical decisions. *MCN: The American Journal of Maternal Child Nursing, 11,* 161–162.

Schubert, P. E., & Lionberger, H. J. (1995). Mutual connectedness: A study of client-nurse interaction using the grounded theory method. *Journal of Holistic Nursing, 13,* 102–116.

Schultz, P. R., & Meleis, A. I. (1998). Nursing epistemology: Traditions, insights, questions. *Image: Journal of Nursing Scholarship, 20,* 217–221.

Schvaneveldt, R. W., Durso, F. T., Goldsmith, T. E., Breen, T. J., Cooke, N. M., Tucker, R. G., et al. (1985). Measuring the structure of expertise. *International Journal of Man-Machine Studies, 23,* 699–728.

Schwartz-Barcott, D., & Kim, H. S. (2000). An expansion and elaboration of the hybrid model of concept development. In B. L. Rodgers & K. A. Knafl (Eds.), *Concept development in nursing: Foundations, techniques, and applications* (2nd ed., pp. 129–159). Philadelphia: W.B. Saunders.

Scott, T. H., Bexton, W. H., Heron, W., & Doane, B. K. (1959). Cognitive effects of perceptual isolation. *Canadian Journal of Psychology, 13,* 200–209.

Segal, J. Z. (2007). "Compliance" to "concordance": A critical view. *Journal of Medical Humanities, 28,* 81–96.

Segall, A. (1976). The sick role concept: Understanding social behavior. *Journal of Health and Social Behavior, 17,* 163–170.

Selye, H. (1956). *The stress of life.* New York: McGraw-Hill.

Selye, H. (1976). *The stress of life* (rev. ed.). New York: McGraw-Hill.

Shapere, D. (1977). Scientific theories and their domains. In F. Suppe (Ed.), *The structure of scientific theories* (2nd ed., pp. 518–579). Urbana, IL: University of Illinois Press.

Shattell, M. (2004). Nurse–patient interaction: A review of the literature. *Journal of Clinical Nursing, 13,* 714–722.

Shilling, C. (2002). Culture, the 'sick role' and the consumption of health. *British Journal of Sociology, 53,* 621–638.

Shirk, S. R., Gudmundsen, G., Kaplinski, H. C., & McMakin, D. L. (2008). Alliance and outcome in cognitive-behavioral therapy for adolescent depression. *Journal of Clinical Child and Adolescent Psychology, 37,* 631–639.

Silva, M. C., Sorrell, J. M., & Sorrel, C. D. (1995). From Carper's patterns of knowing to ways of being: An ontological philosophical shift in nursing. *Advances in Nursing Science, 18,* 1013.

Simon, H. (1957). *Models of man.* New York: John Wiley.

Simon, H. (1979). *Models of thoughts.* New Haven, CT: Yale University Press.

Skalski, C. A., DiGerolamo, L., & Gigliotti, E. (2006). Stressors in five client populations: Neuman systems model-based literature review. *Journal of Advanced Nursing, 56,* 69–78.

Skinner, B. F. (1953). *Science and human behavior.* New York: Macmillan.

Smart, A. (2008). Social capital. *Anthropologica, 50,* 409–428.

Smith, M. J., & Liehr, P. R. (Eds.). (2003). *Middle range theory for nursing.* New York: Springer Publishing Company.

Smith, M. J., & Liehr, P. R. (Eds.). (2008). *Middle range theory for nursing* (2nd ed.). New York: Springer Publishing Company.

Sochaslski, J., Estabrooks, C. A., & Humphrey, C. K. (2009). Nurse staffing and patient outcomes: Evolution of an international study. *Canadian Journal of Nursing Research, 41,* 320–339.

Sooman, A., & Macintyre, S. (1995). Health and perceptions of the local environment in socially contrasting neighbourhoods in Glasgow. *Health and Place, 1,* 15–26.

Spielberger, C. D. (1975). Anxiety: State-trait-process? In C. D. Spielberger & I. G. Sarasen (Eds.), *Stress and anxiety* (Vol. 1). Washington, DC: Hemisphere.

Staats, A. W. (1989). Unificationism: Philosophy for the modern disunified science of psychology. *Philosophical Psychology, 2,* 143–164.

Stagno, D., Gibson, C., & Breitbart, W. (2004). The delirium subtypes: A review of prevalence, phenomenology, pathophysiology, and treatment response. *Palliative Support Care, 2,* 171–179.

Stainton, M. C., Lohan, M., Fethney, J., Woodhart, L., & Islam, S. (2006). Women's responses to two models of antepartum high-risk care: Day stay and hospital stay. *Women and Birth: Journal of the Australian College of Midwives, 19*, 89–95.

Stetler, C. B. (2001). Updating the Stetler model of research utilization to facilitate evidence-based practice. *Nursing Outlook, 49*, 272–279.

Stevens, B. J. (1979). *Nursing theory: Analysis, application, evaluation*. Boston: Little, Brown.

Stevenson, J. S. (1983). Adulthood: A promising focus for future research. In H. H. Werley & J. J. Fitzpatrick (Eds.), *Annual review of nursing research* (Vol. 1, pp. 55–74). New York: Springer Publishing Company.

Stevenson, J. S., & Woods, N. F. (1986). Nursing science and contemporary science: Emerging paradigms. In *Setting the agenda for the year 2000: Knowledge development in nursing* (pp. 6–20). Kansas City, MO: American Academy of Nursing.

Stevenson, L. (1987). *Seven theories of human nature*. New York: Oxford University Press.

Strauss, A. (1978). *Negotiations: Varieties, contexts, processes, and social order*. San Francisco: Jossey-Bass.

Suedfeld, P. (1969). Introduction and historical background, and theoretical formulations II. In J. P. Zubek (Ed.), *Sensory deprivation: Fifteen years of research* (pp. 3–15, 433–448). New York: Appleton-Century-Crofts.

Sullivan, T. J. (1998). *Collaboration: A health care imperative*. New York: McGraw-Hill.

Sumner, J. (2001). Caring in nursing: A different interpretation. *Journal of Advanced Nursing, 35*, 926–932.

Suppe, F. (Ed.). (1977). *The structure of scientific theories* (2nd ed.). Urbana, IL: University of Illinois Press.

Suppe, F. (1996). Middle range theory—Role in nursing theory and knowledge development. In *Proceedings of the sixth Rosemary Ellis Scholar's retreat, nursing science implications for the 21st century*. Cleveland, OH: Frances Payne Bolton School of Nursing, Case Western Reserve University.

Suppe, F., & Jacox, A. K. (1985). Philosophy of science and the development of nursing theory. In J. J. Fitzpatrick (Ed.), *Annual review of nursing research* (Vol. 3, pp. 241–267). New York: Springer Publishing Company.

Svenaeus, F. (2003). Hermeneutics of medicine in the wake of Gadamer: The issue of phronesis. *Theoretical Medicine & Bioethics, 24*, 407–431.

Svendsen, G. L. H. (2006). Studying social capital in situ: A qualitative approach. *Theory and Society, 35*, 39–70.

Swain, M. A., & Steckel, S. B. (1981). Influencing adherence among hypertensives. *Research in Nursing and Health, 4*, 213–222.

Tanner, C. A., Benner, P., Chesla, C., & Gordon, D. R. (1993). The phenomenology of knowing the patient. *Image: Journal of Nursing Scholarship, 25*, 273–280.

Tarlier, D. (2005). Mediating the meaning of evidence through epistemological diversity. *Advances in Nursing Inquiry, 12*, 126–134.

Taylor, C. (1985). *Philosophy and the human sciences. Philosophical papers 2*. Cambridge, UK: Cambridge University Press.

Taylor, C. (1987). Interpretation and the sciences of man. In P. Rabinow & W. M. Sullivan (Eds.), *Interpretive social science: A second look* (pp. 33–81). Berkeley, CA: University of California Press.

Tees, R. C., Midgley, G., & Bruinsma, Y. (1980). Effect of controlled rearing on the development of stimulus-seeking behavior in rats. *Journal of Comparative Physiological Psychology, 94*, 1003–1018.

Thompson, J. L. (1985). Practical discourse in nursing: Going beyond empiricism and historicism. *Advances in Nursing Science, 7,* 59–71.

Thompson, J. L., Allen, D. G., & Rodrigues-Fisher, L. (Eds.). (1992). *Critique, resistance, and action: Working papers in the politics of nursing.* New York: National League for Nursing.

Thorne, S. E. (1993). *Negotiating health care: The social context of chronic illness.* Newbury Park, CA: Sage.

Toulmin, S. (1953). *The philosophy of science: An introduction.* London: Hutchinson.

Toulmin, S. (1972). *Human understanding* (Vol. 1). Princeton, NJ: Princeton University Press.

Toulmin, S. (1977). Postscript: The structure of scientific theories. In F. Suppe (Ed.), *The structure of scientific theories* (pp. 600–614). Urbana, IL: University of Chicago Press.

Travelbee, J. (1964). *Interpersonal aspects of nursing.* Philadelphia: F. A. Davis.

Treharne, G. J., Lyons, A. C., Hale, E. D., Douglas, M. J., & Kitas, G. D. (2006). "Compliance" is futile but is "concordance" between rheumatology patients and health professionals attainable? *Rheumatology, 45,* 1–5.

Tullmann, D. F., & Dracup, K. (2000). Creating a healing environment for elders. *AACN Clinical Issues, 11,* 34–50.

Turnbull, A. (1976). Measurement of health. *American Journal of Nursing, 76,* 1985–1987.

Turner, J. H. (1986). *The structure of sociological theory.* Chicago: Dorsey Presss.

Turner, J. H. (1990). The misuse and use of metatheory. *Sociological Forum, 5,* 37–42.

Turner, R. J. (1981). Social support as a contingency in psychological well-being. *Journal of Health and Social Behavior, 22,* 357–367.

Twaddle, A. C. (1969). Health decisions and sick role variations: An exploration. *Journal of Health and Social Behavior, 10,* 105–114.

Twaddle, A. C. (1974). The concept of health status. *Social Science and Medicine, 8,* 29–38.

Twaddle, A. C. (1979). *Sickness behavior and the sick role.* Cambridge, MA: Schenkman Publishing Company.

University of Rhode Island. (1996). *Building a cumulative knowledge base for nursing: From fragmentation to congruence of philosophy, theory, methods of inquiry and practice: Invited papers of the 4th & 5th symposia of the knowledge development series.* Kingston, RI: University of Rhode Island College of Nursing.

Uzarewicz, C. (1999). The concept of culture and transculturality. In H. S. Kim & I. Kollak (Eds.), *Nursing theories: Conceptual and philosophical foundations* (pp. 71–86). New York: Springer Publishing Company.

Van der Zahm, J., & Bergum, V. (2000). Hermeneutic-phenomenology: Providing living knowledge for nursing practice. *Journal of Advanced Nursing, 31,* 211–218.

Vasquez, M. J. (2007). Cultural difference and the therapeutic alliance: An evidence-based analysis. *American Psychologist, 62,* 875–885.

Veenstra, G. (2002). Social capital and health (plus wealth, income inequality and regional health governance). *Social Science & Medicine, 54,* 849–868.

Voda, A. M., & George, T. (1986). Research on nursing practice: Menopause. In J. J. Fitzpatrick, H. H. Werley, & R. Taunton (Eds.), *Annual review of nursing research* (Vol. 4, pp. 55–75). New York: Springer Publishing Company.

Wade, D. T., & Halligan, P. W. (2007). Social roles and long-term illness: Is it time to rehabilitate convalescence? *Clinical Rehabilitation, 21,* 291–298.

Wainwright, P. (2000). Towards an aesthetics of nursing. *Journal of Advanced Nursing, 32*(3), 750–756.

Waitzkin, H. (1991). *The politics of medical encounters: How patients and doctors deal with social problems.* New Haven, CT: Yale University Press.

Walker, L. O., & Avant, K. C. (2000). *Strategies for theory construction in nursing* (4th ed.). Norwalk, CT: Appleton & Lange.

Wan, T. (1976). Predicting self-assessed health status: A multivariate approach. *Health Services Research, 11,* 464–477.

Watson, J. (1979). *Nursing: The philosophy and science of caring.* Boston: Little, Brown.

Watson, J. (1985a). *Nursing: Human science and human care: A theory of nursing.* Norwalk, CT: Appleton-Century-Crofts.

Watson, J. (1985b). Reflections on different methodologies for the future of nursing. In M. Leininger (Ed.), *Qualitative research in nursing.* Orlando, FL: Grune & Stratton.

Watson, J. (1988). *Nursing: Human science and human care. A theory of nursing* (NLN Publication No. 15-2236, pp. 1–104). New York: National League for Nursing.

Watson, J. (1994). Poeticizing as truth through language. In P. L. Chinn & J. Watson (Eds.), *Art & aesthetic in nursing* (pp. 3–17). New York: National League for Nursing.

Watson, J. (1999). *Postmodern nursing and beyond.* New York: Churchill Livingstone.

Watson, J. (2007). Theoretical questions and concerns: Response from a caring science framework. *Nursing Science Quarterly, 20,* 13–15.

White, J. (1995). Patterns of knowing: Review, critique, an update. *Advances in Nursing Science, 17,* 73–86.

Whittemore, R. (2000). Consequences of not "knowing the patient." *Clinical Nurse Specialist, 14,* 75–81.

Wiedenbach, E. (1964). *Clinical nursing: A helping art.* New York: Springer Publishing Company.

Wills, E. M. (1996). Nurse-client alliance: A pattern of home health caring. *Home Healthcare Nursing, 14,* 455–459.

Wilson, H. S. (1977). Limiting intrusion and social control of outsiders in a helping community: An illustration of qualitative comparative analysis. *Nursing Research, 26,* 103–111.

Wittgenstein, L. (1968). *Philosophical investigations* (3rd ed., G. E. M. Anscombe, Trans.). New York: Macmillan.

Wolf, S. (1981). *Social environment and health.* Seattle, WA: University of Washington Press.

Wolff, H. G. (1962). A concept of disease in man. *Psychosomatic Medicine, 24,* 25–30.

Wolinsky, F. D., & Wolinsky, S. R. (1981). Expecting sick-role legitimation and getting it. *Journal of Health and Social Behavior, 22,* 229–242.

Woods, N. F. (1980). Women's roles and illness episodes: A prospective study. *Research in Nursing & Health, 3,* 137–145.

Woods, N. F. (1985). New models for women's health care. *Health Care for Women International, 6,* 193–208.

Woods, N. F. (1993). *Midlife women's health: There's more to it than menopause* (NLN Publication No. 19-2546). New York: National League for Nursing.

Woods, N. F., & Earp, J. A. (1978). Women with cured breast cancer: A study of mastectomy patients in North Carolina. *Nursing Research, 27,* 279–285.

Woodward, J. (1989). Data and phenomena. *Synthese, 79,* 393–472.

World Health Organization. (1996). *Nursing practice* (WHO Technical Report Series, No. 860). Geneva: Author.

World Health Organization. (2003). *Adherence to long-term therapies: Evidence for action* (E. Sabate, Ed.). Geneva: Author.

Worrell, J. D. (1971). Nursing implications in the care of the patient experiencing sensory deprivation. In C. K. Kintzel (Ed.), *Advanced concepts in clinical nursing* (pp. 130–143). Philadelphia: J. B. Lippincott.

Wright, B. W. (2007). The evolution of Rogers' science of unitary human beings: 21st century reflections. *Nursing Science Quarterly, 20,* 64–67.

Wuest, J. (2000). Concept development situated in the critical paradigm. In B. L. Rodgers & K. A. Knafl (Eds.), *Concept development in nursing: Foundations, techniques, and applications* (pp. 369–386). Philadelphia: W. B. Saunders.

Wuest, J. (2001). Precarious ordering: Toward a formal theory of women's caring. *Health Care Women International, 22,* 167–193.

Yura, H., & Torres, G. (1975). Today's conceptual frameworks within baccalaureate nursing programs. In *Faculty-curriculum development part III: Conceptual framework—Its meaning and function* (pp. 17–25). New York: National League for Nursing.

Zartman, I. W. (Ed.). (1976). *The fifty percent solution.* Garden City, NY: Doubleday.

Zigmond, D. (1987). Three types of encounter in the healing art: Dialogue, dialectic and didacticism. *Holistic Medicine, 2,* 69–81.

Zubek, J. P. (1969). Sensory and perceptual-motor effects. In J. P. Zubek (Ed.), *Sensory deprivation: Fifteen years of research* (pp. 207–253). New York: Appleton-Century-Crofts.

Zuckerman, M. (1969). Hallucinations, reported sensations and image; and theoretical formulations I. In J. P. Zubek (Ed.), *Sensory deprivation: Fifteen years of research* (pp. 85–125, 407–432). New York: Appleton-Century-Crofts.

Index